CARDIAC HYPERTROPHY IN HYPERTENSION

Perspectives in Cardiovascular Research

Volume 8

Perspectives in Cardiovascular Research

Series Editor

Arnold M. Katz

Chief, Division of Cardiology
University of Connecticut School of Medicine
Farmington, Connecticut

Vol. 1: Developmental and Physiological Correlates of Cardiac Muscle, *edited by M. Lieberman and T. Sano.* 322 pp., 1975.

Vol. 2: Neural Mechanisms in Cardiac Arrhythmias, *edited by P. J. Schwartz, A. M. Brown, A. Malliani, and A. Zanchetti.* 460 pp., 1978.

Vol. 3: Ischemic Myocardium and Antianginal Drugs, *edited by M. M. Winbury and Y. Abiko.* 256 pp., 1979.

Vol. 4: Prophylactic Approach to Hypertensive Diseases, *edited by Y. Yamori, W. Lovenberg, and E. D. Freis.* 606 pp., 1979.

Vol. 5: Mechanisms of Cardiac Morphogenesis and Teratogenesis, *edited by Tomas Pexieder.* 526 pp., 1980.

Vol. 6: Central Nervous System Mechanisms in Hypertension, *edited by Joseph P. Buckley and Carlos M. Ferrario,* 432 pp., 1981.

Vol. 7: Myocardial Hypertrophy and Failure, *edited by Norman R. Alpert,* 704 pp., 1983.

Vol. 8: Cardiac Hypertrophy in Hypertension, *edited by Robert C. Tarazi and John B. Dunbar,* 368 pp., 1983.

Cardiac Hypertrophy in Hypertension

Perspectives in Cardiovascular Research
Volume 8

Editors

Robert C. Tarazi, M.D.
Vice Chairman
Research Division
Cleveland Clinic Foundation
Cleveland, Ohio

John B. Dunbar, Dr.P.H.
Health Scientist Administrator
National Heart, Lung, and Blood
  Institute
National Institutes of Health
Bethesda, Maryland

Raven Press ∎ New York

Raven Press, 1140 Avenue of the Americas, New York, New York 10036

Made in the United States of America

International Standard Book Number 0-89004-871-1
Library of Congress Catalog Card Number 82-40288

The material contained in this volume was submitted as previously unpublished material, except in the instances in which credit has been given to the source from which some of the illustrative material was derived

Great care has been taken to maintain the accuracy of the information contained in the volume. However, Raven Press cannot be held responsible for errors or for any consequences arising from the use of the information contained herein.

Materials appearing in this book prepared by individuals as part of their official duties as U.S. Government employees are not covered by the above-mentioned copyright.

Library of Congress Cataloging in Publication Data
Main entry under title:

Cardiac hypertrophy in hypertension.

   (Perspectives in cardiovascular research ; v. 8)
   Includes bibliographical references and index.
   1. Heart--Hypertrophy--Addresses, essays, lectures.
2. Hypertension--Complications and sequelae--Addresses,
essays, lectures. I. Tarazi, Robert C. II. Dunbar,
John B. III. Series. [DNLM: 1. Heart enlargement--
Complications--Congresses. 2. Hypertension--Compli-
cations--Congresses. W1 PE871AL v.8 / WG 200 C262 1982]
RC685.H9C373 1983   616.1'2   82-40288
ISBN 0-89004-871-1

Preface

The study of cardiac hypertrophy in hypertensive diseases has acquired new momentum in recent years because of the conversions of developments in many areas, both clinical and basic. The risks associated with development of left ventricular hypertrophy in hypertension were highlighted dramatically by the conclusions of the Framingham study. "Within three years of the development of left ventricular hypertrophy in man, 30 percent will sustain a major cardiovascular accident." This unsimilar finding took on an added dimension as echocardiography allowed a more direct evaluation of left ventricular dimension than was hitherto possible by noninvasive repeatable techniques. Increased left ventricular mass and wall thickness was documented in adolescents 14 to 16 years old, who had only borderline hypertension.

On the other hand, studies in experimental models of hypertension—now beginning to be confirmed by echocardiographic studies in man—demonstrated the reversibility of ventricular hypertrophy by medical therapy. The relative rapidity with which hypertrophy could develop and regress under appropriate conditions was surprising; the structural cardiac lesions of hypertension did not represent, therefore, a late fixed irreversible complication but could indeed be an early and dynamically significant part of the evolution of hypertension. The observation that regression of hypertrophy did not occur equally with all antihypertensive agents spurred intensive investigation of the factors modulating the hypertrophic response to an increased pressure load. The possibility of influencing cardiac muscle mass thus, lent a new urgency to the still unanswered questions of the functional consequences of hypertrophy and of the advantage or drawback of its regression.

The symposium held under the auspices of the National Heart, Lung, and Blood Institute proposed to reexamine these questions, outline the present state of the art, and summarize the major recent advances in the field; it also aimed at identifying particularly significant lines of research that could eventually prove the therapeutic approach to the problem of left ventricular hypertrophy in hypertensive patients. Whenever possible, the conclusions derived from the studies of left ventricular hypertrophy due to other courses were compared with the results obtained in the study of hypertension. This publication is an attempt to share the large amount of information made available at that meeting. Its purpose is also to stimulate further investigations, both clinical and fundamental and to improve patient care. To the extent that left ventricular hypertrophy is the most common antecedent of heart failure and because of the ultimately poor prognosis associated with the development of cardiac decompensation, it is evident that a better understanding of hypertrophy and of its modulation by treatment would represent significant advance in the prevention of heart failure.

The Editors

Acknowledgments

In 1980, the National Heart, Lung, and Blood Institute, through its Arteriosclerosis, Hypertension, and Lipid Advisory Committee, determined that a symposium be undertaken on the subjects of hypertension and left ventricular hypertrophy. The meeting took place in Bethesda, Maryland on September 21 to 22, 1981, and was the source of this volume.

It was judged that recent advances in molecular, cellular, and clinical studies would make for productive, even controversial, presentations and viewpoints about needed research emphases. To this end a Steering Committee to plan and conduct the symposium was appointed: Robert C. Tarazi, M.D.—Chairman; L. Maximilian Buja, M.D.; Charles K. Francis, Jr., M.D.; William B. Hood, Jr., M.D.; Howard E. Morgan, M.D.; Edmund H. Sonnenblick, M.D.; Joseph Wiener, M.D.; and John B. Dunbar, D.M.D.

The last session of the symposium was devoted to a roundtable discussion of the potential for reversing cardiac hypertrophy and the clinical implications of such an outcome. The editors regret that space limitations precluded publication of the roundtable session. The discussion was full and rich, and special gratitude is due Dr. William Hood, Jr. for organizing and moderating, and to the following scientists who led off the discussion with brief presentations: Dr. Sanford Bishop, Dr. Anthony Cutilletta, Dr. Edward Frohlich, Dr. Nathaniel Reichek, and Dr. Richard Devereux.

Further, the editors wish to acknowledge the dedication and patience of the individual authors, and to express gratitude for the support of many others, including Dr. Robert Levy, formerly Director of the National Heart, Lung, and Blood Institute; Dr. Barbara Packard, Director of the Division of Heart and Vascular Diseases; Dr. Gardner McMillan, Associate Director for Atherosclerosis and Hypertension; and Dr. Barbara Orlans of the Cardiac Functions Branch. A special note of thanks is extended to Ms. Ruby Dunbar and Ms. Brenda Ackley for critical help behind the scenes.

Contents

Introduction

1 Growth Characteristics of Cardiac Hypertrophy
Radovan Zak

13 Ventricular Hypertrophy: Models and Methods
*Edmund H. Sonnenblick, John E. Strobeck,
Joseph M. Capasso, and Stephen M. Factor*

21 What Is the Stimulus to Myocardial Hypertrophy?
Jay N. Cohn and Karl A. Nath

Morphometry of Hypertrophy

27 Morphometric Studies of Left Ventricular Hypertrophy
Piero Anversa, Giorgio Olivetti, and Alden V. Loud

41 Cell Size in Experimental Cardiomegaly
Karel Rakusan and Borivoj Korecky

49 Alterations in Cardiac Collagen with Hypertrophy
James B. Caulfield

59 Structural Characterization of Coronary Arteries and
Myocardium in Renal Hypertensive Hypertrophy
Joseph Wiener and Filiberto Giacomelli

Biochemistry

73 Myosin Isozymes in Cardiac Hypertrophy: A Brief Review
Eugene Morkin

83 Relationship of Changes in Molecular Forms of Myosin Heavy
Chains to Endogenous Level of Thyroid Hormone During
Postnatal Growth
*Alan W. Everett, Richard A. Chizzonite, William A. Clark, and
Radovan Zak*

93 Control of RNA Synthesis in the Normal and Hypertrophied
Myocardium
Constantinos J. Limas

111   Alteration in Sarcoplasmic Reticulum in Cardiac Hypertrophy
        James Scheuer

123   Model Dependence of Contractile and Energetic Function of
        Hypertrophied Myocardium
        George Cooper, IV

145   Changes in Creatine Kinase System During the Transition from
        Compensated to Uncompensated Hypertrophy in the
        Spontaneously Hypertensive Rat
        Joanne S. Ingwall

157   Myocardial Myosin Isoenzymes and Thermomechanical
        Economy
        Norman R. Alpert and Louis A. Mulieri

Functional Consequences of Hypertrophy

167   Myocardial Mechanics in Two Models of Pressure Overload
        Hypertrophy
        Oscar H. L. Bing, Wesley W. Brooks, and Allen W. Wiegner

179   Myocardial Contractile Alterations Induced by Hypertensive
        Hypertrophy and Its Reversal
        *John E. Strobeck, Joseph M. Capasso, Ashwani Malhotra, and
        Edmund H. Sonnenblick*

193   Cardiac Hypertrophy in the Spontaneously Hypertensive Rat:
        Adaptation or Primary Myopathy?
        Marc A. Pfeffer and Janice M. Pfeffer

201   Mechanical and Structural Aspects of the Hypertrophied
        Human Myocardium
        Karl T. Weber, Joseph S. Janicki, and Sanjeev Shroff

211   Influence of Cardiac Hypertrophy on Myocardial Compliance
        William Grossman and Beverly H. Lorell

219   Electrical Properties of Hypertrophied Ventricular Muscle of
        Rats with Renal Hypertension
        R. S. Aronson and E. C. H. Keung

235   Cardiac Reflexes
        Vernon S. Bishop and Eileen M. Hasser

Coronary Perfusion and Ventricular Hypertrophy

249   Capillary Reserve and Tissue O_2 Transport in Normal and
         Hypertrophied Hearts
         Carl R. Honig and Thomas E. J. Gayeski

261   Myocardial Blood Flow in Experimental Left Ventricular
         Hypertrophy
         Robert J. Bache and Thomas R. Vrobel

273   Abnormalities in Coronary Circulation Secondary to Cardiac
         Hypertrophy
         *Melvin L. Marcus, Samon Koyanagi, David G. Harrison,
         Loren F. Hiratzka, Creighton D. Wright, Donald B. Doty,
         and Charles L. Eastham*

287   Cardiac Hypertrophy in Chronic Ischemic Heart Disease
         *L. Maximilian Buja, Kathryn H. Muntz, Kirk Lipscomb, and
         James T. Willerson*

Factors Modulating Cardiovascular Hypertrophy

295   Abnormalities of the Cardiac Sympathetic Nervous System in
         the Hypertrophied and Failing Heart
         James F. Spann

309   Myocardial Catecholamines in Hypertensive Ventricular
         Hypertrophy
         Subha Sen and Robert C. Tarazi

319   Adaptation of Arterial Vasculature to Increased Pressure and
         Factors Modifying the Response
         Rosemary D. Bevan

337   Angiotensin and Myocardial Protein Synthesis
         Philip A. Khairallah and Jan Kanabus

349   Conclusion and Future Directions
         Robert C. Tarazi and John B. Dunbar

353   *Subject Index*

Contributors

Norman R. Alpert, Ph.D. *University of Vermont, College of Medicine, Department of Physiology and Biophysics, Given Building, Burlington, Vermont 05405*

Piero Anversa, M.D. *Department of Pathology, New York Medical College, Valhalla, New York 10595*

Ronald S. Aronson, M.D. *Albert Einstein College of Medicine, 1300 Morris Park Avenue, Bronx, New York 10461*

Robert J. Bache, M.D. *Department of Medicine, Cardiovascular Section, University of Minnesota Medical School, Box 338, Mayo Memorial Building, Minneapolis, Minnesota 55455*

Rosemary D. Bevan, B.S. *Department of Pharmacology, School of Medicine, University of California, Los Angeles, California 90024*

Oscar H. L. Bing, M.D. *ACOS R&D, Veterans Hospital, 150 South Huntington Avenue, Boston, Massachusetts 02130*

Sanford P. Bishop, D.V.M., Ph.D. *Department of Pathology, University of Alabama in Birmingham, University Station, Volker Hall—Room G-024, Birmingham, Alabama 35294*

Vernon S. Bishop, Ph.D. *Department of Pharmacology, The University of Texas Health Science Center, 7703 Floyd Curl Drive, San Antonio, Texas 78284*

Wesley W. Brooks, M.D. *Thorndike Laboratory and Department of Medicine, Harvard Medical School and Department of Medicine, Boston Veterans Administration Medical Center, Boston, Massachusetts 02115*

L. Maximilian Buja, M.D. *Department of Pathology, The University of Texas Health Science Center at Dallas, 5323 Harry Hines Boulevard, Dallas, Texas 75235*

Joseph M. Capasso. *Albert Einstein College of Medicine, Division of Cardiology, 1300 Morris Park Avenue, Bronx, New York 10461*

James B. Caulfield, M.D. *Department of Pathology, School of Medicine, University of South Carolina, Columbia, South Carolina 29208*

Richard A. Chizzonite, M.D. *Department of Medicine and the Department of Pharmacological and Physiological Sciences, The University of Chicago, Chicago, Illinois 60637*

William A. Clark, M.D. *Department of Medicine and the Department of Pharmacological and Physiological Sciences, The University of Chicago, Chicago, Illinois 60637*

Jay N. Cohn, M.D. *Cardiovascular Division, University of Minnesota Hospital, Box 488, Minneapolis, Minnesota 55455*

George Cooper, IV, M.D. *Department of Internal Medicine and Physiology, Temple University Health Science Center, Philadelphia, Pennsylvania 19104*

Anthony F. Cutilletta, M.D. *Division of Pediatric Cardiology, Johns Hopkins Hospital School of Medicine, Halsted 408, 600 North Wolfe Street, Baltimore, Maryland 21205*

Richard B. Devereux, M.D. *Cornell University Medical College, 1300 York Avenue, New York, New York 10021*

Donald B. Doty, M.D. *University of Iowa and Veterans Administration Hospitals, Iowa City, Iowa 52242*

John B. Dunbar, Dr.P.H. *National Heart, Lung, and Blood Institute, National Institutes of Health, Bethesda, Maryland 20205*

Charles L. Eastham, M.D. *University of Iowa and Veterans Administration Hospitals, Iowa City, Iowa 52242*

Alan W. Everett, M.D. *Department of Medicine, The University of Chicago, Chicago, Illinois 60637*

Stephen M. Factor, M.D. *Albert Einstein College of Medicine, Division of Cardiology, 1300 Morris Park Avenue, Bronx, New York 10461*

Charles K. Francis, Jr., M.D. *Cardiology Division, Yale University School of Medicine, 333 Cedar Street, New Haven, Connecticut 06504*

Edward D. Frohlich, M.D. *Education in Research, Alton Ochsner Medical Foundation, Division of Hypertension Diseases, Ochsner Clinic, New Orleans, Louisiana 70121*

Thomas E. J. Gayeski, M.D. *Department of Physiology, University of Rochester Medical Center, Rochester, New York 14642*

Filiberto Giacomelli, M.D. *Department of Pathology, Wayne State University School of Medicine, Detroit, Michigan 48201*

William Grossman, M.D. *Cardiovascular Division, Beth Israel Hospital, 330 Brookline Avenue, Boston, Massachusetts 02215*

David G. Harrison, M.D. *University of Iowa and Veterans Administration Hospitals, Iowa City, Iowa 52242*

Eileen M. Hasser, M.D. *Department of Pharmacology, The University of Texas Health Science Center at San Antonio, San Antonio, Texas 78284*

Loren F. Hiratzka, M.D. *University of Iowa and Veterans Administration Hospitals, Iowa City, Iowa 52242*

Carl R. Honig, M.D. *Department of Physiology, School of Medicine and Dentistry, University of Rochester, 601 Elmwood Avenue, Rochester, New York 14642*

William B. Hood, Jr., M.D. *Cardiology Department, Boston City Hospital, 818 Harrison Avenue, Boston, Massachusetts 02118*

Joanne S. Ingwall, Ph.D. *Department of Medicine, Physiology, Brigham and Women's Hospital, Harvard Medical School, 75 Francis Street, Boston, Massachusetts 02115*

Joseph S. Janicki, Ph.D. *Cardiovascular–Pulmonary Division, Department of Medicine, University of Pennsylvania, Philadelphia, Pennsylvania 19104*

Jan Kanabus, M.D. *Department of Cardiovascular Research, Division of Research, Cleveland Clinic Foundation, Cleveland, Ohio 44106*

E. C. H. Keung, M.D. *Albert Einstein College of Medicine, Department of Medicine, Division of Cardiology, 1300 Morris Park Avenue, Bronx, New York 10461*

Philip A. Khairallah, M.D. *Department of Cardiovascular Research, Cleveland Clinic Foundation, 9500 Euclid Avenue, Cleveland, Ohio 44106*

Borivoj Korecky. *Department of Physiology, Department of Physiology, School of Medicine, University of Ottawa, Ottawa, Ontario, Canada*

Samon Koyanaqi, M.D. *University of Iowa and Veterans Administration Hospitals, Iowa City, Iowa 52242*

Constantinos J. Limas, M.D. *Department of Medicine, University of Minnesota, School of Medicine, Box 19, Mayo Memorial Building, Minneapolis, Minnesota 55455*

Kirk Lipscomb, M.D. *Departments of Pathology and Internal Medicine, The University of Texas Health Science Center at Dallas, Veterans Administration Hospital, Dallas, Texas 75235*

Beverly H. Lorell, M.D. *Department of Medicine, Harvard Medical School, Beth Israel Hospital and Brigham and Women's Hospital, Boston, Massachusetts 02115*

Alden V. Loud, Ph.D. *Department of Pathology, New York Medical College, Valhalla, New York; and University of Parma, Parma, Italy*

Ashwani Malhotra, Ph.D. *Cardiovascular Research Laboratories, Division of Cardiology, Albert Einstein College of Medicine, 1300 Morris Park Avenue, Bronx, New York 10461*

Melvin L. Marcus, M.D. *University of Iowa, Department of Internal Medicine, Iowa City, Iowa 52242*

Howard E. Morgan, M.D. *Department of Physiology, Penn State University, College of Medicine, Hershey, Pennsylvania 17033*

Eugene Morkin, M.D. *Department of Internal Medicine, Arizona College of Medicine, 1501 North Campbell Avenue, Tucson, Arizona 85724*

Louis A. Mulieri. *Department of Physiology and Biophysics, University of Vermont, College of Vermont, Burlington, Vermont 05405*

Kathryn H. Muntz, Ph.D. *The Departments of Pathology and Internal Medicine (Cardiac Division), The University of Texas Health Science Center at Dallas, Veterans Administration Hospital, Dallas, Texas 75235*

Karl A. Nath. *Cardiovascular Division, Department of Medicine, University of Minnesota Medical School, Minneapolis, Minnesota 55455*

Giorgio Olivetti, M.D. *Department of Pathology, New York Medical College, Valhalla New York; and University of Parma, Parma, Italy*

Marc A. Pfeffer, M.D. *Department of Medicine, Brigham and Women's Hospital, 75 Francis Street, Boston, Massachusetts 02115*

Karel J. Rakusan, M.D. *Department of Physiology, University of Ottawa, 275 Nicholas Street, Ottawa, Ontario, KIN 9A9, Canada*

Nathaniel Reichek, M.D. *951 Gates, Hospital of the University of Pennsylvania, 3400 Spruce Street, Philadelphia, Pennsylvania 19104*

James Scheuer, M.D. *Albert Einstein College of Medicine, Montefiore Hospital and Medical Center, 111 East 210th Street, Bronx, New York 10467*

Subha Sen, Ph.D. *Research Division, Cleveland Clinic Foundation, 9500 Euclid Avenue, Cleveland, Ohio 44106*

Sanjeev Shroff, Ph.D. *Cardiovascular Pulmonary Division, Department of Medicine, University of Pennsylvania, Philadelphia, Pennsylvania 19104*

Edmund H. Sonnenblick, M.D. *Division of Cardiology, Albert Einstein College of Medicine, 1300 Morris Park Avenue, Bronx, New York 10461*

James F. Spann, M.D. *Cardiology Section, Temple University Health Science Center, Philadelphia, Pennsylvania 19140*

John E. Strobeck, M.D. *Division of Cardiology, Albert Einstein College of Medicine, Room G39, Forchheimer Building, 1300 Morris Park Avenue, Bronx, New York 10461*

Robert C. Tarazi, M.D. *Research Division, Section of Clinical Science, Cleveland Clinic Foundation, 9500 Euclid Avenue, Cleveland, Ohio 44106*

Thomas R. Vrobel, M.D. *The Department of Medicine, Cardiovascular Section, University of Minnesota Medical School, Minneapolis, Minnesota 55455*

Karl T. Weber, M.D. *Cardiovascular Pulmonary Division, 987 Maloney Building, Hospital of the University of Pennsylvania, 3600 Spruce Street, Philadelphia, Pennsylvania 19104*

Allan W. Wiegner. *Thorndike Laboratory and Department of Medicine, Harvard Medical School, and Department of Medicine, Boston Veterans Administration Medical Center, Boston, Massachusetts 02115*

Joseph Wiener, M.D. *Department of Pathology, School of Medicine, Wayne State University, Detroit, Michigan 48201*

James T. Willerson, M.D. *Departments of Pathology and Internal Medicine, The University of Texas Health Science Center at Dallas, Veterans Administration Hospital, Dallas, Texas 75235*

Creighton D. Wright. *University of Iowa and Veterans Administration Hospitals, Iowa City, Iowa 52242*

Radovan H. Zak, Ph.D. *Department of Medicine, The University of Chicago, 950 E. 59th Street, Chicago, Illinois 60637*

*Perspectives in Cardiovascular
Research, Vol. 8,*
edited by R. C. Tarazi and J. B. Dunbar.
Raven Press, New York © 1983.

Growth Characteristics of Cardiac Hypertrophy

Radovan Zak

*Cardiology Section of the Department of Medicine and the Department of
Pharmacological and Physiological Sciences, The University of Chicago,
Chicago, Illinois 60637*

The growth of the heart, similar to that of most other organs, is closely related to the work it is required to perform. The effect of hemodynamic load on heart size can be seen both in the individuum as well as in a comparison of animals with different life-styles. In the individuum, the effect of functional demands is evident in the increased growth rate of the left ventricle following birth and in the cardiac enlargement that accompanies pressure and volume overload due to disease. In a comparison of animal species, the biggest hearts relative to body size are found in those animals whose survival requires endurance exercise rather than short bursts of activity. Moreover, breeding for speed is accompanied by large cardiac size even in the absence of training; domestication, on the other hand, results in decreased heart size compared to that of wild animals.

The response of the heart to hemodynamic challenge occurs at two levels. First, adenosine triphosphate (ATP) synthesis is activated in the mitochondria. When energy requirements are increased acutely and intermittently, such as during exercise, they are adequately met by myocardial tissue due to the large capacity of its mitochondria for oxydative phosphorylation. Even during strenuous exertion, the reserve pathway of ATP generation, the glycolysis, is not activated (provided that the heart is well oxygenated). Second, myocardial growth is stimulated. When the increased energy utilization is sustained, and exceeds some as yet unspecified limit, another more slowly responding mechanism is activated: the expression of specific genes.

The growth response of the heart can take several forms: (a) cardiac enlargment (cardiac hypertrophy), which can be accomplished either by proliferation of heart cells (cellular hyperplasia), enlargement of existing cells (cellular hypertrophy), or a combination of both processes; (b) change in the relative amounts of cellular constituents, such as preferential synthesis and accumulation of mitochondria in the phase of developing hypertrophy; and (c) change in the complement of cellular proteins, such as replacement of one myosin isozyme by another. In most situations, all three of these forms of gene activation participate in the cardiac response to altered physiological demands. Depending on the nature and extent of the overload, however, one form of response will be activated more readily than another.

1

Identifying the correlations between functional requirements and gene expression in the heart is a great challenge to clinicians and cell biologists. For the clinician, the main tasks are to evaluate the functional correlates of various forms of cardiac growth and to define the distinction between physiological and pathological hypertrophy. The challenges to the biologist, on the other hand, are to delineate the physiological mechanisms that, by regulating the contractile function, also regulate gene expression, and to identify the feedback signal(s) that couples physical and genetic activities of cardiac cells.

This article presents an analysis of cardiac hypertrophy in an attempt to understand the causal relationship between fuction and growth. Cardiac hypertrophy is thus viewed as an extreme stage of cellular differentiation and development of the heart. Consequently, three stages of cardiac development will be discussed: cytodifferentiation, embryogenesis, and postnatal growth.

DIFFERENTIATION OF HEART CELLS

Cardiac Histogenesis

The scheme of cell differentiation leading to histogenesis of cardiac tissue is shown in Fig. 1. Because of experimental convenience, the earliest stages of cardiac development have been studied most thoroughly in the chicken. However, a similar description applies to mammals and to other amniotic embryos (1).

The myogenic cells of the developing vertebrate heart are derived from splanchnic mesoderm (2). During the first 30 hours of incubation of the fertilized egg, the myogenic cells appear rounded or spindle-shaped. The structure and abundance of various cell organelles are those typical of any undifferentiated cell. Although no muscle-specific structures are present at this stage, all of the cells will eventually acquire myofibrils. At this stage, the cells are referred to by different investigators as premyoblasts, or presumptive myocytes. During the subsequent 6 hours, the premyoblasts begin to synthesize cell-specific proteins such as myosin and actin and, as a consequence, the first thick and thin filaments appear within their cytoplasm. The cells are now referred to as developing myocytes. At approximately 30 hours of incubation, the first contractions can be detected. Because the circulatory system has not yet developed, it is apparent that the earliest stage of cardiac morphogenesis occurs independently of hemodynamic forces. This conclusion is strengthened by the finding that an identical sequence of events occurs when cardiac cells are grown in culture (3).

EMBRYOGENESIS

Process of Looping

As the cardiac myocytes develop, the myofilaments become more abundant and demonstrate greater orientation, and by approximately 35 hours they begin

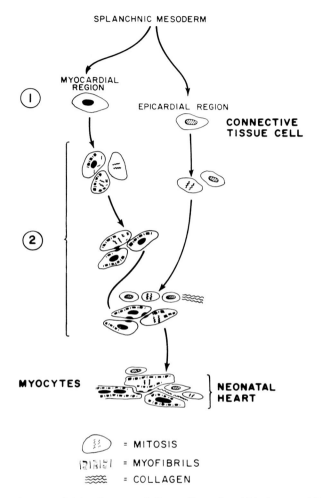

FIG. 1. Scheme of myocardial development. **1:** Precardiac cells, which do not exhibit the cardiac muscle cell phenotype ("premyoblasts," or "presumptive myocytes"). **2:** Overtly differentiated muscle cells, which contain muscle-specific proteins ("developing myocytes"). The connective tissue cells represent a broad category of cells other than myocytes.

to resemble myofibrils. The continuing formation of myofibrils is correlated with changes in cell shape. As a consequence, the bilaterally symmetric heart is transformed into an asymmetric C-shaped structure; this process is referred to as looping (4).

Although this morphologic change coincides with the onset of contractions, the hemodynamic forces are clearly shown not to be the morphogenetic factors that trigger looping. When the heartbeat, already present at this stage of normal embryogenesis, is prevented by placing the embryo explant into a medium containing a high concentration of potassium ions, the progression of looping remains similar to that seen *in vivo* (5). Several lines of evidence obtained by Manasek et al. (6) indicate that looping requires a critical mass of myofibrils. It was shown that looping does not occur when myofibrillar assembly is prevented by cytochalasin B, when synthesis of total proteins is inhibited by cycloheximide, or when synthesis of contractile proteins is preferentially blocked by bromodeoxyuridine. It thus appears that both the information required for synthesis of cell-specific proteins and the forces responsible for the first major morphologic transformation of the primitive heart are intrinsic properties of the heart itself.

Postlooping Stage

At the looping stage, the heart consists of a myocardium composed of a pure population of developing myocytes. The endocardium is still a simple endothelium, and no epicardium, coronary vessels, or nerves are present. After looping, however, cardiac morphogenesis becomes a progressively more complex process. During this period, a variety of non-muscle cells invade the myocardium, which gradually becomes composed of heterogeneous cell populations. In the 7-day-old chick embryo, for example, in addition to myocytes, the following types of cells can be distinguished: vascular endothelial and smooth muscle cells, epithelial and mesenchymal cells of the epicardium, nerve cells, blood cells (including phagocytes), and endothelial fibroblasts. The non-muscle cells proliferate rapidly, so that in the heart of the adult rat they outnumber muscle cells three to one (7,8).

Another change in the myocardium that occurs after looping is in the myofilaments, which eventually form a substantial fraction of the cell volume. As a consequence, at a certain point of development, the cells lose their plasticity and cannot change their shape as readily as they could during looping. The morphologic transformations in the developing heart from this state onward become much more complex and are carried out mainly by two processes: differential growth and cell death.

Differential Regional Growth

The principal feature of cardiac growth during the embryonic period is a combination of hyperplasia and hypertrophy. Both myoblasts and developing myocytes divide mitotically. In contrast to skeletal muscle, however, the synthesis of deoxyribonucleic acid (DNA) and that of cell-specific proteins are not mutually exclusive processes in cardiac myocytes. Cinematographic recordings of cultured embryonic heart muscle cells, for example, have clearly shown actively contracting cells in the process of division (9). At first, the frequency of mitoses is high; however, as development progresses, especially during the late gestation period, the number of dividing cells decreases, and the enlargement of existing myocytes becomes the major mode of cardiac growth.

Myocardial Cell Death

In addition to preferential regional growth, death of myocardial cells has been implicated in morphologic transformations of the developing heart. Degeneration and death of cells are common phenomena that accompany normal ontogeny in many tissues (10). The ultrastructural features of degenerative changes in the myocardial cells are likewise similar to those in other tissues (11). As degeneration proceeds, the typical spindle or cylindrical shape of myocytes is lost, and the cells gradually become rounded. The loss of shape is accompanied by the loss of normal myofibrillar architecture. Moreover, during the process of rounding, the intracellular junctions become disrupted, and the dead cells are eventually moved out into the intercellular space. Once the cells are separated from the surrounding normal tissue, their degradation proceeds by the usual pathway within the phagocytes. There is general agreement among investigators about the universal occurrence of cell death. However, its frequency and distribution in various regions of the developing heart have not yet been causally related to the observed changes in cardiac shape.

Role of Hemodynamic Factors

The available experimental evidence, obtained for the most part in studies of cardiac malformations, indicates that, in contrast to early morphogenesis, cardiac embryogenesis after looping is affected by hemodynamic factors. For example, the decreased inflow of blood created by occlusion of the atrioventricular (A-V) canal in the chick embryo was shown to result in an abnormally small left atrium and ventricle (hypoplasia) and in simultaneous enlargement of the right heart chambers (12,13). Somewhat different results were obtained when the blood flow was modified by selective occlusion of various aortic arches (14). As a result of such intervention, the size of the left atrium was diminished as in occlusion of the A-V canal, and in addition, a marked narrowing of the aortic arch was present. However, the left ventricle did not enlarge as would be expected after aortic coarctation; instead, its growth was suppressed and a variety of ventricular septal defects was observed.

In addition to its effect on cardiac growth, manipulation of intracardiac blood flow alters the topography and frequency of cell death in the developing chick myocardium (15). Despite rather limited information, the foregoing results indicate that after looping, hemodynamic factors can be causally related to the growth and development of the heart.

POSTNATAL DEVELOPMENT

During the late embryonic period, the mitotic activity of cardiac myocytes declines rapidly; consequently, at birth, only about 2% of the rat heart cells are dividing. During the neonatal period, mitotic activity continues to decline, and at approximately 2 months of age, mitoses in the rat heart are noted infrequently, if at all. Nevertheless, the number of myocytes in the rat heart doubles during the first 3 to 4 weeks of life (16–18).

Factors Influencing Proliferation of Cardiac Myocytes

Two points concerning the proliferation of myocytes must be emphasized. First, the exact timing of the development mentioned here applies to the rat only. The maturity and size of the heart relative to body weight vary among species depending on their life-style. At birth, the heart size of animals such as sheep, goats, and cattle is about one-third the adult size. In contrast, the heart of rabbits, dogs, or cats, whose survival does not depend on their ability to run soon after birth, is only about one-sixth the adult size (19). Second, the rapid decrease in mitotic activity during the late embryonic and early neonatal periods is by no means exclusively typical of cardiac myocytes. A similar decline occurs in all cells except those of renewing tissues, e.g., epidermis, mucosal epithelium of the gut, and blood cells. In contrast to most other cells, however, the myocytes of the adult myocardium have never been shown unequivocally to resume mitosis secondary to injury (17) or induced growth (7,8,21,22).

Hemodynamic Function and Cardiac Growth

In the postnatal period, the importance of hemodynamic function in the regulation of cardiac growth is clearly documented by several lines of evidence, including comparison of the growth rates of the right and left ventricles. During prenatal life, the work load of both ventricles is equal, as is their size (23). However, closure of the *foramen ovale* after birth results in rapid growth of the left ventricle, whereas the decreased function of the right ventricle is accompanied by a drastic reduction in its rate of growth (24).

There is further evidence in the common observation that an increase in hemodynamic load on the heart, due either to pathologic changes in the cardiovascular system or to increased physiologic activity, promptly induces cardiac growth. The resulting ratios of heart weight to body weight exceed values typical for normal animals of a given species. The observed growth—compensatory hypertrophy—can be viewed as an adaptive process because it allows the individual to survive. The term hypertrophy in this case is understood as enlargement of the entire organ rather than of its constituent cells, as is implied in the definition of hypertrophy used by cell biologists. The cell features of compensatory cardiac hypertrophy vary depending on the age of the animal at the time of onset of the work overload. Thus, if the growth stimulus is applied during the period when mitoses are still present (i.e., during the first 3 to 4 postnatal weeks), autoradiographic (21,22,25–27) and histometric (28) data indicate that accelerated nuclear divisions accompany cardiac enlargement. In contrast, similar experimental procedures applied to adult animals do not lead to increased DNA synthesis in cardiac myocytes (7,8,21,25,26), and accordingly, the observed cardiac enlargement can be explained by an increase in the volume of existing myocytes. [In the human heart, however, if there is extreme enlargement due to disease, cell hypertrophy is supplemented by the addition of new muscle cells (29)].

An example of the compensatory hypertrophy produced by constriction of the ascending aorta of the mature rat is shown in Fig. 2. The adaptive nature of the growth response is best demonstrated if the weight of the hypertrophic heart is superimposed on the growth curve of the normal myocardium. After the operation, the heart enlarges very rapidly, approximately in exponential fashion, until the compensatory stage is reached, when the new hemodynamic load is matched by the enlarged myocardium. When the constricting band is removed, heart size returns to typically normal values (30). The rate of regression of cardiac hypertrophy is as rapid as its development.

Factors Regulating Processes of Cardiac Growth

Although similar correlations between hemodynamic load and cardiac growth have been observed in a great variety of experimental models, very little is known about the factors that regulate the processes of growth. One very important question, recently addressed by Hollenberg and co-workers (31) and Rakusan et al. (32), is whether the number of cell divisions of cardiac myocytes is genetically programmed, or can be modified in normal animals by factors that affect body growth. Both groups of investigators manipulated the rate of body growth by adjusting the number of newborn animals per litter; the smaller the litter, the greater was the rate of postnatal growth. The cell proliferation was assessed by two methods. First, it was determined using the following histometric measurements: cell diameter, the fraction of the total volume of the sample occupied by myocytes, and ratios of myocyte length to width. Second, the rate of nuclear proliferation was derived from the radioautographically determined decrease in the density of nuclear labeling with ^{3}H-thymidine (31). [However, not every nuclear division necessarily leads to cell division. Because it is well known that the number of cells with more than

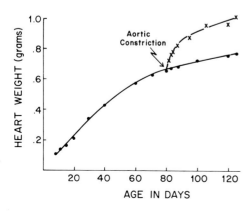

FIG. 2. Normal (*closed circles*) and compensatory (*crosses*) growth of rat myocardium. The heart weight refers to combined ventricular weight of Sprague-Dawley female rats. To induce cardiac hypertrophy, the ascending aorta was constricted to approximately 30% of the original diameter of the lumen by means of a hemostat clip.

one nucleus increases after birth (33), the second method provides information only about the nuclear activity and not about the total number of muscle cells.] In both cases, the data are consistent with the interpretation that the rate of myocyte proliferation is increased when body growth is enhanced during the weaning period. On the basis of this evidence, it is reasonable to assume that a genetically programmed finite number of mitotic divisions in the myocardium does not exist.

REGULATION OF DNA SYNTHESIS AND CARDIAC GROWTH

Our knowledge of the molecular mechanisms responsible for the regulation of DNA synthesis, and growth in general, is still limited. It has been established that the decline in mitotic activity correlates in time with the loss of activity of both DNA polymerase-α (34) and thymidine (dThd) kinase (35). However, most measurements of enzyme activity reported thus far have only limited value because no distinction was made between nuclei of muscle cells and those of nonmuscle cells. Recently, a procedure was developed that allows separation of muscle and nonmuscle cells (36). Using this technique, we demonstrated that muscle cell DNA polymerase-α, which normally decreases to low levels during the neonatal period, is activated when cardiac enlargement is induced in 25-day-old rats by aortic constriction (37).

In several studies, attempts were made to identify the factors regulating DNA replication. For example, adenosine diphosphate (ADP) ribosylation of chromosomal proteins [sequential transfer of ADP ribosome moiety of nicotinamide adenine dionucleotide (NAD) to chromosomal protein] was reported to be inversely related to the rate of DNA synthesis measured in mixed nuclei of growing hearts (38). The appearance of functional adrenergic innervation was also implicated in the control of DNA replication, with norepinephrine and cyclic adenosine monophosphate (cAMP) acting as the chemical modulators (39). In another study, radioautographic assessment of DNA synthesis in neonatal hearts suggested that a low oxygen environment similar to that found in utero increases the incorporation of ^{3}H-dT into muscle nuclei (40). It is likely that the low partial pressure of oxygen reduces the synthesis of poly(ADP)-ribose, which has been shown in a variety of experimental systems (41) to act as an inhibitor of DNA synthesis.

CONTROL OF GENE EXPRESSION IN THE HEART

The experiments described in the preceding paragraphs are examples of growth regulation by functional demands. We are, however, only at the beginning in the analysis of the causal relationship between function and the pattern of growth at the genetic level. In the past, studies of gene activity in higher organisms have been hampered by the presence of several types of cells within the same organ. In the heart, for example, non-muscle and smooth muscle cells are more abundant than myocytes. Even typical muscle proteins, such as myosin and actin, cannot be considered unequivocal markers of specific genes, since molecular variants of these proteins are present in a great variety of cells (e.g., fibroblasts). Consequently, a given muscle protein is one member of a family of closely related proteins that have identical general structure and function, but are products of different genes and therefore have different amino acid sequences. This molecular polymorphism is not only characteristic of enzymes, such as creatine phosphokinase or myosin, but characteristic also of proteins that do not have catalytic function, such as actin and tropomyosin. The proteins of the same biological function, but of different catalytic and/or structural characteristics, are referred to variously as isoproteins, isoforms of a given protein, or, more specifically, as myosin isozymes, isomyosins, isoactins, etc.

In the last several years, considerable progress has been made in the identification, isolation, and characterization of cardiac isoproteins particularly of isomyosin (42). It has been known for some time that atrial and ventricular myosin within the same heart have different properties, and that the ATPase activities of ventricular myosin of various animals are not the same. Of great interest is the distinction of multiple molecular forms of myosin within the atria and ventricles themselves. Thus, in the rabbit, there are two isomyosins in the atria (A1 and A2), and three in the ventricle (V1, V2, and V3). The molecular basis of this polymorphism is currently under investigation, and some uncertainties still remain. The prototype of the myosin molecule consists of two heavy chains, each containing one set of two dissimilar light chains. In the atria, it appears that the two isomyosins, A1 and A2, contain identical heavy chains but different light chains. In contrast, in the ventricle, myosin diversity is the result of two heavy chains (HC_α and HC_β). The three isomyosins are produced by the formation of two homodimers of HC_α and HC_β, respectively (V_1 and V_3), and one heterodimer of HC_α–HC_β (V_2). The complement of light chains is the same in each case. The structural polymorphism of myosin is reflected in its ATPase activity. For example, in the rabbit ventricle V_1, isomyosin has the highest ATPase activity, V_3 has the lowest, and V_2 ranges in the middle. Although the relationship between myosin ATPase and muscle function is certainly more complex in cardiac muscle than in skeletal muscle, the generalization appears to hold true for both muscles that there is a correlation between the actin-activated ATPase activity of myosin and the maximal speed of shortening.

This much has been learned about myosin polymorphism in studies of rabbits and rats. As far as other species are concerned, the identification and characterization of isomyosins are incomplete. Nevertheless, it appears true that each animal species has its own characteristic pattern of isomyosin. The expression of a particular form of myosin, however, is not static throughout an animal's life, but is determined by the developmental, physiological, and hormonal state of the animal. For example, shortly after birth, V_1 isomyosin is the most abundant form in the rabbit ventricle. Its relative amount, however, declines with aging, as it is continuously replaced by the V_3 form. Administration of thyroid hormone in an amount sufficient to induce thyrotoxicosis, shifts the balance toward the V_1 form; within two weeks of treatment, practically all V_3 isomyosin is eliminated both in young and old animals. In contrast, a treatment that decreases the shortening velocity of the heart, such as production of hypothyroidism or pressure overload, results in a shift towards the V_3 form.

Compared to myosin, much less has been learned to date about polymorphism of other contractile proteins of the heart, and muscle in general. It appears, nevertheless, that cardiac-specific variants exist for actin and for the subunits TN-I and TN-T of troponin. In contrast, cardiac tropomyosin appears identical to that of fast muscle, and troponin TN-C to that of slow muscle. Although with advancing analysis this picture is likely to change, it appears at this time that the gene family of a given protein has its own pattern of expression; the theme of isomyosin is not necessarily repeated in the case of other contractile proteins.

So far, our understanding of the polymorphism in the structure and function of muscle proteins has not been reflected in studies of the factors that control cardiac growth. Only nonspecific indices of the structure of genetic apparatus and its transcription rate have been examined. For example, the acidic non-histone proteins have frequently been implicated in regulation of the transcription process. One possibility is that the activity of acidic proteins is modulated by phosphorylation catalyzed by cAMP-dependent nuclear protein kinase (43,44). Another possibility is that the chromatin proteins are covalently modified by ADP ribose by way of an enzymatic transfer from poly(ADP)-ribose. ADP ribosylation has been shown to accompany repression of chromatin activity (45). Moreover, polyamines, which are present in elevated amounts in growing organs including the hypertrophic heart (46) serve as a trap for an intermediate in the ADP-ribosylation reaction.

The second level of transcriptional control involves the amount or activity, or both, of ribonucleic acid (RNA) polymerase, a variety of humoral factors including norepinephrine (47), and muscle-growth-stimulating RNA (48). A recent report (49) suggests that extracts from the hypertrophic heart enhance the translational activity of RNA prepared from the normal heart.

The isolation and characterization of molecular variants of cardiac proteins will eventually make possible the preparation of probes for transcription of specific genes. For now, we are only able to assess the activity of the entire genome. When specific probes become available, we will be able to follow the activity of individual genes. It is conceivable that the same growth stimulus results in activation of one set of genes, and in inactivation of another. These advances will, in turn, make it possible to search in a more meaningful way for the still elusive mechanisms that couple the physiological activity of an organ with its rate of growth.

ACKNOWLEDGMENTS

This treatise on cardiac hypertrophy is based on an article published for the Symposium on Cardiac Hypertrophy, held on May 1–2, 1979 in Cleveland, Ohio (*Am. J. Cardiol.* 44: 941, 1979). A different title, however, has been given to this paper to indicate that substantial revision has been made, mostly to reflect the profound impact made on cardiovascular research by the rapidly advancing field of molecular biology.

This study was supported in part by grants HL16637 and HL20592 from the National Heart and Lung Institute and by a grant from the Muscular Dystrophy Association of America.

REFERENCES

1. Sisman, N. J. (1970): *Am. J. Cardiol.*, 25:141–149.
2. Manasek, F. (1970): *Am. J. Cardiol.*, 25:149–168.
3. Haray, I., and Farley, B. (1963): *Exp. Cell Res.*, 29:451–465.
4. Manasek, F. J., Burnside, M. B., and Waterman, R. E. (1972): *Dev. Biol.*, 29:349–371.
5. Manasek, F., and Monroe, R. G. (1972): *Dev. Biol.*, 27:584–588.
6. Manasek, F. J., Kulikowski, R., and Fitzpatrick, L. (1978): In: *Morphogenesis and Malformation of Cardiovascular System*, edited by G. C. Rosenquist and D. Bergsma, pp. 161–178. A. R. Liss, New York.
7. Grove, D., Nair, K. G., Zak, R., and Aschenbrenner, V. (1969): *Circ. Res.*, 25:473–485.
8. Morkin, E., and Ashford, T. P. (1968): *Am. J. Physiol.*, 215:1409–1413.
9. Mark, G. E., and Strasser, F. F. (1966): *Exp. Cell Res.*, 44:217–233.
10. Saunders, J. W., Jr. (1966): *Science*, 154:604–612.
11. Manasek, F. J. (1969): *J. Embryol. Exp. Morphol.*, 21:271–284.
12. Clark, E. B. (1969): *Anat. Rec.*, 163:170–176.
13. Hark, J. Y., Paul, M. H., Gallen, W. J., Friedberg, D. Z., and Kaplan, S. (1973): *Am. J. Cardiol.*, 31:51–56.
14. Rychter, Z. (1962): *Adv. Morphogenesis*, 2:333–369.
15. Pexieder, T. (1975): *Adv. Anat. Embryol. Cell Biol.*, 51:fasc. 3.
16. Hort, W. (1953): *Arch. Pathol. Anat. Physiol.*, 323:223–247.
17. Klinge, O. (1967): *Z. Zellforsch.*, 80:488–517.
18. Sasaki, R., Moshiaki, T., and Yamagata, S. (1968): *Tohoku J. Exp. Med.*, 96:405–411.
19. Zak, R. (1974): *Circ. Res.*, (Suppl. II) 34,35:II-17–II-26.
20. Zak, R., and Rabinowitz, M. (1979): *Ann. Rev. Physiol.*, 41:539–552.
21. Meerson, F. Z., and Alekhina, G. M. (1967): *Dokl. Acad. Sci. USSR*, 173:122–125.
22. Neffgen, J. F., and Korecky, B. (1972): *Circ. Res.*, 30:104–113.
23. Latimer, H. B. (1965): *Anat. Rec.*, 152:225–232.
24. Emery, J. L., and Mithal, A. (1961): *Br. Heart J.*, 23:313–319.
25. Crane, W. A. J., and Dutta, L. P. (1963): *J. Pathol. Bacteriol.*, 86:83–97.
26. Dowel, R. T., and McManus, R. E. (1978): *Circ. Res.*, 42:303–310.
27. Wachtlova, M., Mares, V., and Ostadal, B. (1977): Virchow's Archiv. [Cell Pathol.] 24:335–342.
28. Korecky, B., and Rakusan, K. (1978): *Am. J. Physiol.*, 234:H123–H128.
29. Linzbach, A. J. (1952): *Arch. Kreislaufforsch.*, 41:641–658.
30. Cutilletta, A. F., Dowel, R. T., Rudnik, M., Arcilla, R. A., and Zak, R. (1975): *J. Mol. Cell. Cardiol.*, 7:767–781.
31. Hollenberg, M., Honbo, N., and Samorodin, A. J. (1977): *Am. J. Physiol.*, 233:H356–H360.
32. Rakusan, K., Raman, S., Layberry, R., and Korecky, B. (1978): *Circ. Res.*, 42:212–218.
33. Bishop, S. P., and Hine, P. (1975): In: *Recent Advances in Studies on Cardiac Structure and Metabolism, Vol. 8,* edited by P. E. Roy, and P. Harris, pp. 77–98. University Park Press, Baltimore.

34. Doyle, C. M., Zak, R., and Fischman, D. A. (1974): *Dev. Biol.*, 37:133–145.
35. Claycomb, W. C. (1975): *J. Biol. Chem.*, 250:3229–3235.
36. Cutilletta, A. F., Aumont, M. C., Nag, A. C., and Zak, R. (1977): *J. Mol. Cell. Cardiol.*, 9:399–407.
37. Bugaisky, L., Zak, R., and Rabinowitz, M. (1978): *J. Cell. Biol.*, 79:333a.
38. Claycomb, W. C. (1976): *J. Biochem.*, 154:387–393.
39. Claycomb, W. C. (1976): *J. Biol. Chem.*, 251:6082–6089.
40. Hollenberg, M., Honbo, N., and Samorodin, A. J. (1976): *Am. J. Physiol.*, 231:1445–1450.
41. Roberts, J. H., Stark, P., and Smulson, M. (1974): *Proc. Natl. Acad. Sci. USA*, 71:3212–3216.
42. Zak, R. (1981): *Cell and Muscle Motility*, 1:1–33.
43. Chiu, J. F., Brade, W. P., Thompson, J., Tsai, Y. H., and Hnilica, L. S. (1975): *Exp. Cell Res.*, 91:200–206.
44. Limas, C. J., and Chan-Stier, C. (1978): *Circ. Res.*, 42:311–336.
45. Kun, E., Chang, A. C. Y., Sharma, M. L., Ferro, A. M., and Nitecki, D. (1976): *Proc. Natl. Acad. Sci. USA*, 73:3131–3135.
46. Russel, D. N., Shiverick, K. T., Hamrell, B. B., and Alpert, N. R. (1971): *Am. J. Physiol.*, 221:1287–1291.
47. Caldadera, C. M., Casti, A., Rossoni, C., and Visioli, O. (1971): *J. Mol. Cell. Cardiol.*, 3:121–126.
48. Desphande, A. K., Jakowlew, S. B., Arnold, H. H., Crawford, P. A., and Siddiqui, M. A. G. (1977): *J. Biol. Chem.*, 252:6521–6527.
49. Hammond, G. L., Weiben, E., and Market, C. L. (1979): *Proc. Natl. Acad. Sci. USA*, 76:2455–2459.

*Perspectives in Cardiovascular
Research, Vol. 8,*
edited by R. C. Tarazi and J. B. Dunbar.
Raven Press, New York © 1983.

Ventricular Hypertrophy: Models and Methods

Edmund H. Sonnenblick, John E. Strobeck,
Joseph M. Capasso, and Stephen M. Factor

Albert Einstein College of Medicine, Division of Cardiology, Bronx, New York 10461

Hypertrophy of the adult heart is characterized largely, if not solely, by myocyte enlargement with hyperplasia presenting only in interstitial cells and microvasculature (1,9). While the causes of hypertrophy are multiple (Table 1), it generally occurs in response to an overload. The load per individual myocardial cell may be increased secondary to deviations of systolic pressure, ventricular volume, or as a result of loss of myocardial cells, whether segmental or diffuse.

Many studies have shown that when systolic pressure is increased in a sustained manner, whatever the cause, the myocardial cells enlarge until the load stabilized per unit of myocardium (stress) returns to normal (2–8). This process can be expressed by the simplest form of the LaPlace equation (Fig. 1). How the mechanical message of increased stress is translated by the myocyte into increased synthesis of contractile proteins, and how the process is then self-limited, remains one of the most intriguing and fundamental problems in the biology of hypertrophy and growth.

The response of the heart to a volume overload differs from that of a pressure overload (10–12); an increased volume load is accommodated for initially by the Starling mechanism of increased cell length and, therefore, sarcomere length. In compensated volume overloads, tension is slightly altered—or even reduced—during the course of systole, since peripheral impedance tends to be lower in these conditions, and the heart empties more rapidly and completely. In pressure overloads, stress remains normal until failure ensues with ventricular dilatation; but the stress increases when a further concomitant volume increase occurs, outstripping the increase in wall thickness (13–17) (Fig. 2). This provides a secondary pressure load on an already overloaded and compromised ventricle. In volume overloads, a decrease in myocardial contractility occurring late in the course of myocardial hypertrophy will result in decreased speed and extent of ventricular emptying. This ultimately leads to an increased ventricular volume throughout systole, causing an increase in wall stress so that an additional pressure load becomes superimposed on the initial volume load, and wall thickening occurs (Fig. 3).

TABLE 1. *Etiology of hypertrophy*

Overloads
  Systolic pressure: hypertension, aortic stenosis
  Volume: aortic and mitral regurgitation, atrial septal defect, A-V shunt

Reactive (loss of myocardium)
  Segmental: myocardial infarction
  Diffuse: myocarditis, cardiomyopathy

Myopathies
  Primary: idiopathic
  Secondary: $\downarrow$contractility $\rightarrow$ $\uparrow$load $\rightarrow$ $\uparrow$mass

Physiological and hormonal
  Normal growth
  Thyroid excess or hyperthyroidism
  Exercise
  Catecholamines

Changes in myocardial contractility that occur in the presence of hypertrophy may be affected by many factors (Table 2). In studies in the cat (16), in which the pulmonary artery was acutely narrowed by a band so as to produce a pressure overload, myocardial contractility [measured as maximum speed of unloaded muscle shortening (V_{max})] fell. Normalized force development (P_O) was reduced to a lesser muscle-shortening (V_{max}) fall in relation to the severity of the hypertrophic response, so that the rate of force development (dp/dt) declined. Force development and shortening tend to be sustained; they diminish only when the contractility has fallen to the point where ventricular failure occurs. The decline in V_{max} is paralleled by a decrease in actomyosin

$$T = \frac{PR}{2}$$

$$S = \frac{PR}{2h}$$

Pressure overload	Volume overload
$\uparrow S = \dfrac{\uparrow PR}{2h}$	$\uparrow S = \dfrac{P \cdot R\uparrow}{2h}$
$\updownarrow h$	$\downarrow$
$S = \dfrac{\uparrow PR}{2h\uparrow}$	$S = \dfrac{\downarrow P \cdot R\uparrow}{2h}$

FIG. 1. Pressure- and volume-overload states of myocardial hypertrophy analyzed according to the LaPlace relation. *T*, tension; *S*, stress; *P*, pressure; *R*, radius; *h*, wall thickness. In pressure overload, myocardial stress increases as the pressure exposed to the left ventricle increases during systole. This could be expected to induce a secondary increase in wall thickness accompanying the development of myocardial hypertrophy. The overall effect of a concomitant increase in myocardial thickness would be to normalize myocardial stress despite persistance of the elevated systolic pressure. In volume overload, myocardial stress is increased directly as a result of increased left ventricular radius. As ventricular dilatation ensues, and peripheral vascular resistance declines, pressure during systole declines, normalizing overall myocardial stress.

(1) $\uparrow S = \dfrac{\uparrow P \cdot R}{2h}$

$\Downarrow\uparrow h$

(2) $S = \dfrac{\uparrow P \cdot R}{2h\uparrow} = \text{normal}$

(3) $S = \dfrac{\uparrow P \cdot R\uparrow}{2h\uparrow} = \pm\uparrow$

$\downarrow \text{ as } h/R \downarrow$

$\uparrow S = \dfrac{\uparrow P \cdot R\uparrow\uparrow}{2h\uparrow}$

FIG. 2. The interrelationships of ventricular pressure (**P**), ventricular radius (**R**), and wall thickness (**h**) during (**1**) the initial, (**2**) compensatory, and (**3**) late stages of pressure overload, myocardial hypertrophy, and failure. In the initial stage, myocardial stress is increased because of the exposure to elevated systolic ventricular pressure. This results in compensatory hypertrophy and increases in wall thickness, tending to normalize myocardial stress. With persistance of the pressure overload, myocardial contractility declines, producing a late stimulus for ventricular dilatation. As ventricular radius increases, the ratio of wall thickness to radius decreases, producing a late increase in myocardial stress, which severely affects left ventricular pump performance.

adenosine triphosphatase (ATPase) (18), which now appears to be due to the shift in myosin enzymes from a faster isoenzyme (V_1) to a slower (V_3) enzymatic form (18).

In contrast to a pressure overload, volume overload—at least in early phases—does not produce a decrease in $V_{\max}$ despite ventricular enlargement (10–12). However, since the increase in mass is due to a primary increase in chamber circumference while wall thickness is maintained, it is unclear whether myocardial cell enlargement is as great in volume overload as it is in pressure overload states (Table 3).

(1) $\uparrow S = \dfrac{P \cdot R\uparrow}{2h}$

$\downarrow$

$S = \dfrac{\pm \downarrow P \cdot R\uparrow}{2h \pm \uparrow}$

$\downarrow \text{ as } P\uparrow, R\uparrow$

(2) $\uparrow S = \dfrac{\uparrow P \cdot R\uparrow}{2h\uparrow}$

FIG. 3. The interrelationships of myocardial stress (**S**), ventricular pressure (**P**), ventricular radius (**R**), and wall thickness (**h**), in (**1**) the early and (**2**) late stages of volume overload, myocardial hypertrophy, and failure. With induction of volume overload, left ventricular radius increases, increasing myocardial stress in both systole and diastole. This results, in the early stage, in slight decreases in ventricular pressure and slight increases in wall thickness. These changes serve to normalize myocardial stress during the compensatory stage. Late decompensation, however, associated with decreases in myocardial contractility, is associated with increasing end diastolic and systolic pressure, which in combination with the increased left ventricular radius, further increases myocardial stress and depresses left ventricular pump performance.

TABLE 2. *Variables in induction of hypertrophy*

Overload
    Type
    Location—RV vs LV, proximal vs distal
    Acuteness
    Severity
    Increase in resistance
    Duration
    Variability of load with time
    Time of measurement
    Initial induction of failure with recovery
    Progression of load (e.g., elevated BP with time)

Model
    Species and strain
    Age of lesion and study
    Sex

Confounding variables
    Diabetes
    Thyroid status
    Concurrent coronary artery disease
    Salt and water balance
    Combined lesion (e.g., renal lesion and volume load)
    Loss of myocardium
    Diastolic properties of myocardium

Less well understood are what we would call the reactive hypertrophies, illustrated best by the hypertrophy that occurs in the non-infarcted part of the heart following an acute myocardial infarction. While one may assume that the extent of hypertrophy is proportional to the amount of myocardial cell loss so that the stress on the remaining heart is increased, extensive modeling of infarction—induced hypertrophy—has not been done. Moreover, it is unclear whether the contractility of the hypertrophied myocardium remains normal or declines with time, adding a further increase in stress to the functioning myocardium. This problem is of great clinical importance when one considers the end-stage dilated hypertrophic myopathy in coronary disease. Further, it is not clear whether this type of reactive hypertrophy represents a response to a pressure or a volume overload.

The same considerations may pertain to conditions where myocardial cells are lost in a more diffuse or focal manner, as is commonly the case in various cardiomyopathies and myocarditis. We have recently developed evidence that in certain experimental cardiomyopathies, microvascular spasm causes myocytolytic necrosis and subsequent focal myocardial fibrosis (19). This diffuse focal loss of cardiac cells would leave a larger stress on the remaining viable cells, which then undergo reactive hypertrophy in response to the increased load. In a similar fashion, a diffuse decrease in myocardial contractility, even in the absence of cell loss, could create an increase in wall stress during systole and result in a hypertrophied ventricle. The former condition would yield a dilated hypertrophic myopathy, while the latter state might yield a non-dilated

TABLE 3. Changes in myocardial structure and function with hypertrophy and failure

Cause of stress	Wall thickness (h)	Diastolic volume (R)	R/h	Cell size	Sarcomere length	Slippage	Actomyosin ATPase	V_{max}
Pressure overload								
Early	↑↑	normal	↓	↑↑	normal	0	±↓	±↓
Late	↑↑↑	↑↑	↑↑	↑↑↑	↑	±↑	↓↓	↓↓
Volume overload								
Early	normal	↑↑	↓↓	normal	↑↑	0	normal	normal
Late	↑↑	↑↑↑	↓±↑	normal	↑↑↑	↑	↓	↓
Dilated myopathy	↑	↑	normal to ↑	↑↑	?	?	↓↓	↓↓
Diabetes	normal	normal	normal	normal	normal	normal	↓	↓
Hyperthyroidism	↑	normal	normal	normal	normal		↑↑	↑↑
Exercise	↑	↑	normal	↑	±↑	0	↑	↑

↑ = increase; ↓ = decrease; 0 = no change.

hypertrophic myopathy. Viewed in this way, reactive hypertrophies are pressure overloads despite the presence of a normal pressure. Ultimately, reactive hypertrophic states are complicated by potential further cell loss and a secondary decrease in contractility that results from the hypertrophy itself. When and within what limits these processes occur requires further study and definition.

In general, pressure overload hypertrophy results in a decrease in V_{max} that correlates with a decline in actomyosin ATPase (20–24). Both of these changes are reversible, within limits, when the load is removed and the hypertrophy regresses (21). Might the same benefits occur were pressure to be lowered within tolerable limits in reactive hypertrophic states? If so, this would be an argument for early and vigorous unloading with reduction of the arterial pressure as tolerated, even in the absence of congestive failure.

During exercise, hypertrophy of mild degree occurs, but contractility tends to increase and actomyosin ATPase is enhanced (25,26). Hyperthyroidism produces similar changes (27). Whether or not this is so when hypertrophy is induced by the chronic administration of catecholamines, in amounts insufficient to induce hypertension, is not known.

Experimental diabetes mellitus produced in rats results in the same mechanical and biochemical abnormalities as those that occur with hypertension induced by renal artery stenosis: a decrease in V_{max} in isolated papillary muscles, accompanied by a prolongation of contraction, with decreased rates of relaxation and sustained force development (28). A parallel decrease in actomyosin ATPase occurs, which, with the mechanical changes, is reversible by insulin administration (29). Since diabetes commonly complicates human pathology, its concomitant role may be a very important consideration. A further complication is our finding that microvascular spasm occurs in the diabetic hypertensive rat, leading to focal myocytolytic necrosis and subsequent focal scarring, resulting in the picture of a cardiomyopathy.

Given the moderate depression of contractility that occurs in response to pressure overload hypertrophy, a depression that is readily reversible under certain conditions, a major and substantive question arises: Why and when does irreversibility and further decline in contractility occur, with resultant heart failure in all clinically relevant models of hypertrophy studied to date? One important factor may be the actual loss of myocardial cells, possibly in progressive fashion, a loss that cannot be replaced and that serves to amplify the overload (19,30). Another factor may be the "plastic" changes that occur in the ventricular wall when dilatation ensues (31); still another is the possibility that hypertrophy-induced depression of contractility leads to further relative pressure-overload, creating a vicious cycle that ultimately depresses pump function beyond a reversible stage.

Consideration of these important concepts, particularly in light of several currently available clinically relevant experimental models of myocardial hypertrophy, should result in a re-focusing of our efforts in the field of a myocardial hypertrophy and failure toward the questions of (a) why irreversible left ventricular dysfunction and failure develop in patients with hypertrophic myocardial disease, and (b) how the onset of irreversibility might be delayed or prevented with specific forms of therapy. By addressing these highly important questions, we hope to define fruitful, future directions of research in myocardial hypertrophy and failure.

ACKNOWLEDGMENTS

This research was supported in part by NIH grants HL18824-06 and HL20426-05.

REFERENCES

1. Salerno, T. A., Shizgal, H. M., and Dobell, A. R. C. (1979): *Ann. Thorac. Surgery*, 27:141–143.
2. Meerson, F. Z. (1965): *Am. J. Cardiol.*, 15:755–760.
3. Mehmel, H. C., Mazzoni, S., and Krayenbuehl, H. P. (1975): *Am. Heart J.*, 90:236–240.
4. Braunwald, E., and Selwyn, A. (1975): The Myocardium: Failure and Infarction. HP Publishing Co., New York.
5. Braunwald, E., Chidsey, C. A., Pool, P. E., Sonnenblick, E. H., Ross, J., Mason, D. T., Spann, J. F., and Covell, J. W. (1966): *Ann. Int. Med.*, 64:904–941.
6. Siegel, J. H., and Sonnenblick, E. H. (1964): *Arch. Surgery*, 89:1026–1036.
7. Braunwald, E., Ross, J., and Sonnenblick, E. H. (1976): *Mechanisms of Contraction of the Normal and Failing Heart*. Little Brown, Boston.
8. Gunther, S., and Grossman, W. (1979): *Circulation*, 59:679–688.
9. Spotnitz, H. M., and Sonnenblick, E. H. (1976): In: *Congestive Heart Failure*, edited by B. D. Mason, pp. 13–24. York Medical Books, New York.
10. Turina, M., Bussmann, W. D., and Krayenbuhl, H. P. (1969): *Cardiovasc. Res.*, 3:486–495.
11. Taylor, R. R., Covell, J. W., and Ross, J. (1968): *J. Clin. Invest.*, 47:1333–1342.
12. Cooper, G., Puga, F. J., Zujko, K. J., Harrison, C. E., and Coleman, H. N. (1973): *Circ. Res.*, 32:140–148.
13. Jouannot, P., and Hatt, P. Y. (1975): *Am. J. Physiol.*, 229:355–364.
14. Kammereit, A., and Jacob, R. (1979): *Basic Res. Cardiol.*, 74:389–405.
15. Meerson, F. Z., and Kapelko, V. I. (1972): *Cardiology*, 57:183–199.
16. Spann, J. F., Buccino, R. A., Sonnenblick, E. H., and Braunwald, E. (1967): *Circ. Res.*, 21:341–354.
17. Spann, J. F., Covell, J. W., Eckberg, D. L., Sonnenblick, E. H., Ross, J., and Braunwald, E. (1972): *Am. J. Physiol.*, 223:1150–1157.
18. Scheuer, J. and Bhan, A. K. (1979): *Circ. Res.*, 45:1–12.
19. Factor, S. M., Minase, T., Cho, S., Dominitz, R., and Sonnenblick, E. H. (1982): *Circulation*, 66:342–354.
20. Capasso, J. M., Strobeck, J. E., and Sonnenblick, E. H. (1981): *Am. J. Physiol.*, 10:H435–H441.
21. Capasso, J. M., Strobeck, J. E., Malhotra, A., Scheuer, J., and Sonnenblick, E. H. (1981): *Am. J. Physiol.*, 242:H882–H889.
22. Cooper, G., Tomanek, R. J., Ehrhardt, J. C., and Marcus, M. L. (1981): *Circ. Res.*, 48:488–497.
23. Pool, P. E., Chandler, B. M., Spann, J. R., Sonnenblick, E. H., and Braunwald, E. (1969): *Circ. Res.*, 24:313–320.
24. Chandler, B. M., Sonnenblick, E. H., Spann, J. F., Jr., and Pool, P. E. (1967): *Circ. Res.*, 21:717–726.
25. Bhan, A. K., and Scheuer, J. (1972): *Am. J. Physiol.*, 223:1486.

26. Penpargkul, S., Malhotra, A., Schaible, T., and Scheuer, J. (1980): *J. App. Physiol.*, 48:409–413.
27. Skelton, C. L., and Sonnenblick, E. H. (1978): In: *The Thyroid*, edited by S. Werner and S. Ingbar, pp. 861–867. Harper & Row, New York.
28. Fein, F., Kornstein, L., Strobeck, J. E., Capasso, J. M., and Sonnenblick, E. H. (1980): *Circ. Res.*, 47:922–933.
29. Penpargkul, S., Malhotra, A., Fein, F., Strobeck, J., Sonnenblick, E. H., and Scheuer, J. (1979): *Clin. Res.*, 27:441A.
30. Spotnitz, H., and Sonnenblick, E. H. (1973): *Am. J. Cardiol.*, 32:398–406.
31. Factor, S. M., Minase, T., Cho, S., Dominitz, R., and Sonnenblick, E. H. (1982): *Circulation*, 66:342–354.

Perspectives in Cardiovascular Research, Vol. 8,
edited by R. C. Tarazi and J. B. Dunbar.
Raven Press, New York © 1983.

What Is the Stimulus to Myocardial Hypertrophy?

Jay N. Cohn and Karl A. Nath

Cardiovascular Division, Department of Medicine, University of Minnesota Medical School, Minneapolis, Minnesota 55455

The physiologic stresses that commonly induce myocardial hypertrophy are widely recognized clinically and frequently utilized experimentally. The biochemical sequences that characterize the process of early hypertrophy have also been described. Less attention has been directed to the link between the physiologic stimulus and the biochemical response—the signal or signals that turn on the synthetic process. An understanding of the link between the physiologic and biochemical events may be of particular importance, since aberrancies in this "trigger" could contribute to inappropriate hypertrophy, which may impair cardiac function, as well as to inadequate hypertrophy, which may also impair cardiac function in the presence of a heightened load.

Were hypertrophy a homogeneous process, one might be attracted to seek a single common pathway that could be activated by a number of stresses. It has long been recognized, however, that the microscopic nature of hypertrophied myocardium varies according to the inciting stimulus. Recent evidence further indicates that striking molecular differences in myosin result from different hypertrophic stresses (1–3). Therefore, while it may no longer be attractive to seek a single trigger for all processes of hypertrophy, the need for understanding the various potential signals is undiminished.

Table 1 lists the various stimuli that appear capable of inducing hypertrophy. These have been loosely grouped into three separate categories: (a) increased functional demand; (b) loss of muscle mass; and (c) direct effect on the myocardium. The possible signals through which these stimuli may act are listed, as well as the biochemical response which consists of protein synthesis and various metabolic adjustments. Analysis of the possible interactions between the stimuli and the signals is the subject of this chapter.

INCREASED WALL TENSION OR STRESS

Increased preload or afterload, resulting from pressure or volume overload states, increases the tension in the wall of the ventricle and increases the stress on myocardial fibers. Evidence suggests that this mechanical burden could

TABLE 1. *Mechanisms of hypertrophy*

Stimulus	Signal	Response
Increased functional demands	Increased wall tension or stress	Protein synthesis
Afterload	Increased energy requirements	Selective
Preload	Norepinephrine, β-adrenoreceptors,	Non-selective
Exercise	or cyclic AMP	
Anemia	Angiotensin effect	Metabolic adjustments
Heart block	Prostaglandin synthesis	
	Tissue hormone stimulator	
Loss of muscle mass	Chalones	
	Increased blood flow	
Direct effect		
Ischemia		
Hypoxia		
Thyroid hormone		
Catecholamines		
Angiotensin		

directly lead to stimulation of protein synthesis. Both passive stretch and isometric tension development in isolated papillary muscles lead to increased amino acid transport and protein synthesis. Though the transmembrane sodium concentration may be a major factor in amino acid transport there is no evidence to implicate stimulation of the Na^+ K^+ ATPase enzyme (4,5). It has been demonstrated that during the contraction–relaxation cycle there are significant nuclear conformational changes (6), and it is conceivable that such changes could activate synthetic processes (7). More directly, Schreiber et al. (8) have shown that the application of hydrostatic pressure to isolated myocardial nuclei leads to the synthesis of messenger ribonucleic acid (mRNA). In addition, they argued that this was a direct effect and not achieved through a second messenger such as cyclic AMP (cAMP).

Therefore, a direct mechanical effect on the myocardial cells could account in part for the hypertrophy of pressure overload, volume overload, heart block, anemia, and even chronic exercise.

INCREASED ENERGY REQUIREMENTS

Increases in wall stress, as well as tachycardia and increased contractility, all increase myocardial energy requirements. Furthermore, hypoxia and ischemia have been implicated as stimuli for hypertrophy. Meerson and Pomoinitsky (9) have suggested that a deficiency of high-energy phosphate compounds from either increased adenosine triphosphate (ATP) breakdown or inadequate ATP production may be responsible for activation of protein synthesis. They have postulated that the mechanism of this activation is through the accumulation of 3′5′-cAMP or other molecules from increased cellular breakdown due to ATP deficiency. However, Zimmer et al. (10) have shown that there is little correlation between ATP decline and augmented protein synthesis in isoproterenol and pressure-induced hypertrophy, and prevention of the ATP decline did not significantly inhibit the protein synthesis.

An alternative suggestion is that creatine is the stimulus to hypertrophy. This hypothesis is based on both *in vitro* studies (11) and on the observation that changes in the creatine–creatine phosphate system may be a more sensitive guide to energy stores than ATP or adenosine diphosphate (ADP) (12). This has not been confirmed, however, by recent studies (13).

NOREPINEPHRINE, BETA-ADRENORECEPTOR, OR CYCLIC AMP

Several observations have focused on the possibility that norepinephrine (NE) is the hormone that directly stimulates hypertrophy: (a) Laks and Morady (14) have induced hypertrophy with subpressor doses of NE; (b) cardiac NE content is increased in exercise-induced hypertrophy (15); (c) circulating NE rises soon after experimental aortic stenosis (16); (d) an early rise in adenyl cyclase is observed in overload states (17); and (e) cAMP has been implicated as a stimulus for selective protein synthesis (18). All of these observations would be consistent with β-adrenoreceptor activation (19).

Beta-receptor numbers are increased in thyroxine-induced hypertrophy (20) and in the aortic-constriction model in rats (21), whereas β-receptors are decreased in the spontaneously hypertensive rat (22), in rats treated chronically with isoproterenol (ISO) (23), and in desoxycorticosterone-acetate (DOCA)-salt and renal hypertensive rats (24). Both the number and responsiveness of β-receptors may be dependent on changes in the myocardial cell membrane, and Limas (25) has shown evidence for increased phospholipid methylation that could be responsible.

ANGIOTENSIN EFFECT

Although a direct effect of angiotensin on protein synthesis in the myocardium has not been documented, several studies appear to support this possibility. Khairallah and co-workers have presented data suggesting that angiotensin may stimulate protein synthesis (26). Changes in plasma renin activity appeared to correlate with changes in myocardial hypertrophy during treatment of hypertension in SHR rats (27), and Sen, Tarazi, and Bumpus (28) have shown that captopril effectively reverses myocardial hypertrophy in SHR rats. Since angiotensin has striking hemodynamic effects, dissociation between pressure-induced changes in left ventricular mass and possible direct effects of angiotensin is very difficult in the intact animal. Therefore, any role of angiotensin as a signal mechanism for hypertrophy in hypertensive individuals remains highly speculative.

PROSTAGLANDIN SYNTHESIS

Prostaglandin synthesis is stimulated in pressure-overload hypertrophy (29). Myocardial contractility has been reported to correlate with endogenous prostaglandin content (30), and prostaglandin may increase availability of calcium for the contractile process (31). These observations have led to the suggestion that prostaglandin synthesis serves as an intermediary signal for the hypertrophy process.

TISSUE HORMONE STIMULATOR

Hammond et al. (32) showed that an extract from hypertrophied heart tissue was capable of inducing hypertrophy in a normal perfused heart that was beating but performing no work. Enthusiasm for the role of a circulating tissue hormone in the genesis of hypertrophy must be tempered somewhat by an awareness that hypertrophy often tends not to be a generalized myocardial process but one that is localized to the myocardium exposed to an increased load. Nonetheless, a local role to perpetuate hypertrophy, once the process has been initiated, cannot be excluded. The mechanism by which such a tissue factor may induce protein synthesis, and the tissue specificity of such a substance, has not been established.

CHALONES

Normal cells produce substances that exert feedback inhibition on growth or division of these cells (33,34). A chalone has recently been isolated and purified from adult bovine heart (35) and this substance inhibited deoxyribonucleic acid (DNA) synthesis of newborn hamster hearts. Analysis revealed it to be a glycoprotein that fulfilled the criteria for a chalone, in that it was tissue- and not species-specific, and it had no effect on the target cell. Although any role for chalones in myocardial hyperplasia or hypertrophy is highly speculative, a reduction in circulating chalones as a result of a loss of tissue mass or as a response to a stress could be a factor in new growth.

INCREASED BLOOD FLOW

A fascinating but unexplained clinical observation is the remarkable unilateral hypertrophy that develops in an extremity with a congenital arteriovenous fistula or in an organ with an acquired fistula (36). We are aware of no study of this phenomenon; however, since the only stimulus must be related to the blood flow, it is attractive to postulate that a high-flow state may in itself induce protein synthesis and hypertrophy.

UNRESOLVED ISSUES

One or more of the above signals could account for most of the described physiologic stimuli for myocardial hypertrophy. They do not, however, provide any insight into why the synthetic process and its metabolic adjustment may be so different in response to even slightly different stresses.

One form of hypertrophy that has not received much attention is hypertrophy in response to loss of myocardial mass. We have utilized a non-ischemic model of myocardial necrosis in order to study this phenomenon. Repetitive DC shock across the left ventricle of the closed-chest dog produced localized necrosis involving from 12 to 30% of the left ventricular myocardium (37). Four days after the shock procedure, the myocardium in uninvolved areas distant from the necrosis revealed elevated RNA and DNA content indicative of activation of protein and collagen synthesis (38). Arterial pressure and cardiac output in the shocked dogs were similar to that in control dogs, and the left ventricle was not significantly dilated. Therefore, the usual evidence of pressure or volume load as a physiologic stimulus to hypertrophy was absent. The simplest explanation for this phenomenon is that the load per residual myocardial fiber is increased, since the same stroke volume and stroke work are being now generated by a lesser mass. This implies more shortening of the residual fibers, but extent of shortening is not usually viewed as a quantitatively important determinant of energy expenditure of the heart or of myocardial hypertrophy. Furthermore, the net increase in protein synthesis in these animals appears, eventually, merely to replace the mass lost to necrosis, since the heart weight is restored to normal.

Another unresolved issue is whether the synthetic process is graded in response depending on the strength of the stimulus or signal, or is an all-or-none phenomenon. Whereas the traditional view might be that the rate of myocardial hypertrophy varies with the severity of the load, recent studies from our laboratory by Morioka and Simon (39) raise some doubts. These investigators found that left ventricular wall thickness began increasing before there was much increase in blood pressure in dogs subjected to unilateral renal wrapping. The rate of increase in wall thickness appeared to be quite constant, despite an accelerated blood pressure course after contralateral nephrectomy.

Despite extensive experimental work on hypertrophy over the past decade, we remain ignorant of some of the most rudimentary aspects of the process: what turns it on, how the magnitude or duration of the process is determined, and what turns it off. An understanding of these simple questions may provide new insights into the physiologic and pathologic mechanisms of hypertrophy in man.

REFERENCES

1. Flink, I. L., and Morkin, E. (1979): *J. Biol. Chem.*, 254:3105–3110.
2. Schwartz, K., Bouveret, P., Bercovici, J., and Swynghedauw, B. (1978): *FEBS Lett.*, 93:137–140.
3. Rupp, H. (1981): *Bas. Res. Cardiol.*, 76:79–88.
4. Lesch, M., Gorlin, R., and Sonnenblick, E. H. (1970): *Circ. Res.*, 27:445–460.
5. Peterson, M. B., and Lesch, M. (1972): *Circ. Res.*, 31:317–327.
6. Bloom, S., and Cancilla, P. A. (1969): *Circ. Res.*, 24:189–196.
7. Rabinowitz, M., and Zak, R. (1972): *Ann. Rev. Med.*, 23:245–261.
8. Schreiber, S. S., Oratz, M., Rothschild, M. A., and Reff, F. (1978): *Cardiovasc. Res.*, 12:265–268.
9. Meerson, F. Z., and Pomoinitsky, V. D. (1972): *J. Mol. Cell. Cardiol.*, 4:571–597.
10. Zimmer, H. G., Steinkopff, H. I., and Koschine, H. (1980): *J. Mol. Cell. Cardiol.*, 12:421–426.

11. Ingwall, J. S. (1976): *Circ. Res. (Suppl. 38)*, I:115–122.
12. Rabinowitz, M., and Zak, R. (1975): *Circ. Res.*, 36:367–376.
13. Reilly, P. J., and Cooksey, J. D. (1979): *Proc. Soc. Exp. Biol. Med.*, 161:193–198.
14. Laks, M., and Morady, M. (1976): *Am. Heart J.*, 91:674–675.
15. Ostman, I., Sjostrand, N. O., and Swedin, G. (1972): *Acta Physiol. Scand.*, 86:299–308.
16. Caldarera, C. M., Casti, A., Rossoni, C., and Visioli, O. (1971): *J. Mol. Cell. Cardiol.*, 3:121–126.
17. Schreiber, S. S., Klein, I., Oratz, M., and Rothschild, M. A. (1971): *J. Mol. Cell. Cardiol.*, 2:55–65.
18. Wicks, W. D. (1974): In: *Advances in Cyclic Nucleotide Research, Vol. 4*, edited by P. Greengard, and G. A. Robison, pp. 335–438. Raven Press, New York.
19. Laks, M. (1977): *Am. Heart J.*, 94:394.
20. Tse, J., Wrenn, R. W., and Kuo, J. F. (1980): *Endocrinology*, 107:6–15.
21. Limas, C. (1979): *Biochim. Biophys. Acta* 588:174–178.
22. Limas, C. and Limas, C. J. (1978): *Biochem. Biophys. Res. Commun.*, 83:710–714.
23. Tse, J., Powell, J. R., Baste, C. A., Priest, R. E., and Kuo, J. F. (1979): *Endocrinology*, 105:246–255.
24. Woodcock, E. A., Funder, J. N., and Johnston, C. J. (1979): *Circ. Res.*, 45:560–565.
25. Limas, C. J. (1980): *Circ. Res.*, 47:536–554.
26. Khairallah, P. A., Robertson, A. L., and Davil, O. D. (1972): In: *Hypertension '72*, edited by J. Genest and E. Koiev, p. 212–220. Springer-Verlag, New York.
27. Sen, S., Tarazi, R. C., and Bumpus, F. M. (1977): *Cardiovasc. Res.*, 11:427–433.
28. Sen, S., Tarazi, R. C., and Bumpus, F. M. (1980): *Hypertension*, 2:169–176.
29. Chazov, E. I., Pomoinitsky, V. D., Geling, N. G., Orlova, T. R., Nekrasova, A. A., and Smirnov, V. N. (1979): *Circ. Res.*, 45:205–211.
30. Orlova, T. R., Geling, N. G., Shlain, V. A., and Pomoinitsky, V. D. (1980): *Buill. ESKP Biol. Med.*, 90:515–516.
31. Moura, A. M., and Simpkins, H. (1976): *Molecular and Cellular Endocrinology*, 5:349–357.
32. Hammond, G. L., Wieber, E., and Markert, C. (1979): *Proc. Natl. Acad. Sci. USA*, 5:2455–2459.
33. Bullough, W. S. (1962): *Biol. Rev.*, 37:307–342.
34. Rytomaa, E. (1976) *International Review Exp. Pathol.*, 16:156–206.
35. Krick, J. A., Van Der Walt, B. J., and Bester, A. J. (1981): *Proc. Natl. Acad. Sci. USA*, 7:4161–4164.
36. Horton, B. T. (1932): *JAMA*, 98:373–379.
37. Mehta, J., Runge, W., Cohn, J. N., and Carlyle, P. (1978): *J. Lab. Clin. Med.*, 91:272–279.
38. Cohn, J. N., Limas, C. J., and Carlyle, P. F. (1977): *Clin. Res.*, 25:601A.
39. Morioka, S., and Simon, G. (1981): *Am. J. Cardiol.*, 47:478.

Perspectives in Cardiovascular Research, Vol. 8,
edited by R. C. Tarazi and J. B. Dunbar.
Raven Press, New York © 1983.

Morphometric Studies of Left Ventricular Hypertrophy

Piero Anversa, Giorgio Olivetti, and Alden V. Loud

Department of Pathology, New York Medical College, Valhalla, New York 10595; and the University of Parma, Parma, Italy

Several morphometric investigations of pressure-overload hypertrophy have shown that the myocardium responds to a greater work demand by tissue, cellular, and subcellular growth adaptations. In these processes, however, little alteration is observed in the structural composition and organization of the various tissue components of the enlarged ventricle (1–4). Accumulating structural evidence suggests that experimental cardiac hypertrophy may be seen in most aspects as a form of well compensated accelerated growth. To support this point of view, this chapter will examine and compare some of the results from three recent studies (4–7) showing different magnitudes of induced hypertrophic growth in the rat heart. The myocardium is analyzed in terms of its tissue organization, the adaptations of myocyte and interstitial cell populations, and the adaptations of subcellular components in myocytes, endothelial and connective tissue cells.

TISSUE ADAPTATIONS

As shown in Table 1, an overall 30% hypertrophy of the left ventricle was obtained 1 to 4 weeks after the induction of renal hypertension (5). Constriction of the abdominal aorta to less than 40% of its normal diameter in the young adult rat results in an 85% hypertrophy of the free wall of the left ventricle in 8 days, but only 51% hypertrophy in the papillary muscle (4). In addition, tissue hypertrophy was shown to be greater in subepicardial layers of the ventricle wall than in subendocardial layers following renal hypertension (5) and thyroxin administration (8). It is clearly important to recognize the existence of different magnitudes of tissue response in different parts of the left ventricle, especially in evaluating the compensatory capacity of the ventricle and in relating physiological studies of the papillary muscle and trabeculae carnae to the ventricle as a whole (9,10).

After these changes, the volume fractions of myocytes and interstitium (Fig. 1) are practically unchanged in both the endocardial and epicardial regions examined in the renal hypertension model (5) as well as in the mid-region of

TABLE 1. *Myocardial volume hypertrophy*

	Control	Experimental	Hypertrophy (%)
Renal hypertension			
Body weights (gm)	266.1 ± 8.8	203.8 ± 8.1	—
LV volume (mm³)	635 ± 22	824 ± 13	30[a]
Aortic stenosis			
Body weights (gm)	123.7 ± 2.8	119.9 ± 3.7	—
LV free wall volume (mm³)	186 ± 14	345 ± 20	85[a]
Papillary muscle volume (mm³)	3.78 ± 0.18	5.70 ± 0.19	51[a]

[a] $p < 0.005$.

the left ventricular free wall (7) and papillary muscle (4) following aortic stenosis. Soon after the induction of hypertrophy by aortic stenosis, a significant increase of extracellular fluid throughout the myocardium was observed (11). Early hypertrophy is also accompanied by an elevation of protein synthesis restricted primarily to the myocyte compartment of the tissue (12,13). Cardiac hypertrophy of longer duration, however, leads to hyperplasia of connective tissue cells (14–17) and the accumulation of collagen (11,18). In general, after an initial imbalance (12,13), the interstitial increase parallels the enlargement of muscle cells in such a way that the volume fractions of both components maintain a substantially normal ratio (19).

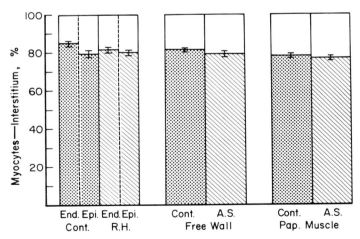

FIG. 1. Volume percent of myocytes (*filled portion of columns*) and interstitium (*empty as indicated*) in rat myocardium. In Figs. 1–5, control tissues (*stipled*) are compared with hypertrophied myocardium (*cross-hatched*) resulting from induced renal hypertension (R.H.) or aortic stenosis (A.S.). In the renal hypertension experiment, morphometric results are shown separately for subendocardial (End.) and subepicardial (Epi.) regions of the left ventricle. Independent studies of the effects of aortic stenosis are given for the mid-region of the left ventricular free wall and the left anterior papillary muscle. Indicated variation = ± SEM.

ADAPTATIONS OF THE CAPILLARY BED

Several structural properties of the microvasculature in muscle tissue are relevant to tissue oxygenation and can be evaluated by applying relatively simple morphometric methods (20):

1. Capillary luminal volume density, which is related to the volume of capillary blood available for gas exchange within the tissue;
2. Capillary luminal surface density, which represents the capillary area available for oxygen transport from the blood to the tissue;
3. The average diffusion distance from the capillary wall to the mitochondria of myocytes, where oxygen is predominantly consumed in generating ATP through the process of oxidative phosphorylation.

The capillary luminal volume fraction in the myocardium is not altered as a result of hypertrophy in either the inner, middle, or outer region of the ventricular wall or in the papillary muscle (Fig. 2). The volume faction of capillary lumen in the myocardium is the product of two factors: the number of capillaries per unit area of tissue (capillary density) and the mean luminal cross-sectional area (Fig. 3). In hypertrophy, capillary density (Fig. 3A) decreases as the individual myocytes increase in diameter. The average size of capillaries (Fig. 3B), however, is consistently larger than that in control animals. Thus, the maintenance of the capillary luminal volume fraction in hypertrophy is accomplished by two mechanisms: An increase in the transverse luminal area of the average capillary that compensates for the decrease in capillary density. These observations agree with measurements showing that coronary blood flow in hypertrophied myocardium increases in proportion to the mass of muscle and the work it must perform (21).

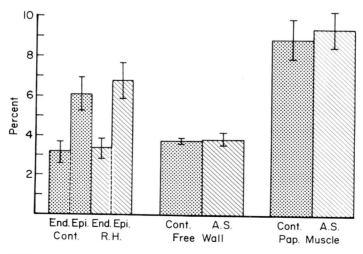

FIG. 2. Volume percent of capillary lumen in the myocardium. See legend to Fig. 1.

A. Capillary Density

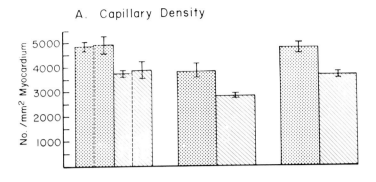

B. Capillary Lumen, Transverse Area

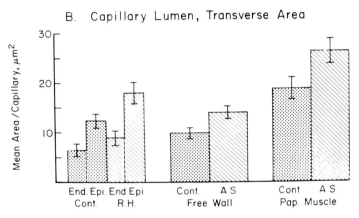

FIG. 3. A: Number of capillary profiles per mm^2 of myocardium sectioned in a plane perpendicular to the long axes of myofibers and capillaries. **B**: Mean transverse cross-sectional area of capillary lumina. See legend to Fig. 1.

Changes in capillary size and number imply corresponding changes in the luminal surface area of capillaries, the area available for oxygen transport. Capillary luminal surface area per unit volume of tissue decreases in proportion to capillary density, but increases with capillary diameter. These two structural modifications are nearly compensating in both endocardium and epicardium of the hypertensive rat and in the papillary muscle, but not so successfully in the midventricular region in the presence of a much greater left ventricular hypertrophy; this change is also not statistically significant (Fig. 4).

Effective tissue oxygenation is finally dependent on the maximum diffusion distance from capillaries to myocyte mitochondria, where oxygen is ultimately consumed. Since mitochondria are uniformly distributed in the interfibrillar compartment of the cell, this diffusion distance can be measured approximately by the radius of a cylinder of muscle tissue supplied by the average capillary,

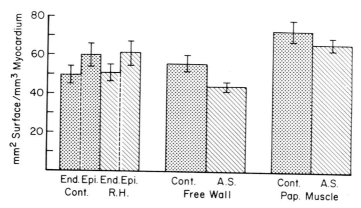

FIG. 4. Area (mm²) of capillary luminal (endothelial) surface per mm³ of myocardial tissue. See legend to Fig. 1.

based on the Krogh's cylinder model for gas exchange in tissue (20,22,23), minus the mean radius of the capillary. Values calculated for this diffusion distance (Fig. 5) are found to be about 6 to 7 μm in control animals, slightly increasing in hypertrophy to 7 to 8 μm. The approximate increase of one μm in this parameter, none of which is statistically significant, seems to be too small a change in the diffusion distance for oxygen to impair cell function (24,25). It should be noted that these morphometric analyses do not reveal the presence or absence of nonpatent capillaries, which constitute the capillary reserve in normal and hypertrophied myocardium (26,27). A small vascular reserve is present in the subendocardial region of adult myocardium (26) and

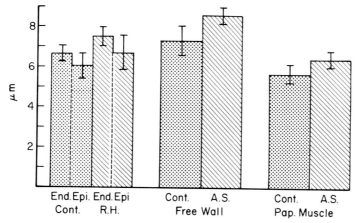

FIG. 5. Mean maximum diffusion distance for oxygen from the capillary wall into the surrounding myocardial tissue. Calculated from the radius of tissue supplied per capillary minus the radius of the average capillary. See legend to Fig. 1.

in the hypertrophied left ventricle (27), possibly causing these tissues to be more susceptible to ischemic injury.

In contrast to normal postnatal development (28,29), the process of capillary proliferation does not occur in pressure-overload hypertrophy of adult myocardium (4,5,7,30). This is evident from the lack of significant changes in the capillary:myocyte ratio and in the total length of capillaries in the left ventricle. On the other hand, adult rats subjected to an exercise regime do show capillary proliferation (30–32) that affords a significant protection of the myocardium following coronary occlusion (32). In addition, capillary proliferation has been demonstrated in severe human myocardial hypertrophy (33,34). In this case, the capillary:myocyte ratio remains essentially constant, but there is evidence that myocyte proliferation also takes place (33,34).

ADAPTATIONS OF THE CELL POPULATIONS

The response of the myocardium to a work overload involves not only the adaptation of the microvasculature but also the simultaneous growth of the three major populations of myocardial cells: myocytes, endothelial cells, and connective tissue cells. It is well established that once myocyte proliferation ceases by the age of weaning in the rat (35) both physiologic and induced myocardial growth occur principally through hypertrophy of myocytes and hyperplasia of interstitial cells (14–16,36,37). Until recently, however, these two growth mechanisms were known only in qualitative terms and the relative contributions of cellular hypertrophy and cellular hyperplasia to the expansion of the interstitial cell populations were unknown. In order to examine these fundamental cellular phenomena, we have developed a morphometric technique that allows the determination of the mean cell volume and number in a specific population of cells within a tissue (4,6). This methodology is based on the observation that the linear increase (slope) in the number of nuclear profiles per unit area of myocardial sections of increasing thickness is equal to the number of nuclei per unit volume of tissue. Such *in situ* analysis can also be performed for a mixed population of mononucleate and binucleate cells, like rat cardiac myocytes, by introducing the more general concept of the mean cell volume per nucleus.

As shown in Table 2, the hypertrophic growth of the papillary muscle was analyzed at four different levels: Whole tissue growth; aggregate enlargement of each cell population; increases in the sizes of the average cells; and changes in the numbers of cell nuclei in the whole papillary muscle. The growth of the myocyte population included an increase in the mean cell volume per nucleus (53%) essentially identical to the increase in muscle cell mass (48%) and to the volume hypertrophy of the whole papillary muscle (51%). In addition, the total number of myocyte nuclei in the whole papillary muscle remained practically constant. Similar results were obtained in the hypertensive rats and in the left ventricular free wall following aortic stenosis (5–7). In hypertensive hypertro-

TABLE 2. *Cellular hypertrophy and hyperplasia in papillary muscle growth*

	Sham-operated	Aortic stenosis	Hypertrophy (%)	Hyperplasia (%)
Volume of papillary muscle (mm³)	3.78 ± 0.18	5.70 ± 0.19	51	—
Myocytes:				
Volume of cell population (mm³)	2.96 ± 0.15	4.38 ± 0.16	48	—
Volume/cell/nucleus (μm³)	7,420 ± 570	11,380 ± 720	53	—
Number of nuclei (thousands)	399 ± 27	385 ± 15	—	−4[a]
Endothelial cells:				
Volume of cell population (mm³)	0.122 ± 0.013	0.244 ± 0.011	100	—
Volume/cell (μm³)	406 ± 18	548 ± 34	35	—
Number of cells (thousands)	300 ± 20	445 ± 32	—	48
Connective tissue cells:				
Volume of cell population (mm³)	0.083 ± 0.011	0.183 ± 0.021	120	—
Volume/cell (μm³)	356 ± 8	584 ± 22	64	—
Number of cells (thousands)	233 ± 12	314 ± 17	—	35

[a] Not significant.

phy, myocyte enlargement in the subepicardial region is greater than that in the subendocardial region, producing a greater tissue growth of the outer layers of the ventricle. The overall 100% growth in the volume of the endothelial cell population is brought about through a 35% hypertrophy of the average cell and a 48% increase in the number of these cells. Similarly, connective tissue cell growth (120%) results from a 64% increase in mean cell size and a 35% increase in cell number.

It can be concluded from these observations that cellular enlargement is the mechanism of myocyte growth in hypertrophy, whereas both cellular hypertrophy and hyperplasia contribute significantly to the growth of the interstitial cell populations. This kind of study shows, further, that myocytes comprise 90% of the volume of myocardial cells but contribute only 43% of the total number of cell nuclei. The latter value drops to 34% 8 days after the induction of myocardial hypertrophy. The overall growth response of interstitial cells is sufficient to increase their volume fraction in the papillary muscle by 40%, while that of the myocytes is unchanged. Some of the altered physiologic characteristics of hypertrophied myocardium have been attributed to changes in the interstitial components of the tissue (9). Since collagen content has little effect on contractility (9), it is possible that changes in the mean cell volumes and numbers of interstitial cells are significant factors in altering the physiologic properties of the myocardium in hypertrophy.

SUBCELLULAR ADAPTATIONS

A remarkably constant property of myocytes is the maintenance of their cell surface to volume ratio in hypertrophy (3–5,7,29,38). Cellular enlargement

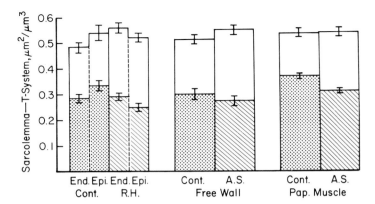

FIG. 6. Ratio of myocyte cell surface to volume, shown as the sum of its external sarcolemma (*filled portion of columns*) and T-system (*empty portion of columns*) components.

decreases the relative surface area of the external sarcolemma (Fig. 6), but this is practically compensated perfectly by the increased surface area of the internalized T-system membranes. A further constant property present in hypertrophied myocytes is the ratio of myocyte cell surface to myofibrillar volume (Fig. 7). It has been suggested that the reduction of the ratio of external cell surface to myofibrillar volume, occurring with cell enlargement in the postnatal period, may elicit the formation of the T-system as this ratio approaches 1 $\mu m^2/\mu m^3$ (38). The compensatory role of the T-system in maintaining a constant cell surface to volume ratio may be related to the speed of conduction of the action potential across the myocardium (39). In general, enlarged cells having less surface area to depolarize per unit volume conduct at a faster rate (40). The constancy of the cell surface to volume ratio suggests that overall increases in cell surface membrane, including the T-system, result in a pro-

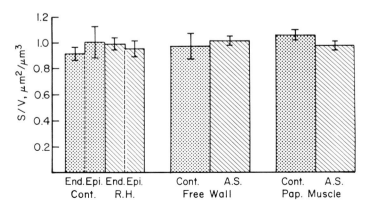

FIG. 7. Ratio of total myocyte cell surface to myofibril volume.

portional increase in total membrane capacitance, minimizing electrophysiological changes during growth and hypertrophy. Although its relative importance may vary from species to species (41), the total cell surface (sarcolemma plus T-system) in cardiac muscle cells has been shown also to have a significant role in calcium metabolism. Since an extracellular calcium source is required in the myocardium, Ca^{2+} movement to the myofilaments occurs through an intermediate binding and exchange region represented by the basement membrane (42,43). This structure is a rather homogeneous appearing layer, approximately 50 nm thick, which coats the sarcolemma and the T-tubules.

The smooth endoplasmic reticulum (SR) in cardiac muscle, like skeletal muscle, functions in excitation–contraction coupling by the release and subsequent uptake of calcium (42). The ratio of SR surface to myofibrillar volume (Fig. 8) increases 20 to 35% during the process of myocyte hypertrophy. This disproportionate growth of SR may be functioning as a compensatory mechanism for the reduced calcium binding capacity of the SR in hypertrophied myocardium (44,45).

The mitochondria represent the primary source of energy for myofibrils through the generation of adenosine triphosphate (ATP) in the mitochondrial cristae. Reduction of the mitochondrial:myofibril volume ratio is a consistent subcellular alteration occurring in myocytes following pressure-overload hypertrophy (1,2). In the models discussed here, this ratio decreases 15 to 20% in all but the subepicardial region of the ventricular wall, where a 7% reduction is not statistically significant (Fig. 9). The general diminishment of this ratio may lead to a relatively deficient energy supply, eventually compromising heart muscle function. Early in the hypertrophic response, however, mitochondrial growth exceeds myofibrillar growth, leading to a transitory elevation of the mitochondrial:myofibril ratio (13), also associated with the synthesis of mitochondrial membranes (46). In contrast to pressure overload hypertrophy,

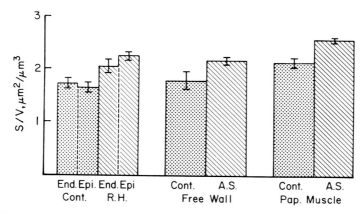

FIG. 8. Ratio of sarcoplasmic reticulum surface to myofibril volume in myocardial myocytes.

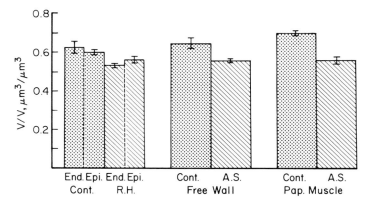

FIG. 9. Ratio of mitochondrial volume to myofibril volume in myocardial myocytes.

the mitochondrial:myofibril ratio is not reduced by a volume overload (47) or by thyroxin administration (3).

Weibel (23) has recently proposed a relevant way to relate the sites of oxygen utilization (mitochondria) to the oxygen source (capillary surface) in tissues. It was found that the ratio of mitochondrial volume to capillary surface is a structural parameter characteristic of different tissues. Figure 10 shows values of this ratio calculated from the present data, ranging from approximately 3 to 5 $\mu m^3/\mu m^2$. None of the values for each tissue region is significantly altered by the process of myocardial hypertrophy. This is then another ratio suggesting the maintenance of structural properties in hypertrophied myocardium.

Looking at the mitochondria of muscle cells as a population of organelles having measurable mean size and number, the adaptation of this population can also be described in terms of the processes of organelle hypertrophy and hyperplasia. Values for the mean mitochondrial size and number per nucleus

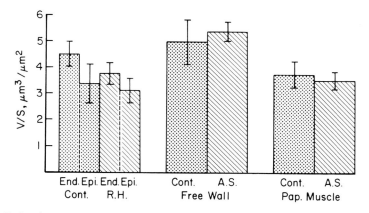

FIG. 10. Ratio of myocyte mitochondrial volume to capillary luminal surface in the myocardium.

TABLE 3. *Mitochondrial adaptation in papillary muscle myocytes*

	Sham-operated	Aortic stenosis	% Change
Volume of mitochondria/cell volume/nucleus (μm^3)	2620 ± 210	3510 ± 230	34[a]
Mean transverse cross-sectional area (μm^2)	0.506 ± 0.023	0.410 ± 0.023	−19[a]
Mean longitudinal length (μm)	1.090 ± 0.023	1.092 ± 0.034	0
Mean mitochondrial volume (μm^3)	0.551 ± 0.028	0.448 ± 0.029	−19[a]
Number per nucleus	4760 ± 440	7830 ± 730	65[a]
μm^2 inner membranes/μm^3 mitochondrion	37.4 ± 3.1	38.8 ± 3.9	4

[a] $p < 0.05$.

obtained in the papillary muscle study (4) are listed in Table 3. Hypertrophy results in a marked (65%) hyperplasia of mitochondria, whose average size is reduced by 19%. It should be noted that the surface density of mitochondrial inner membranes per unit volume of these organelles is not altered in the smaller mitochondria. It has been shown that mitochondrial hypertrophy occurs before mitochondrial multiplication as early as 20 hr after an induced pressure overload (13).

The concepts of hypertrophy and hyperplasia can be similarly applied to the growth of the myofibrillar reticulum in myocytes. Myofibrils are formed of bundles of myofilaments that branch and recombine throughout the length of the cell (4). Detailed quantitative measurements of myofibrillar growth were made in the papillary muscle model of induced hypertrophy. Table 4 shows that the mean transverse cross-sectional area, the surface-to-volume ratio, and sarcomere length are not significantly different 8 days after aortic stenosis. These observations suggest that the size and shape of the average myofibril are essentially unchanged after a 67% increase in the total myofibrillar mass per cell. Thus, the average myofibril exhibits no hypertrophic growth and the increase in contractile substance is accountable entirely by hyperplasia of the myofibrils. This phenomenon is most readily apparent in the 84% increase in the number of myofibrils seen in the mean transverse cross-sectional area of

TABLE 4. *Myofibrillar adaptation in papillary muscle myocytes*

	Sham-operated	Aortic stenosis	% Change
Volume of myofibrils/cell volume/ nucleus (μm^3)	3770 ± 290	6290 ± 400	67[a]
Mean cross-sectional area/myofibril (μm^2)	1.517± 0.041	1.391 ± 0.057	−8
Myofibril surface:volume ratio (μm^{-1})	3.50 ± 0.11	3.26 ± 0.05	−7
Sarcomere length (μm)	1.868 ± 0.039	1.827 ± 0.011	−2
Myofibrils/average cell cross-sectional area	39.6 ± 3.2	72.8 ± 3.9	84[a]

[a] $p < 0.0001$.

myocytes. The mechanism by which such growth occurs is still unknown, although it has been suggested that myofibrils may increase in size by the addition of new contractile proteins at their periphery (19,48) and subsequently split to form two myofibrils (49). The maintenance of myofibrillar size and shape may be due to the existence of a critical perimitochondrial radius for ATP supply of the contractile mass surrounding the mitochondrion, as recently suggested by Page (50).

As previously shown in Table 2, the populations of endothelial cells and connective tissue cells grow by different combinations of cellular hypertrophy and hyperplasia. Their overall organelle growth is nearly proportional to the growth in each population (4). Among endothelial cells of the papillary muscle, there is a 73% increase in the volume and number of pinocytotic vesicles, more than enough to maintain the mechanism for transcapillary exchange for molecules of different sizes (51). Among fibroblasts, the augmentation of the surface area of rough endoplasmic reticulum is 139%, possibly related to the synthesis of extracellular proteins, such as collagen, which accumulates later in hypertrophy (11,18).

In conclusion, the most evident observation from these studies of induced myocardial hypertrophy is the absence of severe relative structural changes. We feel we have looked in detail at a remarkable degree of well balanced compensatory response. Thus, these data probably provide information related more to the compensatory reserve capacity of the myocardium than to changes preliminary to heart failure. Clearly a greater and/or more prolonged stress will be needed to reveal the primary and sequential steps of the pathological uncompensated response.

ACKNOWLEDGMENTS

This work was supported in part by U. S. Public Health Service Research Grants HL-24479 and HL-14713 from the Heart, Lung and Blood Institute, National Institutes of Health; by a Grant-in-Aid from the American Heart Association, with funds contributed in part by the New York Heart Association; and by grants from the Consiglio Nazionale delle Ricerche (C.N.R.).

REFERENCES

1. Anversa, P., Vitali-Mazza, L., Visioli, O., and Marchetti, G. (1971): *J. Mol. Cell. Cardiol.*, 3:213–227.
2. Page, E., Polimeni, P. I., Zak, R., Earley, J., and Johnson, M. (1972): *Circ. Res.*, 30:430–439.
3. Page, E., and McCallister, L. P. (1973): *Am. J. Cardiol.*, 31:172–181.
4. Anversa, P., Olivetti, G., Melissari, M., and Loud, A. V. (1980): *J. Mol. Cell. Cardiol.*, 12:781–795.
5. Anversa, P., Loud, A. V., Giacomelli, F., and Wiener, J. (1978): *Lab. Invest.*, 38:597–609.
6. Loud, A. V., Anversa, P., Giacomelli, F., and Wiener, J. (1978): *Lab. Invest.*, 38:586–596.
7. Anversa, P., Olivetti, G., Melissari, M., and Loud, A. V. (1979): *Lab. Invest.*, 40:341–349.
8. Gerdes, A. M., Callas, G., and Kasten, F. H. (1979): *Am. J. Anat.*, 56:523–532.

9. Bing, O. H. L., Fanburg, B. L., Brooks, W. W., and Matsushita, S. (1978): *Circ. Res.*, 43:632–637.
10. Hamrell, B. B., and Alpert, N. R. (1977): *Circ. Res.*, 40:20–25.
11. Skosey, J. L., Zak, R., Martin, A. F., Aschenbrenner, V., and Rabinowitz, M. (1972): *Circ. Res.*, 31:145–157.
12. Anversa, P., Vitali-Mazza, L., Gandolfi, A., and Loud, A. V. (1975): *Lab. Invest.*, 33:125–129.
13. Anversa, P., Loud, A. V., and Vitali-Mazza, L. (1975): *Lab. Invest.*, 35:475–483.
14. Morkin, E., and Ashford, T. P. (1968): *Am. J. Physiol.*, 215:1409–1413.
15. Grove, D., Nair, K. G., and Zak, R. (1969): *Circ. Res.*, 25:463–471.
16. Grove, D., Zak, R., Nair, K. G., and Aschenbrenner, V. (1969): *Circ. Res.*, 25:473–485.
17. Bishop, S. P., and Melsen, L. R. (1976): *Circ. Res.*, 39:238–245.
18. Lindy, S., Turto, H., and Uitto, J. (1972): *Circ. Res.*, 30:205–209.
19. Anversa, P., Hagopian, M., and Loud, A. V. (1973): *Lab. Invest.*, 29:282–292.
20. Hoppeler, H., Mathieu, O., Weibel, E. R., Krauer, R., Lindstedt, S. L., and Taylor, C. R. (1981): *Respir. Physiol.*, 44:129–150.
21. Nishiyama, K., Nishiyama, A., and Frohlich, E. D. (1976): *Am. J. Physiol.*, 230:691–698.
22. Krogh, A. (1919): *J. Physiol.*, 52:409–415.
23. Weibel, E. R. (1979): In: *Evolution of Respiratory Processes*, edited by S. C. Wood and C. Lenfant, pp. 289–346. Dekker, New York.
24. Rakusan, K. (1971): *Oxygen in the Heart Muscle*. Charles C. Thomas, Springfield.
25. Mueller, T. M., Tomanek, R. J., Kerber, R. E., and Maraes, M. L. (1980): *Am. J. Physiol.*, 239:H731–H735.
26. Myers, W. W., and Honig, C. R. (1964): *Am. J. Physiol.*, 207:653–660.
27. Henquell, L., Odoroff, C. L., and Honig, C. R., (1977): *Circ. Res.*, 41:400–408.
28. Rakusan, K., Jelinek, J., Korecky, B., Soukupova, M., and Poupa, O. (1965): *Physiol. Bohemoslov.*, 14:32–37.
29. Olivetti, G., Anversa, P., and Loud, A. V. (1980): *Circ. Res.*, 46:503–512.
30. Ljungqvist, A., and Unge, G. (1972): *Acta Pathol. Microbiol. (Scand).*, 80:329–340.
31. Leon, A. S., and Bloor, C. M. (1976): *Adv. Cardiol.*, 18:81–92.
32. McElroy, C. L., Gissen, S. A., and Fishbein, M. C. (1978): *Circulation*, 57:958–962.
33. Linzbach, A. J. (1960): *Am. J. Cardiol.*, 5:370–382.
34. Astorri, E., Chizzola, A., Visioli, O., Anversa, P., Olivetti, G., and Vitali-Mazza, L. (1971): *J. Mol. Cell. Cardiol.*, 2:99–110.
35. Claycomb, W. C. (1975): *J. Biol. Chem.*, 250:3229–3235.
36. Katzberg, A. A., Farmer, B. B., and Harris, R. A. (1977): *Am. J. Anat.*, 149:489–500.
37. Korecky, B., and Rakusan, K. (1978): *Am. J. Physiol.*, 234:H123–H128.
38. Page, E., Earley, J., and Power, B. (1974): *Circ. Res. (Suppl.)*, 34/35:12–16.
39. McNutt, N. S., and Fawcett, D. W. (1969): *J. Cell. Biol.*, 42:46–67.
40. Hodgkin, A. L. (1964): *The Conduction of the Nervous Impulse*. Charles C Thomas, Springfield.
41. Bodem, R., and Sonnenblick, E. H. (1975): *Am. J. Physiol.*, 228:250–261.
42. Langer, G. A. (1973): *Ann. Rev. Physiol.*, 35:55–86.
43. Frank, J. S., Langer, G. A., Nudd, L. M., and Seraydarian, K. (1977): *Circ. Res.*, 41:702–714.
44. Sordahl, L. A., McCollum, W. B., Wood, W. G., and Schwartz, A. (1973): *Am. J. Physiol.*, 224:497–502.
45. Ito, Y., Suko, J., and Chidsey, C. A. (1974): *J. Mol. Cell. Cardiol.*, 6:237–247.
46. Albin, R., Dowell, R. T., Zak, R., and Rabinowitz, M. (1973): *Biochem. J.*, 136:629–637.
47. Vitali-Mazza, L., and Anversa, P. (1972): In: *Colloque INSERM*, pp. 55–57. Les Surchanges Cardiaques, Paris.
48. Morkin, E. (1970): *Science*, 167:1499–1501.
49. Bishop, S. P., and Cole, C. R. (1969): *Lab. Invest.*, 20:219–229.
50. Page, E. (1978): *Am. J. Physiol.*, 235:C147–C158.
51. Simionescu, N., Simionescu, M., and Palade, G. E. (1978): *Microvasc. Res.*, 15:17–36.

Perspectives in Cardiovascular Research, Vol. 8,
edited by R. C. Tarazi and J. B. Dunbar.
Raven Press, New York © 1983.

Cell Size in Experimental Cardiomegaly

Karel Rakusan and Borivoj Korecky

Department of Physiology, School of Medicine, University of Ottawa, Ottawa, Ontario, Canada

The basic structural and functional unit of the heart is the cardiac myocyte. The size of cardiac myocyte, which may also influence its function, is increased in most of the cases of experimental cardiomegaly; therefore, this abnormal situation is usually described as cardiac hypertrophy. However, cardiac hyperplasia, i.e., an increase in the number of cardiac muscle cells, is also possible. We have recently analyzed the problem of cardiac hypertrophy as opposed to cardiac hyperplasia (1). In this chapter the methods available for determination of the number of muscle cells in the heart are critically reviewed. As a complement, we present an inventory of available methods for estimation of cell size in cardiac muscle, accompanied with a critical analysis of each. Subsequently, we will review some of our own data concerning cell size in different types of experimental cardiomegaly produced in rats. We will try to determine how the estimated size of the cardiac myocyte is dependent on the method of its measurement, on the site of sampling, on the age of the experimental animal, and on the type of stimulus for accelerated cardiac growth.

METHODS USED FOR ESTIMATION OF CELL SIZE

Size of the myocyte can be estimated either by biochemical analysis of the myocardium or by quantitative morphology. Methods of quantitative morphology may be applied to the isolated myocytes or to the tissue sections.

Biochemical Analysis of the Myocardium

Using biochemical analysis, the size of cardiac myocyte is indirectly estimated by measuring the deoxyribonucleic acid (DNA) content of the tissue and relating cardiac weight or protein to DNA. Indices such as protein:DNA or weight:DNA may serve as a measure of cell size. The tissue is easy to sample, no subjective judgement is involved, and standard biochemical analysis is applied. Nevertheless, this method is useful only as a fast approach in a pilot study for the following reasons. It does not take into account variations in DNA content per nucleus (varying degrees of polyploidy) or variations in the number of nuclei per cell (the percentage of bi- and polynucleated myocytes), and it does not distinguish between the DNA of cardiac myocytes and the DNA of remaining "nonmuscle" cells. Further improvements to this approach have been made by Cheek (2), who suggests correcting the cardiac weight for its extracellular component, e.g., to use muscle weight minus the chloride space as a measure of cellular mass. Furthermore, he proposes the measurement of the DNA unit as a functional replacement of the size of the muscle cell. It was suggested that each nucleus within the myocyte has jurisdiction over a certain volume or mass of cytoplasm to form a DNA unit. On the basis of DNA concentration in the tissue, one can measure the number of diploid nuclei per gram. If one gram of muscle, minus the extracellular fluid in that gram, is divided by the number of nuclei, the size of the DNA unit is obtained. For instance, the DNA unit in the adult rat myocyte would be close to half of the cell size, as 80 to 90 percent of the myocytes are binucleated (3,4). It is of interest that mononucleated cardiac myocytes are approximately one-half of the size of the binucleated cells (5). It should be stressed, however, that even in its improved form, the biochemical approach yields only an estimate of the average size of the myocyte, without any indication of its variability.

Measurements Based on Isolated Myocytes

The isolation technique consists of retrograde perfusion of the coronary vascular tree with hyaluronidase and collagenase and subsequent mechanical separation of adhering cells. In this case, cell width and length are measured either on spontaneously contracting cells observed under phase contrast or on fixed cells using normal microscopy. Cell width can be measured easily, while the subjective element of averaging the irregularities of the intercalated discs is involved in estimations of the cell length. The volume of the myocyte is then calculated using the above parameters and assumed cylindrical configuration. This method is relatively fast and also yields estimates of the variability of cell dimensions. It contains, however, a subjective error and a potential sampling error due to the varying yield of cells. The cell volume is calculated using the cylindrical model which is certainly only a crude approximation of the cell shape (6).

Histometric Methods

The histometric approach to measuring myocytes contains a pleiade of methods which can be subdivided as follows.

Measurements on Cross-Sections

Direct measurement of the cell diameter on cross-sections can be made using a screw micrometer eyepiece. This method presupposes cross-sections precisely perpendicular to the long axis of the cells. Even in this case, however, the cross-sections of the myocytes are not circular but, rather, resemble elipses. If one presumes the cylindrical configuration of the muscle cells, the ellipsoid shape of the cross-section is the result of the distortion due to an angle of the section which is not precisely perpendicular to the long axis. The more this angle differs from 90°, the greater will be the difference between the long and short axes of the ellipsoid on the cross-section. The short axis, however, does not increase, and it corresponds to the diameter of the cylinder.

In a second approach, the departure from the ideal cylindrical configuration is assumed, and the average diameter is determined as a mean of the shortest diameter and one perpendicular to it, or as a mean of the shortest and longest diameters. The best solution of this approach is presented in Aherne's method (7), based on two theorems in geometrical probability. The computing formula is $A = L \times l$, where A is the mean cross-sectional area of the cell, L is the mean value of measurements made across the cell from the most lateral point on one side to the most lateral point on the other side, and l is the mean value of the measurements made at random across the cell profile (i.e., the mean chord).

This methodical approach calls for strictly perpendicular sections, is relatively time consuming, and requires a large number of measurements in order to obtain representative sampling. Calculation of the cell volume assumes the cylindrical model and a constant width-to-length ratio, or, alternatively, additional measurements of the cell length. On the other hand, it provides, in addition to the average values, an estimate of their variability.

With indirect estimation of the cell diameter on a cross-section, it is possible to measure the total cross-sectional area of the muscle cells per unit area and divide it by the number of cell profiles in this area. The result equals the mean cross-sectional area of a single myocyte. The area of the muscle profile may be measured planimetrically, or, more conveniently, by a stereological method of point counting.

An alternative approach is to measure stereologically both volume density and surface density and to derive an average cell diameter as suggested by Arai and co-workers (8). We assume that individual muscle fibers are so transformed as to make geometrical cylinders without changing the surface-to-volume ratio; the diameter of a cylinder is then determined as:

$$S/V = \pi D/\pi(D^2/4) = 4/D, \quad \text{and}$$
$$D = 4V/S$$

This method shares some of the pitfalls of the previous one (the need of exactly perpendicular sections and length measurements, and assumption of the cylindrical model). It is, however, much faster and less subjective than measuring the individual diameters. On the other hand, only average values of the cell diameters are obtained.

Measurements on Longitudinal Sections

The diameter of a muscle cell can be measured accurately on a longitudinal section, only in the situation in which the equatorial plane is located within the slice, since measurements on the remaining sections would yield false low values. It may be possible to detect the presence of the equatorial plane by focusing. If the image of a muscle cell becomes larger and smaller again when focusing up and down, its equatorial plane is located in the slice and may be measured. If by focusing in any one direction (up or down) the image keeps growing until the muscle cell disappears from focus, its equatorial plane lies outside the slice and it is not measured.

A second possible approach is more complicated but less subjective and less tiresome, because it eliminates the need of focusing. In this case, the width of all cells is measured and the result is corrected subsequently for underestimation due to the presence of cells that were cut outside their longitudinal axis. It is possible to calculate the degree of underestimation which depends mainly on the ratio between cell diameter and the thickness of the section (9).

Measurement of the diameter on longitudinal sections with subsequent corrections is faster than direct measurements on a cross-section. The disadvantage is, once again, its dependence on the cylindrical model and the need for access to a computer.

Measurements Based on Tissue Nuclear Profiles

Counts of the number of myocyte nuclear profiles in several histological sections of increasing thickness can be used in order to derive the number of muscle cell nuclei per unit of tissue volume. Finding the myocyte fraction of the tissue volume, independently measured by the point counting technique, it is possible to calculate the average myocyte volume per nucleus that corresponds to the DNA unit as described above (10). The average volume of the myocyte is then estimated taking into account the percentage of bi- and polynucleated cells.

This is a relatively fast method, which therefore enables representative sampling. The subjective component is its need for distinction between muscle and nonmuscle cell nuclei and the ability to estimate the fraction of binucleated cells. Only average values of the volume are obtained.

As may be seen from this review of the available methods for myocyte measurement, each has some strong and weak components. Their main features are summarized in Table 1. The method of choice will depend on the whole experimental protocol and objectives of the study. Whenever possible, only directly measured parameters should be compared. For instance, even a relatively small error in direct measuring of the cell diameter will be amplified when used for computation of three-dimensional volume.

TABLE 1. *Overview of methods used for determination of cell size*

METHOD:	TIME COST	SUBJECTIVITY	SAMPLING	VARIABILITY OBTAINED
BIOCHEMICAL	+	−	−	NO
ISOLATED MYOCYTES	++	++	+	YES
LONGITUDINAL	++	+	+	YES
CROSS-SECTION AVERAGE	++	+	+	NO
CROSS-SECTION INDIVIDUAL	+++	+++	++	YES
NUCLEAR PROFILES	++	+	+	NO

CELL SIZE IN EXPERIMENTAL CARDIOMEGALY

The size of the cardiac myocyte under conditions of accelerated cardiac growth may depend on several factors. It may depend on type of cardiac overload (due to an increase in pressure or in volume), on its rate of development (sudden versus gradual), on the type and age of the organism. The following is a recapitulation of some of our measurements of cell size in experimental cardiomegaly produced in newborn and adult rats by pressure or volume overload with sudden or gradual onset.

The effect of the method of measurement on the estimates of the cell volume is illustrated in Table 2. In this case, aortic banding was produced in adult rats by placing a ring on the abdominal aorta, which resulted in a significant increase in left ventricular weight. The cell size was estimated either by histometric method [indirect estimation on a cross-section (11)] or by measuring cell length and width on isolated myocytes (12). In both situations, a significant increase in the volume of cardiac myocytes has been observed. The absolute values of the cell volume obtained by the cell isolation method, however, seem

TABLE 2. *Two methods of measuring cardiomegaly due to aortic banding in adult rats*

AORTIC BANDING IN ADULT RATS			
ISOLATED MYOCYTES		HISTOLOGY (subendocardial)	
Controls vs Experimental			
LVW mg	752 vs 963	524 vs 781	
Length μm:	120 vs 129	No. of myocytes/mm²	2666 vs 2263
Width μm:	22.2 vs 25.1	Cell profile μm²	300 vs 354
Volume μm³ x 10³	48.4 vs 66.6		30.9 vs 39.7

Data for isolated myocytes are from Korecky and Rakusan, ref.12; data for histometry, from Rakusan and Poupa, ref. 11.

to be higher than those obtained by the histometric method. The isolated myocytes are devoid of interstitium which may have restricted their expansion. There also may be a certain degree of swelling, since their sarcolemmas would be at least temporarily damaged during the separation from neighboring cells (e.g., cleavage of nexuses). All these factors may lead to an increase of cell volume. On the other hand, the preparation of cardiac tissue for histology involves dehydration and shrinkage, which may lead to a decrease of cell volume. The true values of the cell volumes under *in vivo* conditions probably lie between these two extremes.

With the effect of heterogeneity, the values of the cell size are influenced and they depend on the site of sampling as well. There are many reports dealing with heterogeneity of cardiac tissue. Regional differences in the size of cardiac myocytes have been reported, for instance, by Anversa et al. (13), Bishop et al. (14), Gerdes and co-workers (15), and Tomanek (16). In our own study (17), cardiomegaly was produced by chronic aorto-caval fistula in adult rats. Cell width was measured on longitudinal sections with subsequent corrections in two cardiac regions: midwall and subendocardial. While no significant regional differences were found in the normal hearts, a greater increase in the size of myocyte was found in the subendocardial region of the hypertrophic hearts when compared to the midwall region (Table 3). These results underline the importance of sampling for comparison of the results and for general conclusions.

Finally, the effect of age of the organism is illustrated by examples summarized in Table 4 and Fig. 1. Aortic banding in 5-day-old rats resulted in an increase of the left ventricular weight to more than double the values in their sham-operated littermates when both groups were killed at the age of one month (K. Rakusan, B. Korecky, and V. Mezl, *unpublished results*). On the other hand, a similar procedure in the adult animals resulted only in a much smaller increase in left ventricular weight (11). Even life-long spontaneous hypertension resulted in a relatively moderate increase in cardiac weight in 23-month-old rats (K. Rakusan, E. Lakatta, H. A. Spurgeon, and G. Wolfoard, *unpublished results*). The cell size was estimated in the subendocardial region

TABLE 3. *Cardiomegaly reduced by aorto-caval fistula in adult rats*

AORTO-CAVAL FISTULA IN ADULT RATS		
Method: longitudinal measurements		
Controls vs Experimental		
	MIDWALL	SUBENDOCARDIAL
Cell width μm	16.7 vs 18.1	16.9 vs 21.3
Cell volume $\mu m^3 \times 10^3$	22.2 vs 26.3	20.9 vs 42.4

Two regions measured by the same method of longitudinal sections. For more detail, see Hatt et al., ref 17.

TABLE 4. *Cardiomegaly due to pressure overload in neonatal, adult, and senescent rats*

METHOD: Histological sections
CONTROLS vs EXPERIMENTAL

| | AORTIC BANDING | | SHR |
	Neonatal	Adult	Senescent
LVW mg	252 vs 555	524 vs 781	1296 vs 1789
Subendocardial:			
No. of myocytes/mm^2	3626 vs 2706	2666 vs 2263	2162 vs 1772
Volume μm^3 x 10^3	21.2 vs 33.5	30.9 vs 39.7	44.9 vs 58.3
Midwall:			
Diameter μm	15.0 vs 17.0	-	18.2 vs 21.6
Volume μm^3 x 10^3	14.2 vs 20.8	-	24.9 vs 41.8

Data from K. Rakusan, B. Korecky, and V. Mezl (*unpublished results*), Rakusan and Poupa, ref. 11, and K. Rakusan, E. Lakatta, H. A. Spurgeon, and G. Wolfoard (*unpublished results*).

by indirect estimation on cross-sections, while direct measurements were performed on longitudinally cut midwall sections. Generally, the former method yielded higher estimates of the cell volume. Cardiomegaly observed in adult animals is characterized by an increase of the cell volume more or less cor-

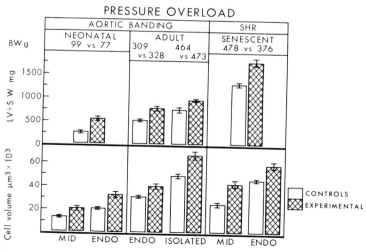

FIG. 1. Body weight, left ventricular weight, and cell volume in different types of cardiomegaly induced by pressure overload. Mean values ±SEM. **Mid**, midwall region; **endo**, subendocardial region; **isolated**, isolated myocytes; **SHR**, rats with spontaneous hypertension. Data from Rakusan et al. (*unpublished results*) (aortic banding in neonates), Rakusan and Poupa, ref. 11, Korecky and Rakusan, ref. 12 (aortic banding in adults), and Rakusan et al. (*unpublished results*) (SHR).

responding to an increase in the left ventricular weight. In contrast, a substantial increase in left ventricular weight due to aortic banding in neonatal animals is accompanied by a relatively small increase in the cell volume, indicating that more than half of the increase in cardiac weight in this experimental situation is due to proliferation of new cardiac muscle cells, i.e., cellular hyperplasia.

We can summarize the results as follows:

1. Cell dimensions and volume can be measured by several methods, each of which has distinct advantages and disadvantages.

2. The absolute values of the cell volume vary, depending on the method used. Usually, the cell volume estimated from the measurements made on isolated cells is higher than the volume estimated from measurements on histological cross-sections, which in turn yield higher values than the method utilizing longitudinal sections.

3. Cell size may vary depending on the sampling site. In our measurements of cell size in cardiomegaly induced by volume overload, the cell volume was greater in the subendocardial than in the midwall region.

4. The growth response of the cardiac myocyte will also depend on the age and developmental stage of the organism. In cardiomegaly induced in newborn rats, cell proliferation still takes place and, therefore, an increase in cell volume is much smaller than expected from the increase in ventricular mass. In contrast, cardiomegaly induced in adult animals is characterized by an increase in cell volume that can account for a proportional increase in cardiac mass.

REFERENCES

1. Rakusan, K., Korecky, B., and Mezl, V. (1983): In: *Hypertrophy and Failure*, edited by N. Alpert, pp. 103–109. Raven Press, New York.
2. Cheek, D. B. (1975): *Fetal and Postnatal Cellular Growth*. Wiley, New York.
3. Katzberg, A. A., Farmer, B. B., and Harris, R. A. (1977). *J. Anat.*, 149:489–500.
4. Korecky, B., Sweet, S., and Rakusan, K. (1979): *Canad. J. Physiol. Pharmacol.*, 57:1122–1129.
5. Bishop, S. P., and Drummond, J. L. (1979): *J. Mol. Cell. Cardiol.*, 11:423–433.
6. Phillips, S. J., Pappas, E. A., Paulosky, M., and Meir-Levi, D. (1981): International Society for Heart Research Meeting, Abstract No. 14. Burlington, Vermont.
7. Aherne, W. (1968): *J. Neurol. Sci.*, 7:519–528.
8. Arai, S., Machida, A., and Nakamura, T. (1968): *Tohoku J. Exp. Med.*, 95:35–54.
9. Rakusan, K., Raman, S., Layberry, R., and Korecky, B. (1978): *Circ. Res.*, 42:212–218.
10. Loud, A. V., Anversa, P., Giacommelli, F., and Wiener, J. (1978): *Lab. Invest.*, 38:586–596.
11. Rakusan, K., and Poupa, O. (1966): *Cardiologia*, 49:293–298.
12. Korecky, B., and Rakusan, K. (1978): *Am. J. Physiol.*, 234:H123–H128.
13. Anversa, P., Loud, A. V., Giacomelli, F., and Wiener, J. (1978): *Lab. Invest.*, 38:597–609.
14. Bishop, S. P., Oparil, S., Reynolds, R. M., and Drummond, J. L. (1979): *Hypertension*, 1:378–383.
15. Gerdes, A. M., Callas, G., and Kasten, F. H. (1979): *Am. J. Anat.*, 156:523–531.
16. Tomanek, R. J. (1979): *Lab. Invest.*, 40:83–91.
17. Hatt, P. Y., Rakusan, K., Gastineau, P., and Laplace, M. (1979): *J. Mol. Cell. Cardiol.*, 11:989–998.

Perspectives in Cardiovascular Research, Vol. 8,
edited by R. C. Tarazi and J. B. Dunbar.
Raven Press, New York © 1983.

Alterations in Cardiac Collagen with Hypertrophy

James B. Caulfield

Department of Pathology, University of South Carolina School of Medicine, Columbia, South Carolina 29208

The myocytes of the ventricles of the heart generate stress in three dimensions. To effect expulsion of blood under pressure, the stresses generated must be transmitted to the ventricular cavity. Similarly, the stress of diastolic filling must be transmitted to the myocytes throughout the ventricular wall. Since most stresses are transmitted via connective tissue, especially collagen, a complex network of collagen can be anticipated for stress distribution in the heart. The actual distribution of the collagen should reflect the stresses at various levels of organization from the cell-to-cell relationships to the entire ventricular wall.

In the presence of abnormal stress, either in amount (as in hypertension) or in direction (as in overdistended ventricles), one can expect the collagen matrix to react in a way quite similar to Wolff's law as developed for stress on bones (1). The reaction could take two forms: a simple increase in the size of individual collagen components, or an alteration in form. A third reaction, the presence of collagen in the form of a scar secondary to loss of tissue, will alter ventricular function severely (2).

Connective tissue is dynamic; turnover has been demonstrated, and the response of interstitial cells to an increased stress—such as aortic banding—is manifest within hours (3). However, following pulmonary artery banding in dogs, the wall stress relationship to volume–mass ratios follows a complex pattern that appears to be biphasic (4). This suggests that alterations of the ventricular form occur over months, and that the final configuration may not have been reached even in the forty weeks of this experiment. Although the connective tissue responds rapidly to pulmonary artery banding, the total effect of this intervention is not complete for much greater periods of time.

In this chapter, some of these contentions will be demonstrated, specifically that there is a complex three-dimensional network of collagen in the heart, and that, under conditions of altered stress, this network will respond. Certain functions can be ascribed to various components of the collagen matrix, and when the matrix is altered, some alteration of function may occur.

MATERIALS AND METHODS

All hearts were examined by standard light microscopy and polarizing optics using paraffin sections. All hearts were examined by scanning electron microscopy (SEM) using standard preparative techniques (5). Some hearts were examined by transmission electron microscopy (TEM) at 60 and 80 kV, and a few at 1,000 kV. In the latter case, epoxy sections .25μ to .5μ were used.

RESULTS AND DISCUSSION

The collagen matrix of the heart is centered around the myocyte (Fig. 1). The three arbitrarily defined components of the matrix of the heart all connect to the myocyte as would be expected if force transmission is a major function. Each myocyte is connected to all contiguous myocytes by numerous collagen struts that in small laboratory animals measure 120 to 150 nm in diameter (5,6). These collagen struts insert nearly perpendicularly into the basal laminae of the myocytes. The number and distribution of the struts would assure that all myocytes are tightly tethered, moving in consonance throughout the cardiac

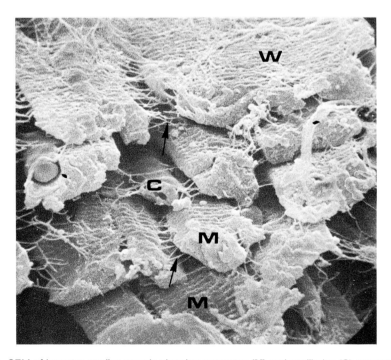

FIG. 1. SEM of hamster cardiac muscle showing myocytes (**M**) and capillaries (**C**) connected by collagen struts (*arrows*). The collagen network (**W**) that surrounds several myocytes is evident but not prominent in hamsters. ×2,000. (From the International Academy of Pathology, American-Canadian Division, with permission.)

cycle. This is particularly important during diastole, since all contiguous cells would be equally stretched and the subsequent contraction of contiguous cells would be equivalent.

Each capillary is connected to all contiguous myocytes by collagen struts 120 to 150 nm in diameter. These insert nearly perpendicularly to the basal laminae of the capillary, but course around the myocyte and insert tangentially (Fig. 2) (6). This geometry would place tension on the strut during myocyte contraction as the radius of the myocyte increases. Thus, during systole the tension on the basal laminae of the capillaries would contribute to the patency of the vessel in the presence of high ventricular wall pressure. At the onset of, and during, isovolumetric contraction there is an increase in coronary artery flow above diastolic flow that is directly related to wall tension (7,8). The systolic flow can amount to 25 to 30% of total coronary flow. This finding is easily explained by the relationship of the struts to the capillaries and myocytes during diastole and systole.

The myocytes of the ventricular wall occur as groups or bundles with varying angular relationships to the ventricular cavity from epicardium to endocardium (9). This grouping is brought about by a situation quite analogous to the perimysium of skeletal muscle, i.e., groups of myocytes are surrounded by a

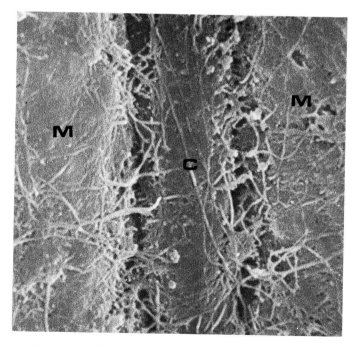

FIG. 2. Hypertrophied human heart demonstrating normal distribution of the capillary (**C**) to myocyte (**M**) struts. ×7,800.

complex reticular structure of collagen that is connected to the collagen fibrils that interconnect the myocytes (Fig. 3) (10). This perimysium that surrounds groups of myocytes is connected to the perimysium of adjacent bundles by thicker collagen fibers, as is seen in skeletal muscles (5,10,11). The perimysium of the heart as seen by SEM consists of a meshwork of collagen bundles (5, 6). The bundles are generally 120 nm or thicker in diameter, with greater variation toward larger diameters than is seen in the intermyocyte struts or capillary-to-myocyte struts. In skeletal muscles, the perimysium has been shown to be a stress-resistant system and to have visco-elastic properties.

In the heart, the extent and complexity of this collagen weave vary markedly in rats and hamsters, the system being much more extensive in rats at all ages, from one to seventeen months, than in hamsters at the same ages (12). This is the only morphologic difference that can reasonably explain the fact that the stiffness constant of rat left ventricles is approximately twice that of hamsters at all ages (12,13,14). Should this observation be confirmed in other systems, it would strengthen the idea that the passive properties of the ventricle are determined to a large extent by the amount and distribution of the weave network of collagen surrounding groups of myocytes.

The collagen network of the heart was first described by Holmgren (15). The optical systems available at that time were incapable of resolving the finer ramifications of the network. With the general availability of SEM, this system can be visualized much more clearly. A complete anatomic description of the development, distribution, and composition of this network is not available as yet, and the functional ramifications are not entirely clear. Consequently, only a few broadly descriptive remarks can be made concerning the alterations

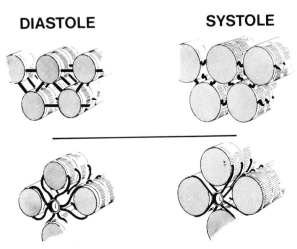

FIG. 3. This diagram represents the relationship of the collagen struts during diastole and systole from rabbit papillary muscle fixed at various lengths as determined from a length tension curve. (From the American Society for Experimental Biology, with permission.)

in various disease states. This lack of data probably correlates with the brief period since the system was first described by SEM in 1979, rather than a lack of significance in disease states (5).

Hearts from hypertensive patients were examined by SEM. The selection criteria included weight between 550 and 650 g, absence of focal scars, and coronary arteries with plaques no more than 60% occlusive. Samples from the anterior and posterior walls midway between the apex and base were prepared for SEM. Alteration of the weave network of collagen took two patterns. The first was a simple increase in the diameter of the struts extending between myocytes and between myocytes and capillaries. The collagen bundles forming the weave were increased in diameter as well. The diameters of the inter-myocyte struts and capillary-to-myocyte struts are approximately 180 to 200 nm in the few (four) normal hearts examined. In the hypertensive hearts, these struts ranged between 250 and 300 nm in diameter. The collagen bundles forming the weave in normal hearts vary in thickness more than the inter-myocyte struts, but seem to measure no more than about 230 nm in diameter. In the hypertensive hearts, the diameters of many bundles forming the weave were well above 300 nm. Since the tensile strength P of a material is a function of its diameter $\left(P = \sigma A; A = \dfrac{\pi D^2}{4} \right)$, an increase in diameter from 200 to 300 nm could support an increase in stress of over 100%. Since these bundles of collagen are formed from intertwined collagen fibrils, the diameter increase, consisting of an increase in the number of fibrils, would not necessarily have a large effect on the bulk properties of the collagen struts and, by extension, the wall itself. Thus, in hypertrophy secondary to a pressure overload, many of the hearts could be expected to have alteration in passive properties, but not necessarily of major proportions. This is a conclusion reached by Grossman et al. (16) regarding aortic stenosis, in which they suggested that "the increased chamber stiffness was simply due to a thicker wall in the group with pressure overload without any change in the material properties of the tissue composing the wall." Small changes in the properties of the wall may not be demonstrable with currently available techniques.

The second pattern appeared in three of the hypertensive hearts. The weave network of collagen surrounding groups of myocytes was replaced by collagen in broad bands and sheets (Fig. 4). No interwoven network was seen in the areas examined. This replacement of a mesh network by broad bands and sheets of collagen would seriously alter the visco-elastic properties associated with a woven network pattern and could easily result in a much stiffer ventricle. This change was present throughout the samples examined, but whether it was present throughout the ventricle was not determined. Hearts with the same disease have quite widely divergent stiffness constants (16, 17). This may reflect a markedly different pattern that the connective tissue might assume, as well as a simple increase in the amount of connective tissue. This is well demon-strated in the data of Fester and Samet (17). They showed that the K values

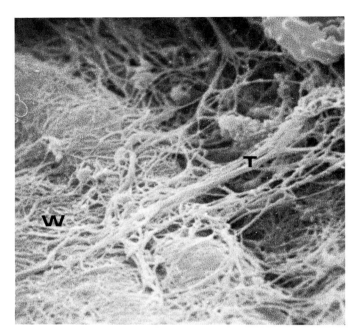

FIG. 4. Hypertrophied human heart with an increase in the diameter of the bundles of collagen forming the weave (**W**). Long tendon-like (**T**) processes that interconnect adjacent weave complexes are evident. ×6,000.

for patients with a specific type myocardial load tended to cluster, but given patients did diverge markedly from the norm of the group. The patients with much stiffer ventricles in a given group could be the ones with altered disposition of the collagen as was seen in three of our patients with hypertrophy. Hydroxyproline total protein ratios may not differentiate the two groups: those with normal distribution and those with abnormal distribution of collagen.

Hypertrophy may involve only one component of an organ. Thus, one could have hypertrophy, i.e., an increase in the amount of collagen, with little or no increase in the size of the cells and no serious enlargement of the heart. This occurs frequently in the subendocardial region of the heart (Fig. 5). A diffuse deposition of collagen that completely encircles myocytes occurs, especially with severe epicardial atherosclerosis. This deposition occurs not only secondary to loss of cells, but in many cases starts by encircling viable cells. By SEM (Fig. 6), the cells surrounded by collagen have lost all intermyocyte and myocyte to capillary struts. The encasement by collagen would effectively isolate the cells as far as lateral impulse conduction is concerned. The stimulus for this type increase in collagen is unknown, but its frequency in ischemic heart disease does suggest some causal relationship, although a similar distri-

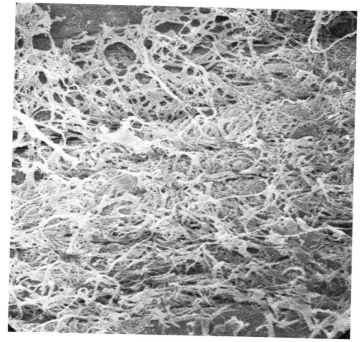

FIG. 5. Hypertrophied human heart with replacement of the weave with broad bands of collagenous material. This should be compared with Fig. 4, which is a far higher magnification. ×1,000.

bution of collagen may be seen with widely patent coronary arteries in various cardiomyopathies.

The functional effects of the deposition of collagen around individual myocytes is not known. The encasement of individual myocytes with collagen would alter the diastolic stretch as well as the distribution of stress generated during cellular contraction. The effect of this distribution of collagen on the ventricular compliance is unknown, although hearts with coronary artery disease may have very stiff ventricles (16).

CONCLUSIONS

There is a complex network of collagen bundles in the heart that interconnects the myocytes, the myocytes to capillaries, and that orders the myocytes into groups. If the weave network around myocytes is analogous to the perimysium of skeletal muscle, it is a stress-resistant system with visco-elastic properties and would contribute to ventricular stiffness. The various components of this system are altered in disease states, but as yet there is no organized body of information to relate abnormalities of the connective tissue to altered ventricular function.

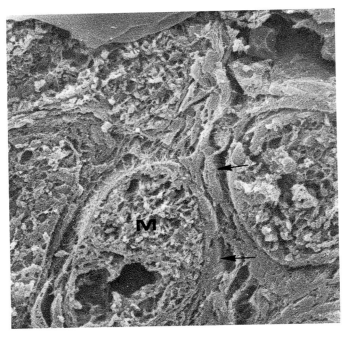

FIG. 6. Human heart showing encasement of myocytes (**M**) by collagen (*arrows*). This is the typical change seen in the subendocardial region in the presence of atherosclerosis, but is also seen in various cardiomyopathies. ×2,200.

ACKNOWLEDGMENTS

This work was partially supported by NIH grants 5R01 HL24935-03 and 1R01 HL27533-01, and AHA grant 79-880.

REFERENCES

1. Wolff, J. (1892): *Das Gesetz der Transformation der Knochen.* Hirschwald, Berlin. Cited in: Englehardt, A., Gull, H., Komitowski, D., Seharbach, H., Heipertz, W., Senear, M., Kooke, D., Zeitz, J., and Bunz, P. (1976): In: *Artificial Hip and Knee Joint Technology,* edited by M. Schaldash and D. Hohmann, p. 475. Springer-Verlag, New York.
2. Hood, W. B., Bianco, J. A., Kumar, R., and Whiting, R. B. (1970): *J. Clin. Invest.,* 49:1316–1327.
3. Turto, H., and Lindy, S. (1976): *Adv. Cardiol.,* 18:41–45.
4. Mirsky, I., and Laks, M. M. (1980): *Circ. Res.,* 46:530–542.
5. Caulfield, J. B., and Borg, T. K. (1979): *Lab. Invest.,* 40:364–370.
6. Borg, T. K., and Caulfield, J. B. (1981): *Fed. Proc.,* 40:2037–2041.
7. Abel, F. L., Borg, T. K., and Caulfield, J. B. (1980): In: *Proc. 28th Int. Cong. of Phys. Sci., (Budapest),* p. 289.
8. Caulfield, J. B., Borg, T. K., and Abel, F. L. (1981): In: *Advances in Myocardiology, Vol. IV.,* edited by E. Chazov, V. Saks, and G. Rona. Raven Press, New York (in press).

9. Spotnitz, H. M., and Sonnenblick, E. H. (1973): *Am. J. Cardiol.*, 32:398–410.
10. Nagel, A. (1935): *Z. Zellforsch. Mikrosk. Anat.*, 22:694–704.
11. Borg, T. K., and Caulfield, J. D. (1980): *Tissue and Cell*, 12:197–207.
12. Borg, T. K., Ranson, W. F., Moslehy, F. A., and Caulfield, J. B. (1981): *Lab. Invest.*, 44:49–54.
13. Mirsky, I., Janz, R. F., Kubert, B. R., Korecky, B., and Taichman, G. C. (1976): *Bull. Math. Biol.*, 38:239–248.
14. Kane, R. L., McMahon, T. A., Wagner, R. L., and Abelmann, W. H. (1976): *Circ. Res.*, 38:74–80.
15. Holmgren, E. (1907): *Arch. Mikr. Anat.*, 71:165–246.
16. Grossman, W., McLaurin, L. P., and Stefadouros, M. A. (1974): *Circ. Res.*, 35:793–800.
17. Fester, A., and Samet, P. (1974): *Circulation*, 50:609–618.
18. Laird, J. D. (1976): *Circulation*, 53:443–449.

*Perspectives in Cardiovascular
Research, Vol. 8,*
edited by R. C. Tarazi and J. B. Dunbar.
Raven Press, New York © 1983.

Structural Characterization of Coronary Arteries and Myocardium in Renal Hypertensive Hypertrophy

Joseph Wiener and Filiberto Giacomelli

*Department of Pathology, Wayne State University School of Medicine,
Detroit, Michigan 48201*

Essential hypertension is a major risk factor for the development of cardiovascular disease, including ventricular hypertrophy (1); however, the number of studies dealing with the ultrastructure of coronary arteries and myocardium in hypertensive hypertrophy is limited (2,3). Classical studies of human material have indicated that myocardial arteries are either intact (4) or infrequently involved (5,6) by hypertension.

The purpose of this chapter is to examine the coronary vasculature and myocardium in short-term ventricular hypertrophy. This was achieved by subjecting rats to 1 to 4 weeks of two-kidney, one clip renal hypertension. The results have previously been reported *in extenso* (7,8) and will only be summarized here. It will be seen that the coronary circuit exhibits the same type of adaptive structural changes as other systemic circuits in hypertension (9).

METHODS

Twenty-one male Wistar-Kyoto normotensive rats weighing about 70 g (4–5 weeks of age) were used in these studies. Hypertension was produced in 12 of these animals by constricting the left renal artery with a silver-wire clip, and their blood pressures monitored before operation and twice weekly thereafter. Blood pressures were also measured in nine unoperated littermates. All animals were sacrificed between the ages of 11 and 14 weeks, at which time the operated group had been hypertensive for 1 to 4 weeks. Following Nembutal® anesthesia (sodium pentobarbital, Abbott Laboratories, North Chicago, Ill.), the abdominal aorta was cannulated, and the hearts arrested in diastole by an intravenous injection of KCl (1 mEq/ml). Following perfusion fixation with 2% buffered glutaraldehyde (Polysciences Inc., Warrington, Pa.) the hearts were excised, weighed, and blocks of tissue including endocardial and epicardial surfaces cut from the midzone of the left ventricular wall. The blocks were then processed for light and electron microscopy and morphometry. Before sectioning the embedded blocks, measurements of wall thickness were made using a magnifier with an incorporated scale accurate to 0.01 mm.

RESULTS

The systolic blood pressures of control animals never exceeded 130 mm Hg and usually ranged between 75 to 100 mm Hg. Severe hypertension (190–220 mm Hg systolic) occurred in three animals, while the remainder exhibited a moderate hypertension with blood pressures ranging between 150 to 170 mm Hg.

Table 1 shows the mean body weights of control and hypertensive animals at time of sacrifice. The average heart weight was increased 24%, and the change of 205 mg was almost completely contained in a 30% increase in left ventricular weight. In contrast, the weight of the right ventricle showed no significant differences. The average thickness of the midzone of the anterior wall of the left ventricle was 42% greater in the hypertensive animals.

Phase Contrast Observations

The epicardial and deeper intramyocardial arteries of hypertensive animals, located in the intermediate and subendocardial layers of ventricular myocardium, were widely patent. There was flattening of endothelium and elongation of medial smooth muscle cells of epicardial arteries (Fig. 1); the adventitial surfaces of intramyocardial arteries were scalloped (Fig. 2). Foci of subendocardial myocardium exhibited vacuolization, contraction zones, and/or bands as well as loss of transverse striations.

Ultrastructural Observations

Morphometry

The volume composition of left ventricular myocardium is shown in Table 2. The volume composition was found to be significantly different in endo-

TABLE 1. *Gross effects of 1 to 4 weeks of renal hypertension*[a]

	Control	Hypertensive	$p<$
No. of rats	9	12	
Wt. of rats (g)	266.1 ± 8.8	203.8 ± 8.1	0.001
Weight (mg)			
Heart	840 ± 24	1045 ± 17	0.001
Right ventricle	168 ± 5	172 ± 5	0.6
Left ventricle	673 ± 23	873 ± 14	0.001
Thickness of left midventricular wall (mm)	2.00 ± 0.09	2.83 ± 0.11	0.0001

[a] Values are means ± SE; p values were determined by Student's *t*-test.

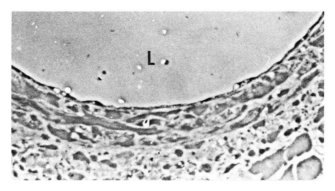

FIG. 1. Phase contrast micrograph of epicardial artery. Note the circumferential elongation of medial smooth muscle cells. L: lumen. ×150.

cardial and epicardial regions in control animals. Hypertension induced a significant change in the relative volumes of endocardial components, but not in those of the epicardium.

The absolute myocyte cell volumes in endocardial and epicardial regions (10) and their response to hypertension are shown in Table 3. It can be seen that epicardial myocytes were larger than endocardial myocytes and that hypertension produced a significant hypertrophy of 37% and 21%, respectively, in these cells.

The interstitial volume in myocardium, which varied from 15.1% to 20.6%, was subdivided morphometrically into the three components listed in Table 4. Significant differences were principally found in the volume percentage of capillary lumen, which is nearly twofold greater in epicardium than in endocardium. The volume percentage of endothelium, however, was not larger proportionately, implying a thinner endothelium lining epicardial capillaries.

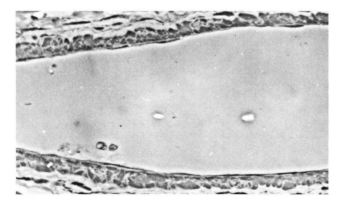

FIG. 2. Phase contrast micrograph of intramyocardial artery discloses scalloping of the adventitial surface of the vessel. ×150.

TABLE 2. *Volume composition of left ventricular myocardium[a]*

		Control	Hypertensive	$p<$
Volume (%) of myocardium				
Interstitium	En	15.1 ± 1.3	18.6 ± 1.3	0.05
	Ep	20.6 ± 1.7	20.2 ± 1.0	0.7
	$p<$	0.025	0.6	
Myocytes	En	84.9 ± 1.3	81.4 ± 1.3	0.05
	Ep	79.4 ± 1.7	79.8 ± 1.0	0.7
	$p<$	0.025	0.6	

[a] En and Ep indicate endocardial and epicardial regions of the left ventricular myocardium, respectively. Values are means ± SE.

The volume of interstitial components per myocyte was calculated from their volume percentages and the mean volumes of myocytes. On this cellular basis, epicardial myocytes were surrounded by 77% more interstitium than endocardial myocytes. Since the number of myocytes in the hypertrophied left ventricular myocardium was unchanged in the hypertensive rats (7), the percentage increases in the volume of interstitium directly indicated the amount of interstitial enlargement in these animals: 55% in the endocardium and 34% in the epicardium. By combining these values of interstitial growth with the corresponding values of myocyte hypertrophy, 21% and 37% (Table 3), the total myocardial hypertrophy was 26% in the endocardium and 37% in the epicardium.

The total luminal area and number of capillary profiles measured in electron micrographs are listed in Table 5. The quotient of these figures yields the mean area of capillary lumen per profile. These transverse capillary areas were significantly larger in the epicardium than in the endocardium. Furthermore, the values in each region of the myocardium were increased in hypertension.

Morphology

Controls

Epicardial arteries of control animals possessed an internal elastic lamella and several layers of medial smooth muscle cells enveloped by basal laminae.

TABLE 3. *Cell volumes (μm^3) of En and Ep populations of myocytes in left ventricular myocardium[a]*

	Control	Hypertensive	$p<$
En	10,370 ± 410	12,520 ± 490 (21)	0.01
Ep	12,600 ± 1,600	17,300 ± 1,100 (37)	0.05
$p<$	0.3	0.005	

[a] Values are means ± SE. Numbers in parentheses indicate the percentage increase produced by hypertension.

TABLE 4. *Volume composition of interstitium in left ventricular myocardium*[a]

		Control	Hypertensive	p<
Volume (%) of myocardium				
Interstitium	En	8.7 ± 1.0	12.7 ± 1.5	0.1
exclusive of	Ep	11.3 ± 2.4	10.8 ± 1.2	0.9
capillaries	p<	0.4	0.4	
Capillary lumen	En	3.2 ± 0.6	3.4 ± 0.5	0.9
	Ep	6.1 ± 0.8	6.8 ± 0.9	0.7
	p<	0.02	0.01	
Endothelial cells	En	3.2 ± 0.2	2.6 ± 0.2	0.1
	Ep	3.2 ± 0.1	2.6 ± 0.1	0.05
	p<	1.0	1.0	
Interstitial volumes/myocyte (μm^3)				
Interstitium	En	1,840 ± 180	2,860 ± 230 (55)	0.005
	Ep	3,270 ± 490	4,380 ± 350 (34)	0.1
	p<	0.02	0.005	
Capillary lumen	En	391 ± 75	523 ± 80 (34)	0.3
	Ep	970 ± 180	1,470 ± 220 (52)	0.2
	p<	0.02	0.001	
Endothelial cells	En	391 ± 29	400 ± 35 (2)	0.9
	Ep	508 ± 66	564 ± 42 (11)	0.6
	p<	0.2	0.02	

[a] Values are means ± SE. Numbers in parentheses indicate the percentage increase produced by hypertension.

The intramural arteries had an internal elastic lamella and 1 to 3 layers of medial smooth muscle cells. The arterioles lacked an internal elastic lamella, and had a single layer of smooth muscle cells in the media.

Hypertensive animals

Prominent morphologic alterations were found in both epicardial and intramyocardial arteries and myocardium. The lumina of epicardial arteries were

TABLE 5. *Capillary distribution in left ventricular myocardium*[a]

		Control	Hypertensive	p<
Area of capillary	En	2,578	4,768	
lumina (μm^2)	Ep	7,715	9,567	
No. of capillary profiles	En	396	529	
	Ep	624	542	
Luminal area/profile	En	6.5 ± 1.2	9.0 ± 1.5	0.3
(μm^2)	Ep	12.4 ± 1.4	17.7 ± 2.2	0.1
	p<	0.01	0.005	

[a] Values are means ± SE.

lined by flattened endothelial cells (Fig. 3). The medial smooth muscle cells of many epicardial arteries were greatly elongated, with their long axes aligned parallel to the circumference of the vessel wall. Peripheral cytoplasmic processes were detached from the main cell bodies and may have undergone lysis.

A less frequent change in the medial smooth muscle cells of epicardial arteries consisted of a range of alterations varying from slight loss of myofilaments to single-cell necrosis. These necrotic cells were restricted to the outer layers of the vessel wall and contained numerous lysosomes and autophagosomes. Spaces in the media of epicardial arteries delimited by the original smooth muscle cell basal laminae may have contained irregularly shaped smooth muscle cell fragments, reduplicated basal laminae, and tubulo-vesicular debris. Collagen fibers were deposited between expanded portions of the interstitial space.

Some of the epicardial arteries exhibited intimal thickening (hyperplastic lesions) characterized by the presence of smooth muscle cells in the subendothelial space (Fig. 4). Smooth muscle cells were also seen within fenestrations of the internal elastic lamella; the media of these vessels appeared thickened.

Intramyocardial arteries also exhibited hyperplastic changes consisting of 1 to 3 layers of smooth muscle cells in the subendothelial space (Fig. 5). The

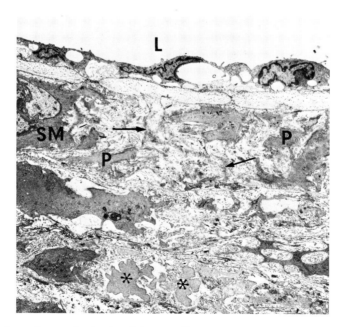

FIG. 3. Electron micrograph of epicardial artery. The endothelium is flattened and vacuolated; the medial smooth muscle cells are elongated. Polar portions of these cells are widely separated from the basal laminae (*arrows*). There is detachment of the processes from the main cell bodies as well as lysis (∗). L: lumen; P: processes; SM: smooth muscle cell bodies. ×3,000.

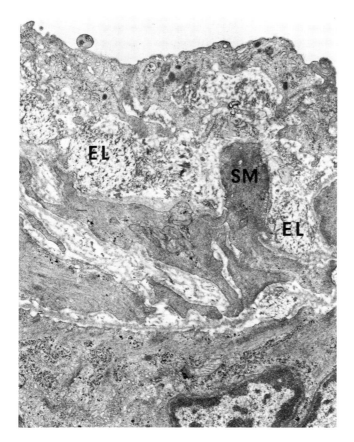

FIG. 4. Electron micrograph of hyperplastic epicardial artery. There is intimal thickening. A smooth muscle cell is present between fenestrations of the internal elastic lamella. EL: internal elastic lamella; SM: smooth muscle cells. ×14,000.

medial smooth muscle cells of many small intramyocardial arteries, as well as smooth muscle cells in the subendothelial space, displayed fragmentation and necrosis. There may also have been fragmentation of the internal elastic lamella.

Endothelial cell nuclei bulge into the lumina of other intramyocardial arteries (Fig. 6). The widened subendothelial space contains acellular electron-dense material resembling plasma, erythrocytes, macrophages, platelets, and polygonal and fibrillar masses of material exhibiting the 11.5 nm periodicity of fibrin (11). The adjacent medial smooth muscle cells exhibited contraction and necrosis; reduplicated basal laminae were also seen in the media.

Constricted arterioles exhibited extensive areas of injury that involved the entire circumference of the vessel in transverse section (Fig. 7). The nuclei of

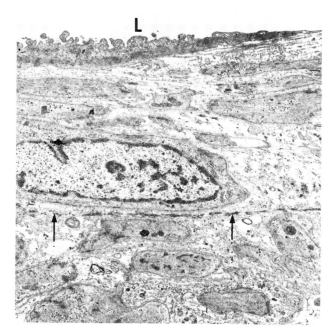

FIG. 5. Intimal thickening of intramyocardial artery with several smooth muscle cells between endothelium and attenuated internal elastic lamella (*arrows*). There are fragmentation and necrosis of subendothelial and medial smooth muscle cells. L: lumen. ×8,000.

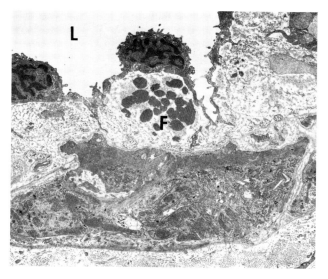

FIG. 6. Endothelial cell nuclei bulge into the lumen. Electron dense material resembling plasma and polygonal masses of fibrin are seen in the expanded subendothelial space. There are contraction and necrosis of adjacent medial smooth muscle cells. L: lumen; F: fibrin. ×3,500.

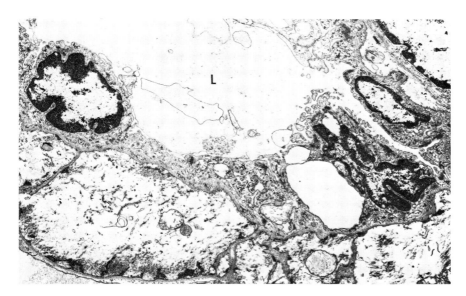

FIG. 7. Intramyocardial arteriole exhibiting pyknosis and rarefaction of endothelial cell nuclei. Endothelial blebs project into the lumen. There is loss of myofilaments and swelling of mitochondria. L: lumen. ×12,000.

the endothelial and smooth muscle cells exhibited pyknosis, or rarefaction and peripheral clumping of chromatin. There was loss of myofilaments from smooth muscle cell cytoplasm and prominence of attachment devices; clusters of thick filaments measuring approximately 15 nm in diameter were visible. Large electron lucent vacuoles were seen in the cytoplasm of some endothelial cells. The lumina of these arterioles also contained large membrane-limited bodies or blebs.

Discrete foci of damage were present in the subendocardial region of the myocardium. The extent of injury ranged from mild disorganization of myofibrillar structure to generalized loss of architecture and severe necrosis. There was depletion of glycogen in myofibrils and peripheral clumping of myocyte nuclear chromatin. Z-lines were thickened, irregular, and out of register. The sarcomeres in such areas were overstretched and may have exhibited asymmetric I-bands. Other sarcomeres displayed severe overcontraction with the formation of contraction zones and/or bands. Mitochondria were dislocated and packed together between overcontracted sarcomeres (Fig. 8). The mitochondria were swollen, possessed a less dense matrix, and exhibited ruptured outer membranes and decreased numbers of cristae that may have been fragmented.

DISCUSSION

The observations presented indicate that two-kidney, one clip renal hypertension of 1 to 4 weeks' duration produces both hyperplastic and necrotic

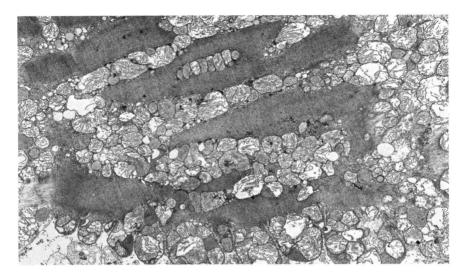

FIG. 8. Electron micrograph of subendocardial region of myocardium. There is severe overcontraction with loss of striated pattern and translocation of swollen mitochondria. ×8,000.

lesions in the epicardial and intramyocardial arteries of rats. Insudative changes were restricted to small intramyocardial arteries. The vascular lesions were associated with foci of myocardial necrosis that were limited to the subendocardial region of the left ventricle. These alterations were found in hearts that exhibited an average 24% increase in weight.

The coronary arterial system consists of two functionally different segments of vessels. The larger and superficial epicardial arteries are conduit channels that respond passively to modifications in intra-arterial pressure, while the smaller intramural arteries tend to autoregulate and maintain constant flow by dilation and constriction (12). Intramyocardial coronary arteries have their caliber affected particularly by mechanical compression from contracting myocardial fibers. While epicardial arteries are exposed to both systolic and diastolic perfusion pressures, intramural arteries and arterioles are primarily perfused during diastole (13).

Two forms of necrosis were found in epicardial arteries. The more frequent change consisted of elongation of smooth muscle cell bodies and subsequent detachment and lysis of their polar extensions in all layers of the media. The less frequent alteration in epicardial arteries involved necrosis of entire smooth muscle cells that was limited to the outer layers of vessel walls. The morphologic features of medial necrosis in epicardial arteries were compatible with the overdistention and stretching of conduit channels by increased intraluminal pressure.

Fragmented medial smooth muscle cells were found only in the media of intramural arterial vessels, despite the fact that these arteries are protected against the elevation in wall stress associated with the systolic pressure rise by the squeezing action of the heart. Similar smooth muscle cell fragmentation has been observed previously in the coronary (14) and mesenteric (15–18) arteries of rats with acute angiotensin-induced hypertension and the medial changes attributed to contraction sustained beyond the metabolic capability of these smooth muscle cells (16). Since short-term, two-kidney, one clip Goldblatt hypertension in the rat is a high-renin state (19,20) and intramyocardial arteries are protected against the elevated systolic pressures, it seems reasonable to suggest that the necrotic lesions of small intramyocardial arteries may be due to smooth muscle contraction provoked by angiotensin II. However, the elevated perfusion (diastolic) pressure may also play a role in the development of these intramural arterial lesions.

A less frequent alteration occurred in intramyocardial arterioles that involved the entire wall. Both endothelial and smooth muscle cells exhibited nuclear and cytoplasmic swelling and lysis. Similar changes as well as endothelial blebs have been observed previously in the intramural coronary arteries and arterioles of rats with acute hypertension due to the infusion of angiotensin II (14). Endothelial blebs have also been found in capillaries associated with the "no-reflow" phenomenon following ischemia (21,22). Ischemia followed by reperfusion may result in the swelling and degeneration of endothelial and smooth muscle cells (23). Thus, the degenerative lesions in intramyocardial arterioles may have an ischemic or anoxic basis. Endothelial cell vacuolization has been attributed recently to the release of free oxygen radicals by prostaglandins in acute angiotensin II induced hypertension (24); angiotensin can mediate the local release of prostaglandins (25–27).

Intimal thickening occurred in both epicardial and intramyocardial arteries. It is now generally accepted that the increased muscle mass of small and large arteries in hypertension is due to both smooth muscle cell hypertrophy and hyperplasia (28–30). Guski et al. (31) have reported a 19% increase in the cross-sectional area of coronary arteries in rabbits with renal compression and neurogenic hypertension. Hyperplastic lesions have also been observed in coronary arteries of rabbits (2) and rats (32) with cellophane perinephritis. The intimal smooth muscle cells originate in the media (29), and represent a structural adaptation that could contribute to the increased coronary vascular resistance in established hypertension. Among the factors that could stimulate the growth of vascular smooth muscle cells are elevated plasma levels of angiotensin II, circumferential stress on the arterial wall, and shear forces or increased permeability to circulating blood constituents (33–35).

Increased vascular permeability is manifested by the accumulation of plasma, fibrin, and hematogenous elements within the subendothelial space of intramyocardial arteries from animals with severe hypertension. Although endothelial discontinuities or separations of interendothelial junctions have not been found in these arteries, such gaps seem the most likely explanation for the insudative changes. Interendothelial gaps and/or endothelial discontinuities are invariably found in hypertensive vessels containing plasma and fibrin when colloidal tracer methodology is applied (15,16,36). Alternatively, the intramural accumulation of plasma, fibrin, and hematogenous elements could result from the transient formation of interendothelial gaps produced by angiotensin-mediated contraction of endothelial cells (37). Their subsequent reclosure ("trap-door" mechanism) could explain the failure to find interendothelial separations. The lack of endothelial discontinuities and localization of plasma constituents to the subendothelial space of intramyocardial arteries may also be related to their protection from the elevated systolic pressures and the bidirectional flux of materials between lumen and wall when permeability is increased (14).

Foci of myocardial injury are restricted to the subendocardium of the left ventricle, the region most vulnerable to ischemic episodes. Although these myocardial lesions bear no consistent relationship to myocardial arteries and arterioles, they do resemble areas of irreversible myocardial injury and reflow after ischemic (38) or anoxic (39) episodes. Similar lesions have been found in myocardium after the intravenous infusion of angiotensin II (14,40).

The foci of myocardial necrosis occurred in hearts that had an average weight increase of 24% over that of normotensive controls. It seems reasonable to suggest that the subendocardial necrosis may have been due at least in part to the development of left ventricular hypertrophy. The morphometric data indicate that while the response of the subendocardial region to the increased work load was limited (26% versus 37% for the epicardial area), interstitial growth was considerably greater in the endocardial region (55% versus 34%). Furthermore, the volume percentage of capillary lumen in the endocardial region was only one-half of that found in the epicardial zone. In addition, wall stresses were considerably greater in endocardium (41,42), and endocardial fibers probably require more oxygen than epicardial fibers because they must develop greater force to generate intraventricular pressure.

Foci of myocardial necrosis, along with proliferative changes in coronary arteries, have also been described in rats following hypertension induced by renal compression and contralateral nephrectomy (43). Focal areas of myocardial necrosis and fibrosis in subendocardial locations have been reported by Hollander et al. (44) in the hearts of cynomulgus monkeys after chronic hypertension due to aortic coarctation. Myocardial fibrosis (45) as well as apical scars (46) have been described in the spontaneously hypertensive rat.

Considerable evidence in animal models and man indicates that the adverse effects of hypertension on cardiac function are due at least in part to the mechanical effects of high blood pressure on both heart muscle and coronary arteries (47,48). An increase in left ventricular systolic pressure caused by hypertension not only increases the oxygen requirement of the heart (49) but also may impair coronary blood flow, especially to the subendocardium, by augmenting coronary vascular resistance. The unfavorable effects of hypertension on myocardial oxygen supply and demand may be aggravated further by myocardial hypertrophy and its attendant interstitial fibrosis, as well as by hypertensive disease of the small coronary arteries. In this regard, it has recently been shown that the myocardial necrosis found in acute angiotensin II induced hypertension does not occur when the pressure rise is prevented by adreno-receptor blockade (40). On the other hand, medial necrosis of intramural arteries can occur in this system in the presence of normal blood pressure.

The occurrence of myocardial injury with structure compatible with myocardial infarction in hypertensive hypertrophy is of interest. Hypertension is a major cause of ventricular hypertrophy, sudden death, and myocardial infarction in man (50). Myocardial infarction remains an important source of morbidity in hypertensive subjects, despite the widespread utilization of antihypertensive therapy. Although some of this cardiac mortality can be attributed to worsening of atherosclerosis by hypertension, the data reported here provide strong evidence that hypertension may have a direct and adverse effect on myocardium that is independent of occlusive coronary artery disease.

ACKNOWLEDGMENT

This study was supported in part by U.S. Public Health Service Grant HL 23603 from the National Heart, Lung, and Blood Institute, National Institutes of Health, Bethesda, Maryland.

REFERENCES

1. Kannel, W. B. (1975): *Angiology*, 26:1–14.
2. Backwinkel, K. P., Schmitt, G., Themann, H., and Hauss, W. H. (1970): *Beitr. Path.*, 141:374–391.
3. Hüttner, I., Rona, G., Theodosis, D., and More, R. H. (1972): *Rec. Adv. Cardic. Metab.*, 1:376–385.
4. Bell, E. T., and Clawson, B. J. (1928): *Arch. Pathol.*, 5:939–1002.
5. Kernohan, J. W., Anderson, E. W., and Keith, N. M. (1929): *Arch. Intern. Med.*, 44:395–423.
6. Fishberg, A. M. (1954): *Hypertension and Nephritis, Fifth Ed.* Lea and Febiger, Philadelphia.
7. Anversa, P., Loud, A. V., Giacomelli, F., and Wiener, J. (1978): *Lab. Invest.*, 38:597–609.
8. Bhan, R. D., Giacomelli, F., and Wiener, J. (1978): *Exp. Mol. Pathol.*, 29:66–81.
9. Noresson, E., Hallbäck, M., and Hjalmarsson, A. (1977): *Acta Physiol. Scand.*, 101:363–365.
10. Loud, A. V., Anversa, P., Giacomelli, F., and Wiener, J. (1978): *Lab. Invest.*, 38:586–596.
11. Wiener, J., Lattes, R. G., and Spiro, D. (1965): *Am. J. Pathol.*, 47:457–485.
12. Cohen, M. V., and Kirk, E. S. (1973): *Circ. Res.*, 33:445–453.
13. Kirk, E. S., and Honig, C. R. (1964): *Am. J. Physiol.*, 207:361–367.
14. Giacomelli, F., Anversa, P., and Wiener, J. (1976): *Am. J. Pathol.*, 84:111–125.
15. Goldby, F. S., and Beilin, L. J. (1972): *Cardiovasc. Res.*, 6:569–584.
16. Wiener, J., and Giacomelli, F. (1973): *Am. J. Pathol.*, 72:221–240.
17. Thorball, N., and Olsen, F. (1974): *Acta Pathol. Microbiol. Scand.*, 82:683–689.
18. Thorball, N., and Olsen, F. (1974): *Acta Pathol. Microbiol. Scand.*, 82:703–713.
19. Brunner, H. R., Kirshman, J. D., and Laragh, J. H. (1971): *Science*, 174:1344–1346.
20. Atkinson, A. B., Brown, J. J., Fraser, R., Lever, A. F., Morton, J. J., Riegger, A. J. G., and Robertson, J. I. S. (1980): *Clin. Exp. Hypertens.*, 2:499–524.
21. Chiang, J., Kowada, M., Ames, A., III, Wright, R. L., and Majno, G. (1968): *Am. J. Pathol.*, 52:455–476.
22. Kloner, R. A., Ganote, C. E., and Jennings, R. B. (1974): *J. Clin. Invest.*, 54:1496–1508.
23. Elemér, G., Kerenyi, T., and Jellinek, H. (1975): *Pathol. Eur.*, 10:123–128.

24. Kontos, H. A., Wei, E. P., Dietrich, W. D., Navari, R. M., Povlishock, J. T., Ghatak, N. R., Ellis, E. F., and Patterson, J. L., Jr. (1981): *Am. J. Physiol.*, 240:H511–H527.
25. Needleman, P., Marshall, G. R., and Sobel, B. E. (1975): *Circ. Res.*, 37:802–808.
26. DeDeckere, E. A. M., Nugteren, D. H., and TenHoor, F. (1977): *Nature (Lond.)*, 268:160–163.
27. Gunther, S., and Cannon, P. J. (1980): *Am. J. Physiol.*, 238:H895–H901.
28. Crane, W. A. J., and Dutta, L. P. (1963): *J. Pathol. Bacteriol.*, 86:83–98.
29. Spiro, D., Lattes, R. G., and Wiener, J. (1965): *Am. J. Pathol.*, 47:19–49.
30. Bevan, R. D., Van Marthens, E., and Bevan, J. A. (1976): *Circ. Res. (Suppl.)* 38:58–62.
31. Guski, V. H., Schmidt, R., and Eckert, H. (1973): *Exp. Pathol. (Jena.)*, 8:168–181.
32. Kunz, V., Keim, U., Braselmann, H., Kreher, C., and Nitschoff, S. (1973): *Exp. Pathol. (Jena.)*, 8:294–302.
33. Pickering, G. W. (1968): *High Blood Pressure (Second Ed.)*. J. and A. Churchill, London.
34. Wolinsky, H. (1970): *Circ. Res.*, 26:507–522.
35. Bevan, R. D. (1976): *Blood Vessels*, 13:100–128.
36. Wiener, J., Lattes, R. G., Meltzer, B. G., and Spiro, D. (1969): *Am. J. Pathol.*, 54:187–207.
37. Robertson, A. L., Jr., and Khairallah, P. A. (1973): *Exp. Mol. Pathol.*, 18:241–260.
38. Herdson, P. B., Sommers, H. M., and Jennings, R. B. (1965): *Am. J. Pathol.*, 46:367–386.
39. Ganote, C. E., Seabra-Gomes, R., Nayler, W. G., and Jennings, R. B. (1975): *Am. J. Pathol.*, 80:419–450.
40. Bhan, R. D., Giacomelli, F., and Wiener, J. (1982): *Am. J. Pathol.*, 108:60–71.
41. Sandler, H., and Ghista, D. N. (1969): *Fed. Proc.*, 28:1344–1350.
42. Giacomelli, F., Anversa, P., and Wiener, J. (1975): *Microvasc. Res.*, 10:38–42.
43. Griffith, R., and Hummel, R. (1973): *Triangle*, 12:75–82.
44. Hollander, W. (1977): In: *Hypertension*, edited by J. Genest, E. Koiw, and O. Kuchel, pp. 945–960. McGraw-Hill, New York.
45. Ooshima, A., Yamori, Y., and Okamoto, K. (1972): *Jpn. Circ. J.*, 36:797–812.
46. Hazama, F., Ooshima, A., Tanaka, T., Tomimoto, K., and Okamoto, K. (1975): *Jpn. Circ. J.*, 39:7–22.
47. Hollander, W. (1973): *Circulation*, 48:1112–1125.
48. Hollander, W. (1976): *Am. J. Cardiol.*, 38:786–800.
49. Braunwald, E. (1969): *Physiologist*, 12:65–93.
50. Roberts, W. C. (1975): *Am. J. Med.*, 59:523–532.

Perspectives in Cardiovascular Research, Vol. 8,
edited by R. C. Tarazi and J. B. Dunbar.
Raven Press, New York © 1983.

Myosin Isozymes in Cardiac Hypertrophy: A Brief Review

Eugene Morkin

Departments of Internal Medicine and Pharmacology, University of Arizona College of Medicine, Tucson, Arizona 85724

Hypertrophied heart muscle may exhibit a decrease in active tension and velocity of shortening (1). The goal of many past and recent studies (2–10) has been to explain these changes in terms of theories of muscle contraction, where the development of force and velocity depends upon the interaction of myosin, actin, Mg-ATP, and Ca^{2+}. Because of the close association between the speed of contraction and the adenosine triphosphatase (ATPase) activity of myosin (11), the question naturally arises as to whether the myosin molecule is defective in hypertrophied and failing hearts (12). The lability of myosin ATPase activity and the size and complexity of the molecule have made this question very difficult to answer definitively.

New insight into the problem has been provided by the recognition that ventricular myosin isozyme composition is altered in cardiac hypertrophy induced by thyroid hormone (13,14). In this unique form of hypertrophy, myocardical performance and myosin ATPase activity are increased, rather than decreased, as in hypertrophy produced by mechanical overload. Under the influence of excess exogenous hormone, a myosin isozyme with high ATPase activity, which is normally only a minor component, becomes the predominant myosin form. A similar change in isozyme composition from a predominance of a low activity form to one of high activity has been found in thyroid-deficient rats treated with triiodothyronine (T_3) (15). These observations may explain, at least in part, the well known effects of thyroid hormone on cardiac performance. Recognition of the existence of cardiac myosin isozymes, and their regulation by thyroid hormone, may also explain some otherwise perplexing observations on cardiac myosin ATPase activity during development, aging, exercise, and in some models of non-thyroidal heart disease.

MYOSIN ISOZYMES AND THYROID HORMONE

The effects of thyroid status on the distribution of ventricular myosin isozymes are shown in Fig. 1. Three major forms of cardiac myosin can be identified by electrophoresis in polyacrylamide gels containing pyrophosphate

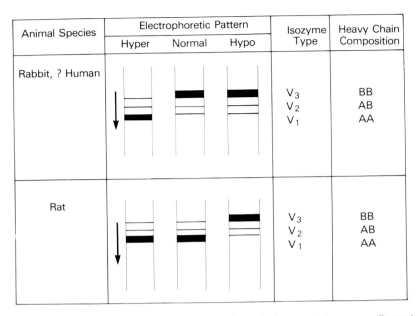

FIG. 1. Effects of thyroid status on the distribution of ventricular myosin isozymes. (Reproduced by permission of *Progress in Cardiovascular Diseases*.)

buffer (15). The isozymes are referred to as V_{1-3}, in order of decreasing electrophoretic ability and ATPase activity. These myosin forms seem to contain the same light-chain components, but differ in their heavy-chain composition. The slowest migrating form, V_3, is thought to contain two similar, if not identical, heavy B chains; the fastest migrating component (V_1) contains two heavy A chains. The intermediate form (V_2) is thought to contain one heavy chain of each type.

In the rat, administration of thyroid hormone has very little influence on rat ventricular myosin isozymes. However, after thyroidectomy or hypophysectomy there is a switch in composition to a predominance of the V_3 type (15). The associated change in myosin ATPase activity following hypophysectomy was observed almost twenty years ago by Lifschitz and Kayne (16); their observations were later confirmed and extended by Rovetto et al. (17).

By contrast, rabbit and several other mammalian species, including man, have a predominance of the V_3 form (18). Administration of thyroid hormone in these species stimulates synthesis of the V_1 form, although the extent of the change has not been documented in all cases. This change in the composition of myosin isozymes was first recognized from differences in one- and two-dimensional peptide maps of CNBr digests of ventricular myosin from normal and thyrotoxic rabbits (13,14). A nearly complete change in myosin isozyme composition occurs in this species when administered excess thyroid hormone (19), a change facilitating recognition of differences in peptide migration patterns.

The possibility that phosphorylation or methylation of histidine residues might be involved in the stimulation of ATPase activity in thyrotoxicosis myosin has been ruled out by the failure to find these substituents upon chemical analysis of the protein (20). More recently, levels of phosphorylation have also been measured in isolated myofibril, myosin light chains, and troponin-I from freeze-clamped thyrotoxic ventricles, and they were found to be the same as in normal controls (21). Additionally, Ca^{2+}-activation of actomyosin and myofibrils from thyrotoxic ventricles have been found normal (20,21).

In addition to ventricular myosin isozymes, there are now known to be distinct myosin forms in atrial muscle (22,23) as well as in fast- and slow-twitch muscle fibers (24). Moreover, there may be embryonic forms of myosin in most, if not all, of these fiber types (25). The possibility exists, therefore, that the myosin isozyme stimulated by thyroid hormone could be the same as one of these other myosin forms. Although this possibility has not been investigated completely, it is known that the V_1 heavy chains are not the same as those found in fast- or slow-twitch skeletal fibers (13). Atrial myosin has a different complement of light chains than any ventricular myosin form (22). However, antigenetic similarities have been described between the heavy chains of rabbit atrial myosin and those of the ventricular myosin isozyme stimulated by thyroxine (26).

The enzymatic properties of myosin from euthyroid and thyrotoxic rabbit ventricular muscle have been summarized in Table 1 (20,27,28). Since there is an almost complete change in isozyme composition, these data can be taken as fairly representative of the enzymatic properties of the V_1 and V_3 forms in the rabbit. Note that the Ca^{2+}-ATPase activity of V_1 myosin is increased, but the K ethylenediaminetetraacetic acetate (EDTA) activity is unchanged.

In addition to this quantitative difference among these isozymes, there also are qualitative differences in their enzymatic properties. For example, V_1-type myosin is not stimulated by sulfhydryl modification with N-ethyl maleimide, and hydrolyzes ATP analogs with a specificity similar to that observed with SH_1-blocked control myosin (20). This initially lead to the suggestion that thyroid hormone might stimulate myosin ATPase activity by blocking the rapidly reacting thiol groups (29). However, these substituents have since been shown to be fully accessible to alkylating reagents (20).

TABLE 1. *Steady state enzymatic properties of myosin from thyrotoxic rabbits*

1. Elevated Ca-ATPase activity
   Unchanged K(EDTA)-ATPase activity
2. Increased actin-activated Mg-ATPase activity
3. Modification of SH_1-thiols with NEM or DTNB does not stimulate Ca-ATPase activity
4. Increased rate of hydrolysis of 6-amino- and 6-oxy-substituted nucleotide triphosphates, resembling SH_1-blocked myosin
5. No change in pH rate profile for Ca-ATPase activity

Myosin from normal and thyrotoxic rabbits has also been compared in a physiological assay system. Figure 2 shows the Mg-ATPase activity of heavy meromyosin (HMM), the soluble 2-headed myosin subfragment, at different actin concentrations. In this method of analysis, the reciprocal of the y-intercept is an estimate of the maximum ATPase activity in the presence of a saturating amount of actin, i.e., V_{max}. The reciprocal of the y-intercept gives a parameter, with the dimensions of actin concentration, that can be taken to represent the apparent dissociation constant for actin as an activator.

As shown in Fig. 2, V_{max} for thyrotoxic HMM is approximately twice the control value. The K_{app} for thyrotoxic myosin was about twice as large as the value for control myosin, indicating a lesser affinity for actin as an activator.

One further way to characterize the actin–myosin interaction is to measure the ATPase activity at varying ionic strengths (28). As shown in Fig. 3, HMM

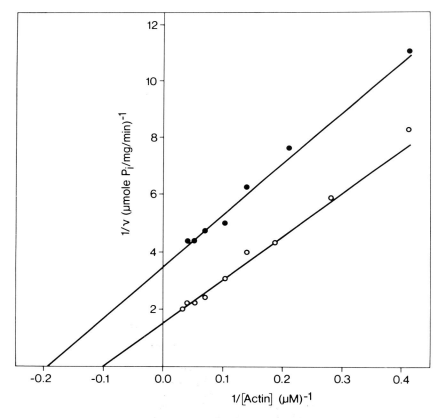

FIG. 2. Double reciprocal plots of actin-activated ATPase activity of euthyroid (*solid circles*) and thyrotoxic (*open circles*) rabbit ventricular myosin-HMM against actin concentration. The reaction medium contained 0.05 M KCl, 1.5 mM $MgCl_2$, 1 mM ATP, and 15 mM Tris-Cl, pH 7.5. The HMM concentration was 0.5 mg/ml. (Reproduced by permission of the *Journal of Biological Chemistry*.)

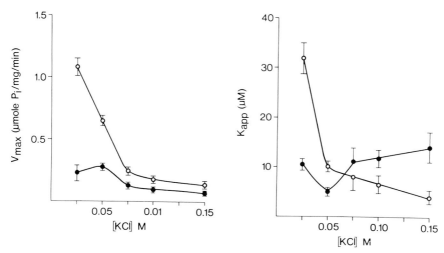

FIG. 3. The effects of variations in KCl concentration on the kinetic parameters for the actin-activated ATPase of ventricular myosin-HMM from euthyroid (*solid circles*) and thyrotoxic (*open circles*) rabbits. The kinetic parameters, V_{max} (**left**) and K_{app} (**right**), were obtained at various KCl concentrations from the intercepts of double reciprocal plots like those shown in Fig. 2. (Reproduced by permission of the *Journal of Biological Chemistry*.)

from euthyroid heart shows a characteristic plateau of activity at low-ionic strength and decreases as the ionic strength is raised. A similar result is obtained with skeletal myosin HMM, which has been attributed to a cooperative interaction between the myosin heads. By contrast, the activity of HMM from thyrotoxic heart shows only a monotonic decrease in activity as the ionic strengths is increased. This type of behavior has been previously described only with S_1, the single-headed myosin subfragment, and suggests that the interaction between the myosin heads in thyrotoxic myosin may be subtly different than normal.

Pope et al. (30) have arrived at similar conclusions regarding the enzymatic properties of cardiac myosin isozymes by comparing V_3 from neonatal rat heart with V_1 from adult animals. They found the Ca^{2+}-ATPase activity of V_1 to be more than three times greater than V_3, while the K(EDTA) activity was fairly similar. Eadie-Hofstee plots of myosin ATPase versus actin concentration were biphasic, with V_1 having a higher V_{max} and a lower K_m than V_3 for both phases.

EFFECTS OF THYROID HORMONE ON THE HEART DURING DEVELOPMENT, AGING, AND IN NON-THYROIDAL ILLNESS

Ventricular myosin isozyme composition has been observed to change in a number of conditions not clearly associated with an alteration in thyroid status. For example, Hoh and co-workers (31) described a switch from V_3 to

V_1 in the rat during the first two weeks after birth. Recently, an early postnatal change from the V_3 form to a predominance of the V_1 form has also been observed in the rabbit (32). This change in myosin isozyme composition appears to coincide with the well known postnatal surge in plasma T_4 (33). In an earlier study (34), the increase in thyroid hormone concentration was held to be responsible for a change in pancreatic amylase isozyme composition in suckling rats.

Further evidence that thyroid hormone levels may mediate changes in myosin isozyme composition in conditions other than overt thyroid disorders is suggested by the gradual change from the V_1 to the V_3 myosin form in the rat during aging (18). This change seems to correlate with decreases in actomyosin ATPase activity and in contractile performance (35–37). Frolkis and co-workers (38) have presented evidence of age-related changes in plasma concentrations of thyroid hormones and in their peripheral metabolism. They found that total plasma T_4 concentration is decreased in aged rats, largely because of a reduction in plasma T_4-binding globulin concentration. Free T_4 remains normal, T_4 binding to tissues is reduced, and tissue deiodinating activity increases. These changes, together with an increase in the distribution space and metabolic clearance of T_4, may result in an increase of the ratio of T_4/T_3 in plasma and tissues.

The combination of reduced myosin ATPase activity, a change from the V_1 to V_3 form of myosin, and depression of cardiac performance also have been reported in streptozocin-diabetes in the rat (39). Plasma thyroxine concentrations are known to be reduced in this model (40), and treatment with thyroid hormone increases myosin ATPase activity, although not to control levels (41).

Finally, a change in cardiac myosin isozymes from the V_1 to the V_3 form has been reported in various rat models of hemodynamic overload (42,43). Plasma thyroid hormone concentrations have not been reported in these models; however, changes in plasma concentration of thyroid hormone and other evidence of disturbances in thyropituitary function following major surgery and in non-thyroidal illnesses are well documented (44). Interestingly, the decrease in myosin ATPase activity that follows aortic coarctation in the rat can be prevented by thyroxine treatment (45). Also, thyroid hormone administration has been found to increase the amount of V_1 isozyme and myosin ATPase activity in hypertrophied left ventricles from rabbits with aortic banding (46). From these examples, it seems reasonable to conclude that thyroid hormone plays at least a permissive role in mediating changes in myosin isozymes in several non-thyroidal cardiac disorders.

It should be emphasized that not all of the experimental evidence cited above may be relevant to clinical heart disease. Although it is tempting to believe that a change in ventricular myosin isozymes similar to that seen in the rabbit may occur in human thyrotoxicosis, the actual extent of this alteration has not been established. Moreover, there would seem to be little potential for "down" regulation of cardiac myosin isozymes in most clinical states associated with hemodynamic overload or in diabetes. This conclusion, however, assumes that a myosin isozyme with lower than normal ATPase activity is not expressed in human ventricular myocardium.

Perhaps the most important clinical implication of the experimental results may be the possibility of inducing the high-activity type myosin isozyme in hypertrophied and failing hearts without significantly altering myocardial oxygen requirements. The potential to regulate myosin isozyme composition in different species is illustrated in Fig. 4. Rat would seem to have a greater potential to "down" regulate to the low-activity V_3 form and only limited ability to "up" regulate to the high-activity V_1 form. On the other hand, humans would have a greater potential for "up" regulation. A goal for future research will be to define how much of this potential can be realized.

SUMMARY

New insight into the question of a "defective" myosin in human and experimental models of cardiac hypertrophy has been provided by recognition of cardiac myosin isozymes and their regulation by thyroid hormone. Three isozymic forms of myosin have been identified in ventricular myocardium,

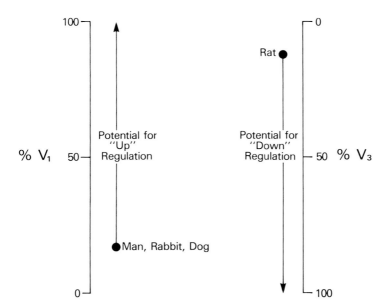

FIG. 4. The potential to regulate the expression of ventricular myosin isozymes is species specific and related to plasma thyroid hormone concentration. Rat has a greater capacity to "down" regulate to the low ATPase activity V_3 form, while man may have a greater capacity to "up" regulate to the high activity V_1 form. (Reproduced by permission of *Progress in Cardiovascular Diseases*.)

which are referred to as V_{1-3} in order of increasing electrophoretic mobility and ATPase activity. These myosin forms have the same light chains, but differ in their heavy-chain compositions. V_1 is thought to contain two A-type heavy chains, V_3 two B-type heavy chains, and V_2 one heavy chain of each type. Rabbit and several other mammalian species, probably including man, normally have a predominance of the low-activity V_3 form. In cardiac hypertrophy induced by administration of excess thyroid hormone, synthesis of the V_1 form is stimulated. By contrast, in the rat ventricle the V_1 form normally predominates, and thyroid ablation procedures lead to expression of the V_3 form. A change from the V_1 to the V_3 form also has been documented in the rat during aging, chemically-induced diabetes, and hypertrophy in response to hemodynamic stress. In some cases, these changes in isozyme composition also seem to be associated with alterations in plasma thyroid hormone concentration.

ACKNOWLEDGMENTS

This work was supported by grants from the Arizona Affiliate of the American Heart Association, the Gustavus and Louis Pfeiffer Research Foundation, and the National Institutes of Health (HL-20984).

REFERENCES

1. Spann, J. F., Buccino, R. A., Sonnenblick, E. H., and Braunwald, E. (1967): *Circ. Res.*, 21:341–354.
2. Hoar, P. F., Shiverick, K. T., Hamrell, B. B., and Alpert, N. R. (1971): In: *Cardiac Hypertrophy*, edited by N. R. Alpert, pp. 333–344. Academic Press, New York.
3. Swynghedauw, B., Douveret, P., Durland, M., Hatt, P-Y., Lemaire, F., and Piquet, V. (1971): *Cardiovasc. Res.*, 4:458–468.
4. Katagiri, T., and Morkin, E. (1974): *Biochim. Biophys. Acta*, 342:262–274.
5. Wikman-Coffelt, J., Fenner, C., Coffelt, R. J., Salel, A., Kamiyama, T., and Mason, D. T. (1975): *J. Mol. Cell. Cardiol.*, 7:219–224.
6. Leclercq, J. F., and Swynghedauw, B. (1976): *Europ. J. Clin. Invest.*, 6:27–33.
7. Shiverick, K. T., Hamrell, B. B., and Alpert, N. R. (1976): *J. Mol. Cell. Cardiol.*, 8:837–851.
8. Raszkowski, R. R., Welty, J. D., and Peterson, M. B. (1977): *Circ. Res.*, 40:191–198.
9. Siemankowski, R. F., and Dreizen, P. (1978): *J. Biol. Chem.*, 253:8659–8665.
10. Carey, R. A., Bove, A. A., Coulson, R. L., and Spann, J. F. (1979): *Biochem. Med.*, 21:235–245.
11. Barany, M. (1967): *J. Gen. Physiol. (Suppl.)*, 50:197–218.
12. Katz, A. M. (1973): *Circulation*, 47:1076–1079.
13. Flink, I. L., and Morkin, E. (1977): *FEBS Lett.*, 81:391–394.
14. Flink, I. L., Rader, J. H., and Morkin, E. (1979): *J. Biol. Chem.*, 254:3105–3110.
15. Hoh, J. F. Y., McGrath, P. A., and Hale, P. T. (1978): *J. Mol. Cell. Cardiol.*, 10:1053–1076.
16. Lifschitz, M. D., and Kayne, H. L. (1966): *Biochem. Pharmacol.*, 15:405–407.
17. Rovetto, M. J., Hjalmarson, A. C., Morgan, H. E., Barret, M. J., and Goldstein, R. A. (1972): *Circ. Res.*, 31:397–409.
18. Lompre, A. M., Mercadier, J. J., Wisnewsky, C., Bouveret, P., Pantaloni, C., D'Albis, A., and Schwartz, K. (1981): *Dev. Biol.*, 84:286–290.
19. Martin, A. F., Pagani, E. D., and Solaro, R. J. (1981): *Fed. Proc.*, 40:1787.
20. Banerjee, S. K., Flink, I. L., and Morkin, E. (1976): *Circ. Res.*, 39:319–326.
21. Litten, R. Z., Martin, B. J., Howe, E. R., Alpert, N. R., and Solaro, R. J. (1981): *Circ. Res.*, 48:498–501.

22. Long, L., Fabian, F., Mason, D. T., and Wikman-Coffelt, J. (1977): *Biochem. Biophys. Res. Comm.*, 76:626–635.
23. Flink, I. L., Rader, J. H., Banerjee, S. K., and Morkin, E. (1977): *FEBS Lett.*, 94:125–130.
24. Sarkar, S., Sreter, F. A., and Gergely, J. (1971): *Proc. Natl. Acad. Sci. USA*, 68:946–950.
25. Price, K. M., Littler, W. A., and Cummins, P. (1980): *Biochem. J.*, 191:571–580.
26. Sartore, S., Gorza, L., Bormioli, S. P., Libera, L. D., and Schiaffino, S. (1981): *J. Cell Biol.*, 88:226–233.
27. Banerjee, S. K., and Morkin, E. (1977): *Circ. Res.*, 41:630–634.
28. Banerjee, S. K., Kabbas, E. G., and Morkin, E. (1977): *J. Biol. Chem.*, 252:6925–6929.
29. Kuczyski, S. F. (1973): Ph.D. Thesis, New York Medical College.
30. Pope, B., Hoh, J. F. Y., and Weeds, A. (1980): *FEBS Lett.*, 118:205–208.
31. Hoh, J. F. Y., and Egerton, L. J. (1979): *FEBS Lett.*, 101:143–148.
32. Zak, R., Chizzonite, R. A., Everett, A. W., and Clark, W. A. (1982): *J. Mol. Cell. Cardiol.*, 14:111–118.
33. Dussalt, J. H., and Labie, F. (1975): *Endocrinol.*, 97:1321–1324.
34. Greengard, O., and Jaindar, S. C. (1971): *Biophys. Biochim. Acta*, 237:476–483.
35. Chesky, J. A., and Rockstein, M. (1977): *Cardiovasc. Res.*, 11:242–246.
36. Heller, L. J., and Whitehorn, W. V. (1972): *Am. J. Physiol.*, 222:1613–1619.
37. Gerstenblith, G., Spurgion, H. A., Froehlich, J. P., Weisfeldt, M. L., and Lakatta, E. G. (1979): *Circ. Res.*, 44:417–423.
38. Frolkis, V. V., and Valueva, G. V. (1978): *Gerontology*, 24:81–94.
39. Dillman, W. H. (1980): *Diabetes*, 29:579–582.
40. Brown, T. J., Bromage, N. E., and Matt, A. (1976): *J. Endocrinol.*, 68:21–22.
41. Malhotra, A., Penpargkul, S., Fein, F., Sonnenblick, E. H., and Scheuer, J. (1981): *Circ. Res.*, 49:1243–1250.
42. Mercadier, J. J., Lompre, A. M., Wisnewsky, C., Samuel, J. L., Bercovici, J., Swynghedauw, K., and Schwartz, D. (1981): *Circ. Res.*, 49:525–532.
43. Rupp, H. (1981): *Basic Res. Cardiol.*, 76:79–88.
44. Chopra, I. H., Chopra, U., Smith, S. R., Reza, M., and Solomon, D. H. (1975): *J. Clin. Endocrinol. and Metab.*, 4:1043–1049.
45. Affito, J. J., and Inchiosa, M. A. (1979): *Life Sci.*, 25:353–364.
46. Litten, R. Z., III, Martin, B. J., Low, R. B., and Alpert, N. R. (1982): *Circ. Res.*, 50:856–864.

Perspectives in Cardiovascular Research, Vol. 8,
edited by R. C. Tarazi and J. B. Dunbar.
Raven Press, New York © 1983.

Relationship of Changes in Molecular Forms of Myosin Heavy Chains to Endogenous Level of Thyroid Hormone During Postnatal Growth

Alan W. Everett, Richard A. Chizzonite, William A. Clark, and Radovan Zak

Department of Medicine, Cardiology Section, and Department of Pharmacological and Physiological Sciences, The University of Chicago, Chicago, Illinois 60637

Ventricles of myocardia of different animals differ in their shortening velocities and properties of myosin adenosine triphosphatase (ATPase) (1). In general, the ventricles of smaller animals have an ATPase activity and shortening velocity higher than those of larger animals; in animals of similar size, the ATPase activity is higher in species whose survival requires sustained exertion rather than short bursts of activity (e.g., hare versus rabbit) (2). Moreover, within the same myocardium, atria and ventricles contain different forms of myosin (3). The ATPase activity, as well as the shortening velocity, is higher in the atria than in the ventricles. Furthermore, several investigators (4,5) have recently shown that both atria and ventricles contain not one, but several, variants of myosin (isomyosin).

In ventricles, which have been examined in more detail than atria, multiplicity of myosin reflects the differences in the primary structure of heavy chains (HC). So far, two classes of HC have been identified: HC_α and HC_β. These two dissimilar heavy chains combine with two sets of identical light chains (LC), LC_1 and LC_2, to form two homodimers, $(HC_\alpha)_2$ and $(HC_\beta)_2$, respectively, and one hybrid molecule HC_α-HC_β. The amino acid composition and sequence of HC_α and HC_β differ. In some species, notably rabbit and rat, the amino acid substitution results in a net charge difference that allows separation of the isomyosins by electrophoresis in native state. Three isomyosins have been detected and labeled according to decreasing electrophoretic mobilities: V_1, V_2, and V_3. The ATPase activity of V_1 is about three times that of V_3, while that of V_2 is intermediate.

The molecular diversity of myosin has recently attracted considerable attention, mostly because previous studies have shown that both contractile and enzymatic properties of the heart change, depending on the hormonal and functional status of the animal. For example, treatment of high doses of thyroid hormone (TH) in rabbits results in elevation of ventricular myosin ATPase with concomitant alteration of its amino acid sequence (6,7). Similarly, in the pressure-overloaded heart, conformational changes have been detected in the myosin molecule that are consistent with amino acid substitution (8).

The alterations in the primary structure of myosin are consistent with changes in the isomyosin composition of thyrotoxic and pressure-overloaded hearts. Thyrotoxicosis, which is accompanied by an increase in the shortening velocity, results in an accumulation of HC_α (9), while the opposite change occurs in the pressure-overloaded heart, where the shortening velocity is decreased (10). The isomyosin composition of the ventricle changes not only as a result of experimentally altered hormonal and hemodynamic states but also as a function of animal age as well. The V_1 variant is the predominant species in young animals and is gradually replaced by the V_3 form as the animal grows older (9).

Since the profile of ventricular isomyosins changes during normal development and also after treatment with TH, we have examined the correlation between the endogenous level of thyroid hormone in the serum and the relative content of HC_α and HC_β in the ventricles of rabbits at various intervals before and after birth. In order to elucidate the factors controlling expression of myosin genes, we have also measured the synthetic rates of HC_α and HC_β.

METHODS

The preparation of ventricular myosin, the immunization protocol, and the procedures for screening of antimyosin-secreting hybridomas have been described previously (11,9). Briefly, myosin was extracted by high salt buffer in the presence of ATP and purified by ammonium sulfate fractionation. Before immunization, myosin was denatured with sodium dodecyl sulfate (SDS).

The monoclonal antibodies (McAb) 25 and 37 were produced by hybridomas resulting from fusion of splenic lymphocytes obtained from Lewis rats immunized with myosin isolated from thyrotoxic rabbits. Antibody 52 was derived from BALB/c mouse lymphocytes after immunization with chicken cardiac myosin. In each case, the myeloma line was P3-X63-Ag8.

To assess antibody affinity for specific types of myosin, we used liquid phase radioimmunoassay. Myosin was iodinated enzymatically (Enzymobead reagent, BioRad) and reacted with antibody at a dilution corresponding to 30 to 60% binding of iodinated myosin. After reaction for 1 hr at 37°C in the presence of 1% DOC and 1% Triton X-100, the immune complex was precipitated using indirect immunoprecipitation (9).

The myosin was fractionated into HC_α and HC_β by affinity chromatography using appropriate McAb coupled to cyanogen bromide activated Sepharose 4B, by standard procedure. Myosin was applied to the immunoabsorbent column in pyrophosphate solution (0.5 M NaCl, 20 mM Na-phosphate, and 20 mM Na-pyrophosphate, pH 7.0). After collecting unabsorbed myosin, the column was washed with the same buffer. Next, the absorbed myosin was eluted with two volumes of 4 M guanidine HCl. Myosin was then collected by ammonium sulfate precipitation (55% saturation) and redissolved by dialysis against pyrophosphate buffer. The unabsorbed myosin was also treated with guanidine HCl.

Electrophoresis of myosin in native state was done according to Hoh et al. (12).

The fractional synthetic rate of myosin HC was determined in unrestrained rabbits which were infused into the ear vein with ^{3}H-leucine for 1 hr (1.5 mC/hr). After infusion, myosin was extracted, passed through an affinity column of the McAb specific for either HC_α or HC_β. Fractionated isomyosins were then subjected to electrophoresis in the presence of SDS. After staining with Coomassie blue, the heavy chains were excised from tube gels and hydrolyzed with 6 N HCl. Leucine-specific radioactivity was determined after its separation and quantitation by dansylchloride method. Plasma leucine was used as precursor, as we have previously shown that its specific radioactivity approximates that of aminoacyl transfer ribonucleic acid (tRNA). Free leucine-specific radioactivity was determined after treatment of plasma with trichloroacetic acid (TCA) followed by its removal by Dowex AG-50W resin. Details of these procedures were published previously (14).

Partial chymotryptic digestion of myosin was done at a myosin:enzyme ratio of 8:1 for 30 min at 37°C. The peptides were separated by electrophoresis in the presence of SDS on 15% acrylamide slab gels using the Laemmli buffer system.

RESULTS

Separation of Myosin HC_α and HC_β

The monoclonal antibodies were screened for their ability to separate the two classes of myosin heavy chains by indirect precipitation of ^{125}I-labeled myosin. The antibody used was that secreted by the hybridoma either into the culture medium or into the ascitic fluid of mice. Two broad categories of McAb were detected: those that reacted preferentially with either HC_α or HC_β and those that reacted equally with both heavy chains. In the first category, McAb 25 and 37 reacted preferentially with myosin V_1 (HC_α), while McAb 52 showed higher binding affinity for myosin V_3 (HC_β) (Table 1).

The McAbs directed against determinants specific for individual isomyosins were then used to construct immunoabsorbent columns. Bulk myosin was extracted from the ventricles and passed over a column of McAb specific for either HC_α or HC_β. Figure 1 shows the separation of individual isomyosins from a myosin preparation containing the three isomyosins, V_1, V_2, and V_3. When an anti-HC_α antibody was used as immunoabsorbent, both V_1 and V_2 were retained by the column, whereas the V_3 isomyosin was excluded in the pure form. With an anti-HC_β column, V_2 and V_3 isomyosins were absorbed

TABLE 1. *Relative specificity of anti-myosin monoclonal antibodies for rabbit cardiac isomyosins*

| | Monoclonal antibodies | | |
| | Anti-V_1 | | Anti-V_3 |
Myosin types	25	37	52
Rabbit ventricle			
Mature adult (V_3)	21	18	2.0
Thyrotoxic adult (V_1)	1.0	1.0	19

Data were derived from competitive radioimmunoassay analysis as described in Methods section. The values given are micrograms of test myosin required to inhibit antibody binding to the ^{125}I-labeled reference myosin to the same degree as 1.0 μg of unlabeled reference myosin. The labeled reference myosins were rabbit V_1 and chicken ventricular for the anti-V_1 and anti-V_3 antibodies, respectively.

and V_1 passed through. The fact that V_2 isomyosin is undetected in the excluded fraction of both columns provides additional support for the claim that V_2 is a heterodimer containing HC_α and HC_β.

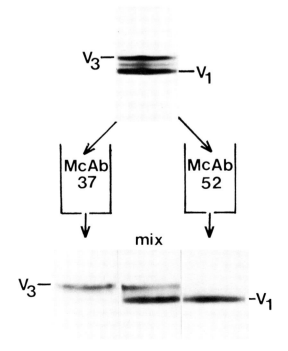

FIG. 1. Separation of rabbit ventricular isomyosins by affinity chromatography using antibodies specific for either HC_α or HC_β. Bulk ventricular myosin containing isomyosins V_1, V_2, and V_3 was passed through two immunoadsorbent columns of McAb 37 (anti-HC_α) and McAb 52 (anti-HC_β). The composition of the original and excluded fractions was determined by electrophoresis in non-denaturing conditions. A mix of the excluded fractions is shown.

Peptide Maps of HC_α and HC_β

The difference in the primary structures of HC_α and HC_β, indicated by differential reactivity with monoclonal antibodies, was further analyzed by comparison of peptide maps produced by partial chymotryptic digestion of V_1 and V_3 isomyosins. The map displayed after one dimensional electrophoresis on SDS polyacrylamide gels is shown in Fig. 2; it is clear that HC_α and HC_β are quite different polypeptides.

Correlation of the Serum Level of TH with the Isomyosin Profile of the Ventricle During Development

We have shown previously that the relative amount of HC_α and HC_β varies according to the age of the rabbit (9). In the late embryonic period, HC_β

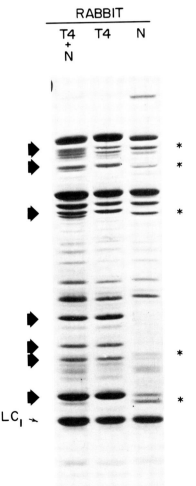

FIG. 2. Polypeptide mapping of chymotryptic fragments of ventricular myosins from adult (**N**) and 21-day thyroxine-treated (**T4**) rabbits. Myosins were partially digested with chymotrypsin, and the digests were analyzed by SDS-polyacrylamide gel electrophoresis as described in the text. An equimolar mixture of myosins from adult and thyroxine-treated rabbits (**N** and **T4**) was made before partial digestion with chymotrypsin. The *arrows* and *asterisks* indicate peptides distinct to ventricular myosins of thyroxine-treated and normal rabbits, respectively. **LC₁** identifies myosin light chain one.

predominates, but after birth is gradually replaced by HC_α, which, in turn, is replaced by HC_β as the rabbit ages. We have also shown that treatment with TH shifts the relative proportion of the two heavy chains in the direction of HC_α. In light of these observations, we have analyzed the correlation between the TH level in the serum of normal rabbits at different stages of development and the isomyosin composition of their hearts. Figure 3 shows that a significant concentration of free T4 is detectable in fetal serum from at least 23 days of gestation. (No total T3 and T4 were detected; this is undoubtedly because the method for measurement of total hormone is much less sensitive than the one used to measure the free hormone.) Around the time of birth, however, there is a great surge in the serum levels of all forms of TH measured; a maximum was reached at approximately 2 weeks of postnatal life. Thereafter, the concentration of T3 remained constant, whereas that of T4 fell over the next 2 weeks to a low concentration which remained stable through the rest of the period analyzed (5 years).

During neonatal life, the relative amount of V_1 isomyosin is closely correlated with the level of serum thyroid hormone. Both V_1 concentration and T4 reached a maximum at 2 weeks of age, and then both declined more or less in parallel. After 4 weeks of age, however, the correlation is lost. While the T4 stabilizes at a constant low level, V_1 is continuously being replaced by V_3 isomyosin. At 4 months of age, V_1 represents approximately 10% of the total. In older animals, the amount is barely detectable.

Rates of Synthesis of Cardiac Isomyosins

As a first step toward elucidating the factors that regulate the accumulation of individual isomyosins during development, we have compared the synthetic rates of HC_α and HC_β after administration of thyroid hormone. Animals of 4 to 5 weeks were selected, as both isomyosins are present in their hearts in approximately a 1:1 ratio.

The rates of synthesis were determined after continuous administration of tracer leucine during a period of 1 hr. After isolation of V_1 and V_3 by affinity chromatography, the leucine-specific radioactivity was determined in the heavy chains and in the serum. From these values and from the rate constant for the time-dependent change in leucine radioactivity in the serum, we have calculated the fractional synthesis rates (k_s). In euthyroid animals, k_s values were similar for both heavy chains. Administration of T4 for 2 days, however, resulted in an approximately threefold increase in k_s of HC_α and a two- to threefold decrease in k_s of HC_β. Similar changes were detected 4 days after treatment with T4 (Table 2).

DISCUSSION

By the use of monoclonal antibodies as immunoabsorbents, we have separated and purified two variants of myosin heavy chain, HC_α and HC_β, from

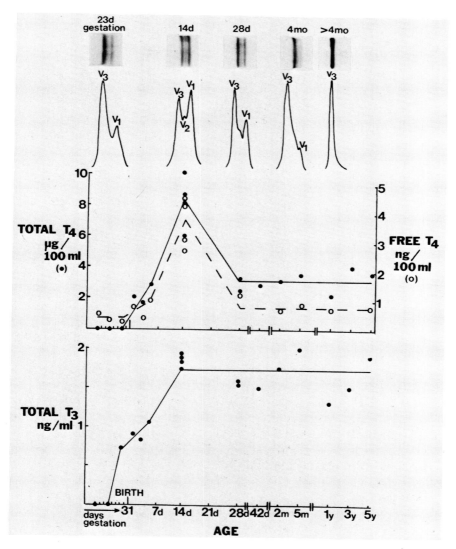

FIG. 3. Isomyosin composition of ventricles and the TH level in the serum of normal rabbits. The relative contents of isomyosins V_1, V_2, and V_3 were determined from densitometric scans of Coomassie blue stained polyacrylamide gels after electrophoretic separation in non-denaturing conditions. Thyroid hormone levels were measured with a standard clinical RIA kit (Clinical Assays).

the hearts of euthyroid rabbits. These two classes of heavy chains are undoubtedly products of different genes, as they differ in peptide maps and antigenic structure. The peptide maps displayed by one dimensional electrophoresis following limited digestion with chymotrypsin contained at least eight different peptide fragments.

TABLE 2. *Fractional rates of synthesis (k_s) of the heavy chains of isomyosins V_1 (HC_α) and V_3 (HC_β) in rabbit hearts before and after treatment with L-thyroxine (T_4)*

Rabbit no.	Weight (g)	Condition	k_s (day^{-1})	
			HC_α	HC_β
1	800	Untreated	0.13	0.10
2	735	Untreated	0.07	0.12
3	585	2 days T_4	0.41	0.04
4	740	4 days T_4	0.24	0.05

Rabbits were infused via an ear vein with 1.5 mCi of ^{3}H-leucine for 1 hr. Rabbits 3 and 4 received 200 μg L-T_4/kg/day. After extraction of myosin from the ventricles, isomyosins V_1 and V_3 were isolated by affinity chromatography (see Fig. 2). The fractional synthesis rate was calculated from the specific radioactivities of leucine both in the heavy chains of V_1 and V_3 and free in the serum.

After characterization of heavy chains and selection of specific antibodies for either HC_α or HC_β, we examined isomyosin transformation in rabbit ventricles during normal development. Our quantitation of heavy chains was based on densitometric tracings of Coomassie blue stained isomyosins separated by electrophoresis of myosin in its native state. The method was verified by radioimmunoassay of isolated ventricular myosin with antibodies specific for individual heavy chains (9). The quantitation of isomyosins was also done by radioimmunoassay using an aliquot of ventricle that was solubilized by sodium dodecyl-sulfate. This is the most rigorous (but also the most laborious) procedure that will yield the amount of isomyosin HC per unit mass of the heart.

The results of our quantitation were as follows: HC_α accumulates from approximately 20% of the total in hearts of 23-day-old embryos to approximately 50% of the total 7 days after birth. For the next 2 weeks, the proportion of HC_α remains relatively constant. Between 4 weeks and 12 months of age, the proportion of HC_α continuously declines until it reaches less than 10% in a 1-year-old animal.

In both young (50% HC_α) and old (10% HC_α) rabbits, the hyperthyroid state is associated with rapid replacement of V_3 (HC_β) isomyosin by V_1 (HC_α). After 21 days of treatment with TH of both old and young rabbits, the shift to 100% HC_α is completed. The heavy chains synthesized under the effect of TH are identical in their peptide maps and immunological properties to HC_α present in the hearts of euthyroid animals. The isomyosin transformation that we have detected in this study is in full agreement with the data of Morkin et al., who analyzed cyanogen bromide peptides (6) and myosin ATPase activity (7), and with the immunofluorescence study of Schiaffino et al. (13), who used polyclonal antibodies specific for V_1 isomyosin to analyze hearts of thyrotoxic animals.

Although TH clearly influences gene expression in the rabbit myocardium, its role during the isomyosin transformation that occurs in normal heart during development is not clear. It is of interest, however, that the burst of HC_α synthesis occurring after birth is correlated with rapid increase in the serum level of TH. At the later period, the change of isomyosins follows its own path, seemingly independent of TH. While the levels of T3 and T4 remain constant, the relative proportion of isomyosin V_1 continues to decline with age. Thus, either factors other than TH regulate gene expression during late adult life, or serum levels of T3 and T4 are inadequate indices of TH action at the cellular level.

As a first step, in order to gain some insight into the processes that control gene expression for individual isomyosins, we have studied the synthesis of HC_α and HC_β after administration of TH. Two days of treatment resulted in a marked increase in fractional synthetic rate of HC_α, while the opposite change occurred in HC_β. In euthyroid animals, where the ratio of HC_α to HC_β was 1:1, their respective synthetic rates were similar. The combined and opposite effects of TH on the synthesis of the two heavy chains in the ventricle would result in substantial redistribution of the isomyosin complement of the myocardium. Moreover, it is quite possible that the alteration in degradation rates plays an additional role in determining the relative concentrations of isomyosins.

SUMMARY

The ventricles of euthyroid rabbits contain three molecular variants of myosin (isomyosins): V_1, V_2, and V_3. The relative concentration of isomyosins varies depending on the developmental stage of the animal. In neonatal animals, the accumulation of the high ATPase V_1 variant is closely correlated with the serum level of thyroid hormone. The concentration of V_1 reaches its maximum at approximately 2 weeks postpartum, when the serum level of T4 is at its peak. After this, both T4 and V_1 concentrations begin to decline; however, the correlation between these two variables is lost. While T4 reaches its constant low level at about 1 month after birth, the relative concentration of V_1 continues to decline throughout the entire first year and is replaced by the V_3 isomyosin. Administration of T4 results in rapid accumulation of V_1 isomyosin, which is associated both with a rapid increase in the fractional synthesis rate of the heavy chain of V_1 (HC_α) and with a marked decrease in the synthesis of the heavy chain of V_3 (HC_β).

REFERENCES

1. Delcayre, C., and Swynghedauw, B. (1975): *Pflugers Arch.*, 355:39–47.
2. Syrovy, I., Delcayre, C., and Swynghedauw, B. (1979): *J. Molec. Cell. Cardiol.*, 11:1129–1135.
3. Flink, I. L., Rader, J. H., Banerjee, S. K., and Morkin, E. (1978): *FEBS Lett.*, 94:125–130.
4. d'Albis, A., and Gratzer, W. B. (1973): *FEBS Lett.*, 29:292–296.
5. Hoh, J. F. Y., Yeoh, G. P. S., Thomas, M. A. W., and Higginbottom, L. (1979): *FEBS Lett.*, 97:330–334.
6. Flink, I. L., and Morkin, E. (1977): *FEBS Lett.*, 81:391–394.

7. Morkin, E. (1979): *Circ. Res.*, 44:1–7.
8. Alpert, N. R., Mulieri, L. A., and Litten, R. Z. (1979): *Am. J. Cardiol.*, 44:947–953.
9. Chizzonite, R. A., Everett, A. W., Clark, W. A., Jakovcic, S., Rabinowitz, M., and Zak, R. (1982): *J. Biol. Chem.*, 257:2056–2065.
10. Lompre, A-M., Schwartz, K., d'Albis, A., Lacombe, G., Van Thiem, N., and Swynghedauw, B. (1979): *Nature (Lond.)*, 282:105–107.
11. Clark, W. A., Everett, A. W., Fitch, F. W., Frogner, K. S., Jakovcic, S., Rabinowitz, M., Warner, A. M., and Zak, R. (1980): *Biochem. Biophys. Res. Commun.*, 95:1680–1686.
12. Hoh, J. F. Y., McGrath, P. A., and Hale, P. T. (1978): *J. Molec. Cell. Cardiol.*, 10:1053–1076.
13. Sartore, S., Gorza, L., Bormioli, S. P., Libera, L. D., and Schiaffino, S. (1981): *J. Cell Biol.*, 88:226–233.
14. Everett, A. W., Prior, G., Zak, R. (1981): *Biochem. J.*, 194:365–368.

Perspectives in Cardiovascular
Research, Vol. 8,
edited by R. C. Tarazi and J. B. Dunbar.
Raven Press, New York © 1983.

Control of RNA Synthesis in the Normal and Hypertrophied Myocardium

Constantinos J. Limas

*Cardiovascular Section, Department of Medicine, University of Minnesota
School of Medicine, Minneapolis, Minnesota 55455*

Increased rate of nuclear ribonucleic acid (RNA) synthesis is one of the earliest biochemical changes during the development of cardiac hypertrophy (1–6); enhanced RNA polymerase activity of myocardial nuclei has been described as early as one hour following acute cardiac overload (3,4). That increased transcriptional activity is a prerequisite for enhancement of protein synthesis is suggested by the fact that actinomycin D, which inhibits RNA synthesis, prevents the development of hypertrophy (5). Since adult cardiac cells have lost their ability to proliferate (6,7), increased functional demands on the heart can only be met by increased cell size (hypertrophy). Interference with this adaptive process (e.g., with RNA or protein synthesis inhibitors) leads to rapid cardiac failure (8). Despite its compensatory nature, cardiac hypertrophy of long duration is accompanied by structural and biochemical changes that directly affect cardiac performance. Chronic pressure overload, for example, is accompanied by altered extent and rate of myocardial fiber shortening (9,10) as well as biochemical changes in the sarcolemma (11), sarcoplasmic reticulum (12), and contractile proteins (13). Despite initially preserved overall pump function, there is a continuum of biochemical changes leading to the eventual development of decompensated cardiac failure (14). In contrast, other forms of hypertrophy, e.g., after thyroxine administration (15) or isotonic exercise (16), are associated with preserved or even enhanced myocardial contractility.

It appears that the nature of the stimulus to hypertrophy, its duration and intensity, dictate the relative amounts and/or quality of proteins involved in the regulation of cardiac contractility. Since the amount and quality of these proteins are, in turn, largely determined at the transcriptional level, elucidation of the mechanisms involved in RNA synthesis regulation is of primary importance in understanding the performance of the hypertrophied myocardium. Surprisingly little is known about these regulatory mechanisms.

A large number of steps are involved in the expression of eukaryotic genes from initiation of transcription to translation of the message into protein (Fig. 1). The most intriguing finding of recent experiments on the organization of

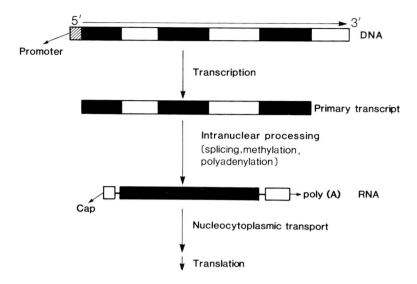

FIG. 1. Steps in the expression of eukaryotic genes.

eukaryotic genes is that, in contrast to bacterial genes, they are fragmented as discrete coding regions (exons) separated by noncoding intervening sequences (introns) (17). Formation of messenger RNA (mRNA) involves the primary synthesis of a large pre-mRNA molecule containing both intervening sequence transcripts and sequences represented in the final, polysomal mRNA. The pre-mRNA molecules are several times larger than the size of the mature mRNA (18). There is convincing evidence pointing toward the 5' end of the mature mRNA being identical with the starting point of transcription. A sequence known as the TATA box (because of the double combination of thymidine and adenosine), approximately 23 nucleotides upstream from the initiation site, has been shown to act as a signal for transcription in several gene systems (19). Other sequences, further upstream, may also play a similar role. The nontranscribed 3' sequence following the coding sequence contains a penta-nucleotide, AAUAA, approximately 10 to 20 nucleotides before the poly(A) starting site. The corresponding diribonucleic acid (DNA) sequences may represent termination signals for transcription (20).

Since transcription produces a faithful copy of the mosaic of coding and noncoding sequences, the RNA message has to be processed before it passes into the cytoplasm: This involves excision of the intervening sequences followed by precise splicing of the coding regions. The regulation of splicing has a crucial role in gene expression, and disease processes may result from splicing errors. Such an example is afforded by cases of thalassemia, in which nuclear globin RNA exists but its processing to functional RNA is defective, resulting in lower globin levels (21).

The following discussion focuses primarily on the steps leading to the formation of the primary transcripts in the normal and hypertrophied myocardium. Intranuclear processing and nucleocytoplasmic transport of RNA have received virtually no attention to date and the relevant control mechanisms are completely unknown.

MECHANISMS FOR SYNTHESIS

In general, study of transcriptional control during the induction of cardiac hypertrophy involves two aspects: (a) mechanisms for the nonselective enhancement of overall RNA synthesis, and (b) pathways for selective readout of unique DNA sequences, including single-gene transcription, which does not necessitate a generalized stimulation of RNA synthesis. Since the complexity of mRNA sequences in eukaryotic cells is considerably less than that of DNA (22), only a fraction of the available sites are actually transcribed. This pattern of RNA synthesis repression is responsible for the presence of tissue-specific protein complements (23). Positive transcriptional control in eukaryotes—defined as the induction of new mRNA species or selective amplification of particular transcripts—is a common event in embryonic development and is largely responsible for the expression of the differentiated state (24,25). Whether or not it also participates in the control of RNA synthesis during cardiac hypertrophy is not known and, in fact, there is virtually no information on RNA sequence complexity in this process.

Synthesis of the primary transcripts in the myocardium, as in other eukaryotic cells, depends on the interaction between the transcribing enzyme (RNA polymerase) and its template (26,27). The simplest level in transcription selectivity is afforded by the multiplicity of the RNA polymerase itself. Indeed, it is known that there are three discrete forms of RNA polymerases each with different localization, properties, and function (Table 1). In addition, each has several subunits, although it is unclear whether variation in subunit composition affects function (28,29). The limited polymorphism of the transcribing enzyme makes it unlikely that it contributes significantly to the complex-

TABLE 1. *Classification and general properties of eukaryotic RNA polymerases*

| Class | Localization | α-Amanitin sensitivity | Conditions for optimal activity | | | |
			Salt	Ions	DNA	Function
I	Nucleolar	Insensitive	0.05 M $(NH_4)_2SO_4$ or 0.17 M KCl	Mg^{2+}	Double-stranded	Ribosomal RNA
II	Nucleoplasmic	Sensitive (1–10 nM)	0.13 M $(NH_4)_2SO_4$ or 0.35 M KCl	Mn^{2+}	Single-stranded	hnRNA (mRNA)
III	Nucleoplasmic (cytoplasmic)	Sensitive (10–100 μM)	Broad optimum	Mn^{2+}	Double- or single-stranded	4S and 5S RNA

ity of synthesized RNAs other than determining the major class (tRNA, mRNA, rRNA).

There are four possible mechanisms through which RNA polymerases may participate in the enhancement of RNA synthesis during the development of cardiac hypertrophy; a brief elucidation follows.

Changes in the Numbers of RNA Polymerase Molecules

Although this is conceptually the most straightforward control mechanism, it has proven difficult to demonstrate unequivocally. The early studies purporting to show increased RNA polymerase activities were performed with intact nuclei and/or exogenous (usually calf thymus DNA) template (1–6). This is clearly unsatisfactory, since it does not allow for variable recoveries because of enzyme leakage during the preparation of nuclei, and the presence of proteases and nucleases in the nuclear pellet can make interpretation of the results difficult. Also, the assay does not distinguish among several steps in the transcription cycle, i.e., binding, initiation, propagation, and release. Finally, the heterogeneity of the cell population in the heart was ignored in early reports, and only recently have isolated myocytes been used in studies of cardiac RNA synthesis (30–33).

An alternative approach is to solubilize the enzyme from nuclear extracts and estimate activities independently of its endogenous template. Since chromatography on DEAE-Sephadex columns is commonly utilized in this approach, care is needed to account for differences in enzymatic recovery. This problem is exemplified by a recent study on the effects of triiodothyronine on myocardial RNA polymerases (30). The activites of the solubilized enzymes (RNA polymerase I and II) were higher in the hyperthyroid animals, but this was largely accounted for by better recovery from DEAE-Sephadex columns (Table 2), probably due to variable ribonuclease activities. In aortic constriction-induced hypertrophy (33), an increase in RNA polymerase activities (solubilized from myocyte nuclei) was detected three days after the induction of pressure overload, while RNA synthesis enhancement was evident at one day. Interestingly, the response pattern of non-muscle cells was distinctly different from that of cardiac myocytes. A more accurate method for quantitating RNA polymerases (34,35) depends on the fact that alkaline hydrolysis of synthesized RNA gives nucleoside monophosphates from internal residues and an unphosphorylated nucleoside from the 3'-hydroxyl end where RNA chain elongation stopped. The two can be conveniently separated by polyethyleneimide cellulose thin-layer chromatography so that elongation rates can be estimated from [³H]UTP/[³H]uridine ratios and the numbers of transcribing RNA polymerase molecules from the radioactivity in uridine. A number of controls are needed to correct for endogenous phosphatases, changes in the recoveries of nucleotides and differences in the size of nucleotide pools. We have applied (31) this methodology to the hypertrophied myocardium of spontaneously

TABLE 2. *Comparison of relative levels and recoveries of polymerases I and II from nuclei of normal and T_3-treated rats*

	Ratio of RNA polymerase activities (polymerase form)							
	I/II		Treated/Untreated					
Group	Fraction IV	DEAE Sephadex	Fraction IV		DEAE Sephadex		Recovery (%) of input	
			(I)	(II)	(I)	(II)	(I)	(II)
Control	0.54	0.34	—	—	—	—	42	35
Hyperthyroid	0.55	0.35	1.19	1.19	1.38	1.51	49	44

Values for polymerase I and II after DEAE-Sephadex chromatography were calculated from the areas under the respective peaks. Input for polymerase I: α-amanitin-insensitive activity in fraction IV; for polymerase II: total activity in fraction IV minus α-amanitin resistant activity. Fraction IV refers to solubilized enzymes prior to DEAE-Sephadex chromatography.
Adapted from ref. 30.

hypertensive rats (SHRs) and found increased numbers of transcribing RNA polymerases (Table 3) without a change in the rate of polyribonucleotide chain elongation (Table 4). It is likely that quantitative changes in RNA polymerase molecules depend on both the model of cardiac hypertrophy and its duration. Studies in other cell systems have indicated that fluctuations in the amounts of RNA polymerases do not always parallel changes in nuclear RNA synthesis (36–38).

Altered Distribution Between Functional Pools

Current estimates (39) of the numbers of RNA polymerase molecules (approximately 2×10^4/cell) and its molecular weight (500,000) (40) lead to the conclusion that only 0.1% of the available sites in the genome can be occupied by the enzyme at any time. Increased transcription must, therefore, involve

TABLE 3. *Quantification of RNA polymerases in nuclei from SHR and WKY controls[a]*

	UMP incorporated as uridine (pmoles)		$10^{-3} \times$ no. of RNA polymerase molecules	
Group	Total	α-Amanitin-resistant	Form I	Form II
Control	1.29 ± 0.07	0.51 ± 0.01	7.3 ± 1.0	11.0 ± 2.0
SHR	1.67 ± 0.08	0.64 ± 0.03	9.1 ± 1.3[b]	14.5 ± 1.6[b]

[a] Reactions were carried at 37°C for 2 min with 60 μg of nuclear DNA. Results represent mean ± SEM for eight experiments.
[b] $p < 0.01$ compared with controls.
Adapted from ref. 31.

TABLE 4. *Polyribonucleotide-elongation rate by RNA polymerases in nuclei of SHR and WKY controls*

	UMP incorporated (pmoles/mg of DNA)		Polyribonucleotide-elongation rate (nucleotide/s)	
	Total	α-Amanitin-resistant	Form I	Form II
Control	23.6 ± 2.1	3.9 ± 1.2	0.13 ± 0.01	0.42 ± 0.11
SHR	33.0 ± 1.9	5.4 ± 1.3	0.14 ± 0.03	0.43 ± 0.10

Adapted from ref. 31.

the recycling of polymerase molecules between several initiation and release sites. This recycling implies that, at any time, a fraction of the RNA polymerases are not engaged in transcription. In fact, there is now ample evidence for two functional pools of the enzyme: The template-engaged, which is actively involved in RNA synthesis, and the "free," which is loosely or not at all attached to the template and synthesizes RNA only with exogenous templates (41–43). The two pools may reflect different stages in the participation of the enzyme in the transcription cycle rather than forms with unique properties. Both pools have to be taken into consideration when estimates of RNA polymerase numbers in different functional states are made. For example, the ratio of engaged to free RNA polymerase is higher in the myocardium of triiodothyronine-treated rats (Table 5). It should be kept in mind that solubilization and extraction of the enzyme with conventional techniques results in variable loss of both free and (mainly) engaged polymerase (43). A shift from the free to the engaged pool (normally 70% and 30% of the total, respectively) (31) may be an important mechanism for quickly mobilizing the enzyme during the induction of cardiac hypertrophy.

TABLE 5. *Comparison of engaged (E) and free (F) RNA polymerases in control and hyperthyroid animals*

	RNA polymerase activity					Ratio (E/F)
	E		F			
Group	I	II	I	II	I	II
Control	210 ± 16	206 ± 11	290 ± 18	260 ± 26	0.72 ± 0.06	0.79 ± 0.06
Hyperthyroid	358 ± 19	329 ± 16	279 ± 20	249 ± 18	1.33 ± 0.09	1.31 ± 0.08

Incubations were carried out at 37°C for 60 min. Results are means ± SE for 6 experiments in each group. Enzymatic activity is expressed as pmoles (^{3}H)UTP/mg DNA/30 min. Free RNA polymerase was assayed with 200 μg poly[d(A-T)], the template, in the presence of 50 μg actinomycin D/ml.
Adapted from ref. 30.

Effect of Stimulators

The structural similarity of RNA polymerase II to the prokaryotic enzyme (44) suggests that similar control mechanisms may exist. Thus, dissociable protein factors such as the sigma factor (45) and other low-molecular weight proteins which are required for proper initiation and specificity of gene expression in prokaryotes may also be present in eukaryotic transcription systems. Factors which specifically stimulate transcription by RNA polymerase II on double stranded DNA templates of chromatin have been identified in extracts of calf thymus (46), rat liver (47), KB cells (48), Novikoff ascites cells (49), and mouse myeloma cells (50). These factors stimulate homologous RNA polymerase II four- to tenfold on native DNA, but do not stimulate the activity of RNA polymerase. Although these stimulators have also been identified in the heart, their function in hypertrophy is not known.

Postsynthetic Modifications

Phosphorylation by endogenous protein kinases has, in particular, been proposed as regulators of RNA polymerase function (51–53).

In summary, there is little evidence to suggest that transcriptional activity during the development of cardiac hypertrophy depends on increased numbers of RNA polymerase molecules. Even when such increases are found in later stages of the hypertrophic process, they probably reflect the participation of the enzyme in the general enhancement of protein synthesis rather than playing a primary role. It is more likely that altered interactions of RNA polymerases with their endogenous templates can account for most of the changes in the rate of myocardial RNA synthesis. In this respect, both the protein composition and the structural organization of chromatin are important. I will summarize only briefly the recent progress in our understanding of this fundamental aspect of gene expression.

HISTONE AND NONHISTONE PROTEINS

In eukaryotes, the genomic RNA is found in association with the histones and nonhistone proteins (NHPs) in a stable complex referred to as chromatin (17). It is widely recognized that chromatin-associated proteins exert both inhibitory and stimulatory influences on the availability of RNA as template for RNA polymerase action (54). It is also known that exogenous histones can inhibit RNA polymerase activity in chromatin (55,56). The observation that selective tryptic digestion of nuclear histones results in a two- to fourfold stimulation of RNA synthesis (57) fits the current view that excision of the aminoterminal region of the histones would make the DNA more accessible to the RNA polymerases. This inhibitory effect can be reversed by postsynthetic modifications of histones, notably phosphorylation (58) and acetylation (59).

In contrast to histone, NHPs represent a heterogeneous group that has attracted considerable attention as possible regulators of positive transcriptive control. Supporting evidence for this concept has been extensively reviewed (60–63) and will only be mentioned briefly here. NHPs have a number of properties that make then likely candidates for transcription control.

Heterogeneity

As determined by their migration on polyacrylamide gels, NHPs exhibit considerable heterogeneity (64–66). High-resolution two-demensional gel electrophoresis has demonstrated about 450 NHP species in HeLa cell chromatin (67), the majority being minor components in quantities less than 10^4 copies per cell. It is likely that many of these proteins are structural components or enzymes concerned with "housekeeping" functions and that only a few represent species involved in gene regulation. NHPs are also found in association with the basic chromatin unit (nucleosome) and are preferentially enriched in the transcriptionally active chromatin fraction (68,69). Mild enzymatic fractionation of rat liver nuclei with micrococcal nuclease has been used to isolate a chromatin fraction preferentially enriched in RNA polymerase II-polynucleosome complexes (70). This fraction is also selectively enriched in NHPs.

Tissue and Species Specificity

A number of NHPs are characteristically found in individual tissues and may represent those with specific gene-control function (71–73). Tissue specificity has also been demonstrated by immunological means (74). On the other hand, a number of NHPs are common to a variety of different tissues and may represent structural protein or ubiquitous nuclear enzymes.

Interaction with DNA and Chromatin

A small subfraction of NHPs binds specifically to homologous DNA, as might be expected for gene regulatory molecules (75,76). Chromatography through DNA-cellulose columns and subsequent elution with salt solutions of increasing ionic strength has been utilized by Kleinsmith (75) to separate specific DNA-binding NHPs. Phenolsoluble nuclear phosphoproteins were similarly shown by Teng et al. (77) to bind preferentially to homologous DNA. More recently, Allfrey et al. (78) have described a comprehensive technique for the fractionation of calf thymus nuclear NHPs by affinity chromatography on aminoethyl sepharose 4B columns charged with fractionated DNA. The method separates NHPs according to their affinities for sequences of DNA with low, intermediate, and high C_0t values.

Gene Regulation

The evidence for the role of NHPs in gene regulation depends, in large part, on experiments with dissociated and reconstituted chromatin, which indicated that transcription specificity is related to the nonhistone fraction (79,80). DNA–RNA hybridization experiments appear to support the conclusion that transcriptional expression of single genes is also dependent upon the nonhistone nuclear proteins (81,82).

Posttranslational Modifications

These include phosphorylation (83), acetylation (84), methylation (85) and poly (ADP) ribosylation (86). Phosphorylation has received most attention; the degree of NHP phosphorylation by endogenous protein kinases seems to regulate their ability to enhance nuclear RNA synthesis *in vitro* (87–89).

Changes

There are numerous reports on quantitative and qualitative changes of NHPs, during the cell cycle and in association with gene activation, in relation to cellular proliferation as well as under conditions where gene transcription is activated (90–92). Nuclear phosphokinase activities parallel these changes. In general, the posttranslational alterations in NHPs support their proposed role in the regulation of specific gene transcription.

STUDIES IN ANIMAL MODELS

Myocardial NHPs have only recently been the subject of systematic study. Suria and Liew (84) described the heterogeneity of NHPs from heart tissue and, more recently, Liew and Sole (93) have fractionated the phenol-soluble nonhistone proteins by two-dimensional polyacrylamide gel electrophoresis. In the cardiomyopathic Syrian hamster, a model of cardiac failure, there were several qualitative differences in the electrophoretic pattern compared to normal controls; in addition, the phosphorylation pattern differed with two phosphorylated components present only in the dystrophic muscle (94). A subsequent report from the same group (95) indicated similar changes in the NHPs from human hearts with muscular subaortic stenosis, but no changes in association with hypertrophy. These findings support the possible involvement of NHPs in cardiac hypertrophy and failure. The importance of NHP phosphorylation for gene transcription prompted Akhtar and Itzhaki (96) to look for nuclear protein kinases. Multiple forms of cyclic AMP-dependent phosphokinases were described in association with NHPs.

We have also isolated multiple forms of nuclear protein kinase activities in association with the NHP fraction (97). Changes in the extent of NHP phosphorylation have been described in association with normal postnatal growth (98), thyroxine-induced hypertrophy (99), and genetic cardiomyopathy (94,95). In thyroxine-induced hypertrophy (99), chromatin dissociation–reconstitution experiments strongly supported a decisive role of NHPs in determining template activity (Table 6). It is not clear whether these changes in nuclear protein phosphorylation reflect *de novo* synthesis or activation of nuclear protein kinases, translocation of cytoplasmic kinases to the nucleus, increased availability of substrate, decreased activity of phosphoprotein phosphatase, or changing amounts of endogenous inhibitors. Any of these mechanisms, alone or in combination, could be operative. The reported multiplicity of nuclear protein kinases is especially intriguing since it may provide for some selectivity in the response to different hypertrophic stimuli. Support for this proposal is given by a recent demonstration that isoproterenol—but not triiodothyronine—induced hypertrophy and nuclear protein activation shows dependence on polyamine biosynthesis (Table 7). This may indicate that isoproterenol stimulates selectively polyamine-dependent protein kinases while T_3 stimulates a broader spectrum of protein kinases.

Any scheme of transcriptional control should take into consideration the structural organization of chromatin. The basic unit of chromatin structure is the nucleosome, a flattened nucleohistone bead about 110 Å in diameter and 57 Å in height (100–102). Electron micrographs of spread chromatin fibers show linear, regularly spaced arrays of nucleosomes distributed along a 30-Å filament at a frequency of approximately 34 nucleosomes/μm (103). The electron microscopic appearance of chromatin as a periodic repeating structure, resembling beads on a string, is confirmed by many biochemical and biophysical studies. It has led to the prevailing view that the DNA strand is periodically wrapped around clusters of histones, each cluster comprising an octamer made up of two molecules each of the four major histone classes: H2A, H2B, H3 and H4.

Coiling of the DNA strand around the histone cores represents the first level of compaction of the genetic material in interphase chromatin. In all species examined, the nucleosomal core particles contain a uniform length of DNA (140–150 nucleotide pairs) (104). Coiling of the DNA around the octameric

TABLE 6. *Transcriptive capacity of myocardial chromatin reconstituted with histones and NHPs of varying origin*

Chromatin preparation	RNA synthesis (pmoles ^{3}H-UMP/mg per minute)
Control histones + control NHPs	106 ± 4.8
Control histones + hyperthyroid NHPs	159 ± 6.7
Hyperthyroid histones + hyperthyroid NHPs	184 ± 7.1
Hyperthyroid histones + control NHPs	111 ± 7.4

Adapted from ref. 39.

TABLE 7. *Effect of cardiac hypertrophy and α-difluoromethylornithine (DFMO)
on nucleoprotein phosphorylation*

Experimental groups	Nucleoprotein phosphorylation (pmoles ^{32}P/mg prot/15 min)		
	Saline-soluble	Histones	NHP
Control	2.30 ± 0.18	0.28 ± 0.02	8.90 ± 0.70
DFMO	2.15 ± 0.17	0.29 ± 0.03	8.75 ± 0.65
Isoproternol	2.49 ± 0.16	0.31 ± 0.02^a	15.8 ± 0.91^a
Isoproterenol + DFMO	2.33 ± 0.20	0.30 ± 0.03	10.7 ± 0.82
T_3	2.51 ± 0.23	0.38 ± 0.04^a	16.10 ± 0.83^a
T_3 + DFMO	2.33 ± 0.21	0.35 ± 0.05^a	14.98 ± 0.91^a

Cardiac hypertrophy was induced in adult Sprague-Dawley rats by four daily injections of either d1-isoproterenol (0.4 mg/kg s.c.) or 3′,3′5′-triiodothyronine (0.1 mg/kg, i.p.). For ornithine decarboxylase inhibition, animals were pretreated with DFMO (0.2 g/kg s.c. daily) for two weeks prior to isoproterenol or triiodothyronine administration. Nuclei were labeled *in vitro* with (γ-^{32}P)ATP and then fractionated. Results represent mean $\pm$ SE for six experiments in each group.
  $^a p < 0.01$.

histone complex results in fivefold shortening of its contour length and also alters its topological state by the introduction of supercoils. Approximately 1.75 turns of DNA of contour length about 425 Å envelop the octameric histone complex (105). On the average, each nucleosome contains one molecule of histone H1 associated with DNA sequences adjoining the nucleosome core. Binding of H1 to a 20-nucleotide pair segment of DNA in the linker region would complete two turns of the double helix around the nucleosome, one turn for each nucleotide pair.

In view of the compactness of chromatin structure, significant changes in its organization must occur before gene readout by the RNA polymerases can be initiated and propagated. The experimental evidence that nucleosomes act to retard passage of RNA polymerase is quite convincing. There is reduction in the rate of RNA chain elongation (106) and in the number of RNA polymerase binding sites in chromatin as compared to deproteinized DNA (107). This restriction of chromatin template function is retained in isolated nucleosomes (107).

The tertiary and quartenary structure of chromatin at the supranucleosomal level may pose further restraints on the action of RNA polymerase and, at the same time, provide sequences for regulatory control. The evidence for altered chromatin structure during gene activation is based, in large part, on the observation that actively transcribed or potentially transcribable genes are more susceptible to digestion by nucleases (108–110). This process has also been utilized to fractionate the active from the inactive chromatin fractions. Such mechanisms also apply to myocardial chromatin. We have recently demonstrated (111) that following phosphorylation of myocyte nuclei, sensitivity to DNase I is significantly enhanced (Fig. 2). In addition, the proportion of chro-

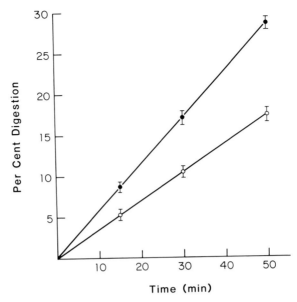

FIG. 2. Time course of DNase I digestion of control (*open circles*) and phosphorylated (*solid circles*) myocardial nuclei. Results represent mean ± SE for six experiments.

matin DNA in the transcriptionally active fraction (P_2) also increases (Table 8). This may indicate that part of the positive transcriptional control of NHPs may be exerted through their influence on chromatin structure.

Changes in the structure of myocardial chromatin also occur in association with cardiac hypertrophy. In spontaneously hypertensive rats (SHRs), sensitivity to DNase I is enhanced compared to age-matched Kyoto Wistar rats (WKYs). Translation of nuclei following incubation with small amounts of DNase I, which nick but do not solubilize active genes, also results in higher nucleotide incorporation in SHRs (Fig. 3). Salt extraction, which removes a

TABLE 8. *Composition of subnuclear fractions obtained through mild micrococcal nuclease digestion of control and phosphorylated myocyte nuclei*

Fraction	DNA (% of total)	Protein/ DNA	Nonhistone/ DNA	RNA/DNA
P_1 control	93.0	2.61	0.84	0.15
phosphorylated	88.2	2.54	0.87	0.14
P_2 control	5.0	3.20	1.24	1.18
phosphorylated	10.0	3.91	1.30	1.20
S control	2.0	9.93	9.30	0.08
phosphorylated	1.5	10.90	9.34	0.09

Adapted from Ref. 111.

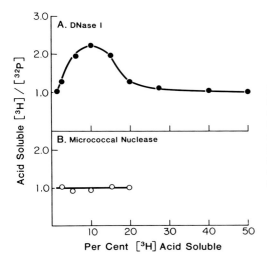

FIG. 3. Nuclease sensitivity of nuclei from SHRs and WKYs. Following "nicking" with 4 μg DNase I, nuclei were translated with *E. Coli* DNA polymerase I in the presence of (^{3}H)TTP (SHRs) or (^{32}P)TTP (WKYs). They were then digested with either DNase I (80 μg) or micrococcal nuclease (100 Units) to different degrees of acid solubility.

number of NHPs, abolished the differences in nuclease sensitivity between SHRs and WKYs. SDS-polyacrylamide gel electrophoresis of 0.35 M NaCl extracts and supernatants from DNase I digestion revealed the presence of high-mobility-group (HMG) proteins (112), which are preferentially released in SHRs. Reconstitution of salt-extracted nuclei with either 0.35 M NaCl extract or HMGs restored nuclease susceptibility to control levels, but did not equalize SHRs and WKYs (Fig. 4). These findings suggest that the altered chromatin structure in SHRs depends, in part, on the HMGs. Additional chromatin components, however, determine the increased nuclease sensitivity. It is likely that NHPs, such as HMGs, may also influence gene transcription indirectly through their effects on histone postsynthetic modifications. In this respect, histone acetylation is of major interest, since recent evidence implies a correlation between gene activity and degree of histone acetylation and a direct correlation between the level of acetylation of histones H3 and H4 and the accessibility of the associated RNA sequences to DNase I (113,114). In most instances, changes in the extent of histone acetylation appear to be modulated through variable inhibition of histone deacetylase. It is particularly important, therefore, that HMGs have been shown to inhibit histone deacetylase in a variety of cells (114) and thus link nonhistone proteins with histone–DNA interactions. Although acetylation of myocardial nucleoproteins has been described (115), its role in cardiac hypertrophy has not been examined.

The relation of chromatin structure and composition in the enhancement of transcriptional activity during the development of cardiac hypertrophy can only be conjectured at present. It would appear that the first step involves a relaxation of the higher order of chromatin, in which NHPs of the "scaffold" regions may play a significant role. This step accounts for increased nuclease sensitivity, but is not sufficient for transcription to occur. It may, however,

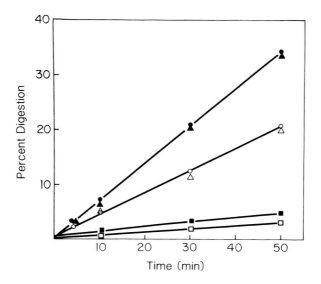

FIG. 4. Effect of HMGs on DNase I sensitivity of cardiac nuclei from SHRs and WKYs. Control nuclei were extracted with 0.35 M NaCl and reconstituted with 50 μg HMGs from cardiac nuclei. Symbols: ●, control SHRs; ■, salt-extracted SRHs; ▲, reconstituted SHRs; ○, control WKYs; □, salt-extracted WKYs; △, reconstituted WKYs.

allow binding of RNA polymerases to their initiation sites. Actual transcription appears to require changes at the level of nucleosomal composition and structures including their transient elimination.

FUTURE DIRECTIONS

It is obvious from the foregoing discussion that very little is known about the specific mechanism for RNA synthesis control in the hypertrophied myocardium. It is expected, however, that increased attention to this fundamental problem, as well as rapidly expanding information from other eukaryotic systems, will result in improved understanding of cardiac hypertrophy. Although these questions are actively pursued in a variety of other cell systems, focus on the myocardial cell is appropriate since it allows study of the hypertrophic process rather than of cell cycle control. A partial agenda of goals for the immediate future would include: (a) evaluation of the sequence complexity of mRNAs from hypertrophied versus normal myocardium; (b) use of probes of chromatin structure during the different stages in the evolution of cardiac hypertrophy; (c) a reevaluation of the role of RNA polymerases, including the possible function of stimulators of specific polymerases; (d) definition of the relationship between qualitative and quantitative changes in NHPs and transcriptive capacity; (e) study of single gene (e.g., myosin) transcription; (f) evaluation of RNA processing from transcription to cytoplasmic transport; and (g) "switching-off" mechanisms during regression of hypertrophy.

ACKNOWLEDGMENT

This study was supported in part by grant HL 24317 from the National Heart, Lung, and Blood Institute, National Institutes of Health, Bethesda, Maryland.

REFERENCES

1. Fanburg, B. L., and Posner, B. I. (1968): *Circ. Res.*, 23:123.
2. Schreiber, S. S., Oratz, M., Evans, C., Silver, E., and Rothschild, N. A. (1968): *Amer. J. Physiol.*, 215:1250.
3. Nair, K. G., Cutiletta, R., Zak, T., Koide, T., and Rabinowitz, M. (1968): *Circ. Res.*, 23:457.
4. Posner, B. I., and Fanburg, B. L. (1968): *Circ. Res.*, 23:137.
5. Morkin, E., Garrett, J. C., and Fischman, A. I. (1968): *Amer. J. Physiol.*, 214:6.
6. Grove, D., Zak, R., Nair, K. G., and Aschenbrenner, V. (1969): *Circ. Res.*, 25:473.
7. Klinge, O., and Stocker, E. (1968): *Experientia*, 24:167.
8. Meerson, E. Z. (1968): *Am. J. Cardiol.*, 22:332.
9. Spann, J. F., Buccino, R. A., Sonnenblick, E. H., and Braunwald, E. (1967): *Circ. Res.*, 21:341.
10. Bing, O. H. L., Matsushita, S., Fanburg, B. L., and Levine, H. J. (1971); *Circ. Res.*, 28:234.
11. Mead, R. J., Peterson, M. B., and Welty, J. D. (1971): *Circ. Res.*, 29:14.
12. Suko, J., Vogel, J. H. K., and Chidsey, C. A. (1970): *Circ. Res.*, 27:235.
13. Luchi, R. J., Kritcher, E. M., and Thyrum, P. T. (1969): *Circ. Res.*, 24:513.
14. Dhalla, N. S., Das, P. K., and Sharma, G. P. (1978): *J. Mol. Cell. Cardiol.* 10:363.
15. Penpargkul, S., Repke, D. I., Katz, A. M., and Scheuer, J. (1977): *Circ. Res.*, 40:134.
16. Levey, G. S., Skelton, C. L., and Epstein, S. E. (1969): *Endocrinology*, 88:1004.
17. Mathis, D., Oudet, P., and Chambon, P. (1980): *Progr. Nucleic Acids Res.*, 24:2.
18. Coutelle, C. (1981): *Biochem. J.*, 197:1.
19. Wickens, M. P., and Laskey, R. A. (1981): In: *Genetic Engineering, I*, edited by R. Williamson, pp. 103–167. Academic Press, New York.
20. Proudfoot, N. J., and Brownlee, G. G. (1976): *Nature*, 263:211.
21. Maquat, L. E., Kinniburgh, A. J., Beach, L. R., Honig, G. R., Lazeron, J., Erschler, W. B., and Ross, J. (1980): *Proc. Natl. Acad. Sci. USA*, 77:4287.
22. Hastie, N. D., and Bishop, J. O. (1976): *Cell*, 9:761.
23. Harding, J. D., and Rutter, W. J. (1978): *J. Biol. Chem.*, 253:8735.
24. Harding, J. D., MacDonald, R. J., Przylbla, A. E., Chirgwin, J. M., Pictet, R. L., and Rutter, W. J. (1977): *J. Biol. Chem.*, 252:2391.
25. Newrock, K. M., Cohen, L. H., Hendricks, M. G., Donnelly, R. J., and Weinberg, E. S. (1978): *Cell*, 14:327.
26. Roeder, R. G. (1976): In: *RNA Polymerase*, edited by R. Losick, and M. Chamberlin, p. 285. Cold Spring Harbor Laboratory, New York.
27. Beebee, T. J. C., and Butterworth, P. H. W. (1977): *Biochem. Soc. Symp.*, 42:25.
28. Sklar, V. E. F., and Roeder, R. G. (1976): *J. Biol. Chem.*, 251:1064.
29. Valenzuela, P., Hager, J. L., Weinberg, F., and Rutter, W. J. (1976): *Proc. Natl. Acad. Sci. USA*, 73:1024.
30. Limas, C. J. (1979): *Amer. J. Physiol.*, 236:H451.
31. Limas, C. J. (1980): *Biochem. J.*, 188:67.
32. Cutilletta, A. F., Rudnik, M., and Zak, R. (1978): *J. Mol. Cell. Cardiol.* 10:677.
33. Cutilletta, A. F. (1981): *Amer. J. Physiol.* 240:H901.
34. Palmiter, R. D., and Haines, M. D. (1973): *J. Biol. Chem.*, 248:2107.
35. Coupar, B. E. H. and Chesterton, C. J. (1977): *Eur. J. Biochem.*, 79:525.
36. Shields, D. and Tata, J. R. (1976): *Eur. J. Biochem.*, 64:471.
37. Gross, K. J., and Pogo, A. O. (1974): *J. Biol. Chem.*, 249:568.
38. Roeder, R. G. (1974): *J. Biol. Chem.*, 249:249.
39. Cochet-Meilhac, M., Nuret, P., Courevalin, J. C., and Chambon, P. (1974): *Biochim. Biophys. Acta*, 353:185.
40. Kedinger, C., Gissinger, F., Gniazdowski, M., Mandel, J. L., and Chambon, P. (1972): *Eur. J. Biochem.*, 28:209.

41. Lampert, A., and Feigleson, P. (1974): *Biochem. Biophys. Res. Commun.*, 58:1030.
42. Fuhrman, S. A., and Gill, G. N. (1975): *Biochemistry*, 14:2925.
43. Yu, F. L. (1975): *Biochim. Biophys. Acta*, 395:295.
44. Hodo, H. G., and Blatti, S. P. (1977): *Biochemistry*, 16:2334.
45. Burgess, R. (1969): *J. Biol. Chem.*, 244:6160.
46. Benson, R. H., Spindler, S. R., Hodo, H. G., and Blatti, S. P. (1978): *Biochemistry*, 17:1387.
47. Legraverend, M., and Glazer, R. E. (1980): *Biochim. Biophys. Acta*, 607:92.
48. Sugden, B., and Keller, W. (1973): *J. Biol. Chem.* 248:3277.
49. Lee, S. C., and Dahmus, M. E. (1973): *Proc. Natl. Acad. Sci. USA*, 70:1383.
50. Lentfer, D., and Lenzius, A. G. (1972): *Eur. J. Biochem.*, 30:278.
51. Martelo, O. J., and Hirsch, J. (1974): *Biochem. Biophys. Res. Commun.*, 58:1008.
52. Jungmann, R. A., Hiestand, P. C., and Schweppe, J. S. (1974): *J. Biol. Chem.*, 249:5444.
53. Jankowski, J. M., and Kleczkowski, K. (1980): *Biochem. Biophys. Res. Commun.*, 96:1216.
54. Allfrey, V. G. (1980): In: *Cell Biology, Vol. 3*, edited by L. Goldstein and D. M. Prescott, p. 342. Academic Press, New York.
55. Huang, R. C. C., and Bonner, J. (1962): *Proc. Natl. Acad. Sci. USA*, 48:1216.
56. Allfrey, V. G., Littau, V. C., and Mirsky, A. E. (1963): *Proc. Natl. Acad. Sci. USA*, 49:414.
57. Allfrey, V. G., (1964): *Proc. Canad. Cancer Res. Conf.*, 6:313.
58. Hohmann, P. (1978): In: *Subcellular Biochemistry, Vol. 5*, edited by D. B. Roodyn, p. 87. Plenum Press, New York.
59. Oberhauser, H., Csordas, A., Puschendorf, B., and Grunicke, H. (1978): *Biochem. Biophys. Res. Commun.*, 84:110.
60. Elgin, S. C. R., and Weintraub, H. (1975): *Ann. Rev. Biochem.*, 44:725.
61. Stein, G. S., Stein, J. L., and Thomson, J. A. (1978): *Cancer Res.*, 38:1187.
62. Wang, T. Y., and Kostraba, N. C. (1978): In: *The Cell Nucleus, Vol. 9*, edited by H. Busch, p. 289. Academic Press, New York.
63. Li, H. J., and Eckhardt, R. H. (1977): *Chromatin and Chromosome Structure*. Academic Press, New York.
64. Elgin, S. C. R., and Bonner, J. (1970): *Biochemistry*, 9:4440.
65. Garrard, W., and Bonner, J. (1974): *J. Biol. Chem.*, 249:1370.
66. Yeoman, L. C., Taylor, C. W., Jordan, J. J., and Busch, H. (1973): *Biochem. Biophys. Res. Commun.*, 53:1067.
67. Peterson, J. L., and McConkey, E. M. (1976): *J. Biol. Chem.*, 257:548.
68. Chan, P. K., and Liew, C. C. (1977): *Canad. J. Biochem.*, 55:847.
69. Neumann, J., Whittaker, R., Blanchard, B., and Ingram, V. (1970): *Nucleic Acids Res.*, 5:1678.
70. Tata, J. R., and Baker, B. (1975): *J. Mol. Biol.*, 118:249.
71. MacGillivray, A. J., Cameron, A., Krause, R. J., Rickwood, D., and Paul, J. (1972): *Biochim. Biophys. Acta*, 277:384.
72. Chiu, J. F., Tsai, Y. H., Sakuma, K., and Hnilica, L. S. (1975): *J. Biol. Chem.*, 250:9431.
73. Wu, F. C., Elgin, S. C. R., and Hood, L. G. (1973): *Biochemistry*, 12:2792.
74. Chytil, F., and Spelsberg, T. C. (1971): *Nature*, 233:215.
75. Kleinsmith, L. J. (1973): *J. Biol. Chem.*, 248:5648.
76. Sevall, J. S., Cockburn, A., Savage, M., and Bonner, J. (1975): *Biochemistry*, 14:782.
77. Teng, C. S., Teng, C. T., and Allfrey, V. G. (1971): *J. Biol. Chem.*, 246:3597.
78. Allfrey, V. G., Inoue, A., Karn, J., Johnson, E. M., Good, R. A., and Hadden, J. W. (1975): In: *The Structure and Function of Chromatin*. p. 199. CIBA Foundation Symposium 28, Elsevier-North Holland, New York.
79. Gilmour, R. S., and Paul, J. (1970): *FEBS Lett.*, 9:242.
80. Harrison, P. R., Hell, A., Birne, G. P., and Paul, J. (1972): *Nature*, 239:219.
81. Gilmour, R. S., and Paul, J. (1973): *Proc. Natl. Acad. Sci. USA*, 70:3440.
82. Streggles, A. W., Wilson, G. N., Kantor, J. A., Picciano, D. K., Flavely, A. K., and Anderson, W. P. (1979): *Proc. Natl. Acad. Sci. USA*, 71:1214.
83. Pumo, D. E., Stein, G. S., and Kleinsmith, L. J. (1975): *Biochim. Biophys. Acta*, 402:125.
84. Suria, D., and Liew, C. C. (1974): *Biochem. J.*, 137:355.
85. Borun, T. W., Pearson, D., and Park, W. K. (1972): *J. Biol. Chem.*, 247:4288.
86. Ueda, K., Omachi, A., Kanhicki, M., and Hayaishi, O. (1975): *Proc. Natl. Acad. Sci. USA*, 72:205.

87. Kisch, V. M., and Kleinsmith, L. J. (1974): *J. Biol. Chem.*, 249:750.
88. Kruh, J., Dastugue, B., Defer, N., Kamiyama, M., and Tichonicky, L. (1974): *Biochimie*, 56:995.
89. Rickaus, L. E., and Ruddon, R. W. (1973): *Biochem. Biophys. Res. Commun.*, 54:387.
90. Bhorjee, J. S., and Pederson, T. (1972): *Proc. Natl. Acad. Sci. USA*, 69:3345.
91. Cohen, M. E., and Hamilton, T. H. (1975): *Proc. Natl. Acad. Sci. USA*, 72:4346.
92. Levy, R., Levy, S., Rosenberg, S. A., and Simpson, R. T. (1973): *Biochemistry*, 12:224.
93. Liew, C. C., and Sole, M. J. (1978): *Circ. Res.*, 42:637.
94. Liew, C. C., and Sole, M. J. (1978): *Circ. Res.*, 42:644.
95. Liew, C. C., Sole, M. J., Silver, M. D., and Wigle, E. D. (1980): *Circ. Res.*, 46:513.
96. Akhtar, R. A., and Itzhaki, S. (1977): *Biochem. J.*, 161:487.
97. Limas, C. J., and Chan-Stier, C. (1977): *Biochim. Biophys. Acta*, 477:404.
98. Limas, C. J. (1978): *Am. J. Physiol.*, 235:H338.
99. Limas, C. J., and Chan-Stier, C. (1978): *Circ. Res.* 42:311.
100. Olins, A. L., and Olins, D. F. (1973): *Science*, 183:330.
101. Hewish, D. R., and Burgoyne, L. A. (1973): *Biochem. Biophys. Res. Commun.*, 52:504.
102. Woodcock, C. L. F., Safer, J. P., and Stanchfield, J. E. (1976): *Exp. Cell. Res.*, 97:101.
103. Oudet, P., Gros-Bellard, M., and Chambon, P. (1975): *Cell*, 4:281.
104. Finch, J. T., and Klug, A. (1978): *Cold Spring Harbor Symp. Quant. Biol.*, 42:1.
105. Miller, D. M., Turner, P., Nienhuis, A. W., Axelrod, D. E., and Gopa-Lakrishnan, T. V. (1978): *Cell*, 14:511.
106. Cedar, H., and Felsenfeld, G. (1973): *J. Mol. Biol.*, 77:237.
107. Williamson, P., and Felsenfeld, G. (1978): *Biochemistry*, 17:5695.
108. Gazit, P., Panet, A., and Cedar, H. (1980): *Proc. Natl. Acad. Sci. USA*, 77:1789.
109. Garel, A., and Axel, R. (1976): *Proc. Natl. Acad. Sci. USA*, 73:3966.
110. Weintraub, H., and Groudine, M. (1976): *Science*, 193:848.
111. Limas, C. J. (1981): *Biochem. Biophys. Res. Commun.* 100:1347.
112. Goodwin, G. H., and Johns, E. W. (1973): *Eur. J. Biochem.*, 40:215.
113. Ruiz-Carillo, A., Wangh, L. S., and Allfrey, V. G. (1975): *Science*, 190:117.
114. Levy-Wilson, B., Watson, D. C., and Dixon, G. H. (1979): *Nucleic Acids Res.*, 6:259.
115. Morgunov, N., and Liew, C. C. (1977): *J. Mol. Cell. Cardiol.*, 9:255.

*Perspectives in Cardiovascular
Research, Vol. 8,*
edited by R. C. Tarazi and J. B. Dunbar.
Raven Press, New York © 1983.

Alteration in Sarcoplasmic Reticulum in Cardiac Hypertrophy

James Scheuer

*Division of Cardiology, Department of Medicine, Montefiore Hospital and Medical
Center of the Albert Einstein College of Medicine, Bronx, New York 10467*

STRUCTURE AND FUNCTION

There are several comprehensive reviews of sarcoplasmic reticulum (SR) (1–3). The sarcoplasmic reticulum is a rich intracellular network of connecting tubes made up of two components: the sarcotubules and the terminal cisternae. The sarcotubules form a branching and interconnecting system of tubules, which intimately surrounds the sarcomere and extends within the cell from one sarcomere to another. The terminal cisternae abut against the invaginations of the extracellular tubular system, the T tubules. It is thought that these junctions between the extracellular T tubules and the intracellular sarcoplasmic reticulum provide the interface through which electrical and rapid ionic exchanges occur during excitation–contraction coupling.

Table 1 shows some of the characteristics of sarcoplasmic reticulum vesicles. These vesicles have a very high content of the ATPase protein. There are two basic types of adenosine triphosphatase (ATPase) associated with sarcoplasmic reticulum: Mg^{2+}-ATPase and Ca^{2+}, Mg^{2+}-ATPase. The vesicles exhibit tight coupling of calcium transport to ATP hydrolysis in heart, usually reported as two moles of calcium transported per mole of ATP. This calcium coupling ratio seems to be constant for the initial velocity of calcium transport, although as calcium transport reaches steady state, coupling ratios may vary. There is a specific membrane orientation so that calcium outside of the vesicle (Ca_o^{2+}) stimulates the ATPase, which results in translocation of the calcium to the inside. Calcium inside the vesicle (Ca_i^{2+}) tends to inhibit these reactions. In the presence of calcium and Mg^{2+}-ATP, a phosphoenzyme intermediate (EP) is formed; this formation is stimulated by external calcium. Dephosphorylation of the phosphoenzyme requires magnesium. The vesicular membrane is permeable to anions that can bind calcium, such as oxalate or phosphate, and these anions are useful in studying enzymatic and transport properties because they sequester calcium on the inside of the vesicle, presumably lowering the concentration of ionized Ca_i^{2+} and permitting calcium transport to proceed. Finally, the reversibility of the ATPase reaction can be studied, the movement

TABLE 1. *Some characteristics of SR vesicles[a]*

1. Membrane maintains a concentration gradient between Ca_o^{2+} and Ca_i^{2+}

2. High content of ATPase protein
   a. Mg^{2+} ATPase
   b. Ca^{2+}-Mg^{2+} ATPase

3. Tight coupling of calcium transport (2 moles) to ATP hydrolysis

4. Specific membrane orientation
   a. Ca_o^{2+} stimulates ATPase from the outside and is translocated to the inside
   b. Ca_i^{2+} is inhibitory

5. EP intermediate formation is stimulated by Ca_o^{2+}; dephosphorylation requires Mg^{2+}

6. Permeability to Ca^{2+} precipitating ions

7. Reversibility of the active transport process—requires Ca_i^{2+}

[a] Ca_o^{2+} = external calcium; Ca_i^{2+} = internal calcium; EP = phosphoenzyme.

of calcium from inside to outside the vesicle requiring a high internal calcium concentration.

Table 2 lists the major chemical constituents of sarcoplasmic reticulum. There are important lipid and protein components that have been characterized. The membranes are rich in phospholipids, which make up approximately 80% of the lipid extracted, and many different types of phospholipids have been identified. Neutral lipids, including cholesterol, may also play an important role in function of sarcoplasmic reticulum. Although many protein bands have been identified, four major bands are seen on SDS gels. The ATPase is a membrane protein with a molecular weight in the range of 100,000 daltons; it makes up the majority of the protein in skeletal muscle sarcoplasmic reticulum but constitutes 35 to 40% in cardiac muscle; the ATPase activity of this protein is observed only in the presence of phospholipids, such as lecithin. Another protein that is associated with the membrane is called proteolipid.

TABLE 2. *Chemical makeup of SR*

Lipids
   a. Phospholipids (80%)
   b. Neutral lipids—cholesterol

Proteins
   a. ATPase (100,000 daltons)[a]
      35–40% of cardiac SR protein (80% of skeletal); a membrane protein
   b. Proteolipid (MW 12,000)
      A membrane protein; role unknown
   c. Calsequestrin (MW 46,500–65,000)
      A luminal protein; role unknown
   d. High-affinity calcium-binding protein (MW 55,000)
      A luminal protein; role unknown

[a] Requires phospholipid to be active.

This has a molecular weight in the range of 12,000, but its role is unknown. There are two proteins that appear to bind calcium and that are found in the luminal portion of the sarcoplasmic reticulum. These are calsequestrin, which was originally thought to be important in controlling internal calcium concentration, but for which no role has been definitely established, and a high affinity calcium binding protein, which might also participate in control of the internal calcium concentration. Electrophoretic analysis of the protein composition of sarcoplasmic reticulum provides a way to monitor the purity of SR preparations and also to study changes that may occur in pathologic or physiologic states. Electrophoresis is also used to isolate the phosphorylated intermediate of the ATPase.

Table 3 lists some of the factors that appear to control calcium transport by the sarcoplasmic reticulum. The concentration of ATP may play a role by altering the K_m and V_{max} of the ATPase. External calcium stimulates transport through a concentration range of approximately 10^{-8} to 10^{-6} M, whereas internal calcium inhibits decompensation of the phosphoenzyme. Higher concentrations of Ca_o^{2+}, in the 10^{-4} M range, can promote calcium release (1); therefore, the balance of internal to external calcium can exert control on calcium uptake and calcium release. Certain ions and ATP influence the kinetics of the ATPase reaction. Potassium and ATP both appear to stimulate decomposition of the phosphoenzyme (3,4) and, as stated previously, magnesium also fosters decomposition. Dephosphorylation promotes more rapid turnover of the enzyme and presumably enhanced calcium transport. Magnesium has other effects in addition to accelerating phosphoenzyme decomposition. These include its requirement for the ATPase reaction and, at high concentrations, Mg^{2+} inhibits phosphoenzyme formation. Finally, phosphorylation of the sarcoplasmic reticulum, particularly through the cyclic AMP (cAMP) and protein kinase (PK) system, but perhaps also through other mechanisms, appears to exert control over sarcoplasmic reticulum function.

As indicated previously, phosphorylation reactions appear to be important in controlling sarcoplasmic reticulum function. Phosphorylation of the sarcoplasmic reticulum proteins has recently been reviewed by Katz (5) and by Barany and Barany (6). As shown in Table 4, in a series of articles (see refs.

TABLE 3. *Control of Ca^{2+} transport*

1. High ATP concentration ↑ K_m and V_{max} of ATPase
2. Ca_o^{2+} stimulates at above 10^{-8} M, at 10^{-6} max
   Ca_i^{2+} inhibits Mg^{2+}, stimulates EP decomposition
   Ca_o^{2+} and Ca_i^{2+} control uptake and release of Ca^{2+}
3. Kinetics of Pi release from ATPase can vary; K^+, Mg^{2+}, and ATP stimulate release
4. Magnesium effects
   a. accelerates EP decomposition
   b. required for optimal ATP action
   c. high concentration inhibits EP formation
5. Phosphorylation increases Ca^{2+} transport and ATPase activity

EP = phosphoenzyme.

TABLE 4. *Phosphorylation of SR*

cAMP-dependent phosphorylation

  1. Phosphorylation of phospholamban (22,000 daltons) by cAMP and PK
  2. Stimulates Ca^{2+} transport and Ca^{2+} ATPase activity
  3. Phospholamban phosphorylation increases rate of dephosphorylation of EP
  4. Kinase modulator inhibits cAMP–PK activity, Ca^{2+} uptake, and phosphorylation of phospholamban

cAMP-independent phosphorylation

  5. Phospholamban phosphorylation by calmodulin-dependent kinase at a phosphorylation site different from the cAMP–PK site is dependent upon Ca^{2+} concentration
  6. Phospholipid dependent-cyclic nucleotide independent phosphorylation

3 and 5 for review) Tada and Katz demonstrated that calcium transport and calcium ATPase activity were enhanced in the presence of cAMP and PK, and they showed further that this stimulation was associated with phosphorylation of a 22,000-dalton portion of the protein that they called phospholamban. Although the reaction occurred with exogenous PK, an endogenous PK also seemed to be present in SR. Phosphorylation of phospholamban resulted in increased phosphoenzyme intermediate formation. Subsequently, there was a phosphoprotein phosphatase found, which appears to be a PK modulator, inhibiting the stimulatory effect of cAMP-PK activity on phosphorylation of phospholamban and calcium uptake. Tada et al. (7) have presented evidence that the mechanism through which phospholamban phosphorylation works is by increasing the rate of dephosphorylation of phosphoenzyme. More recently, it has been demonstrated that phospholamban phosphorylation can be effected by a calmodulin-dependent kinase at a site that differs from the site of cyclic AMP-dependent protein kinase action (8,9). Unlike the cAMP-dependent phosphorylation, calmodulin kinase-dependent phosphorylation is governed by the calcium concentration. Finally, Limas (10) has demonstrated phosphorylation of the sarcoplasmic reticulum by a calcium-activated phospholipid-dependent PK.

The role of phosphorylation of phospholamban in physiologic control of heart function has not been firmly established, but it is obvious that it could have important influence on sarcoplasmic reticulum function. It is likely that the enhanced rate of myocardial relaxation observed with catecholamine stimulation works through this mechanism.

Cyclic GMP also appears to play a role in calcium movement across the sarcoplasmic reticulum membrane (11), but its role is less well elucidated than that of cAMP.

The process of calcium efflux from sarcoplasmic reticulum is also extremely important. This has been reviewed by Fabiato and Fabiato (12) and Endo (13). Reversal of the calcium pump with conversion of adenosine diphosphate (ADP) to ATP occurs when the internal calcium concentration is high and the external calcium concentration is lowered, for instance when EGTA is added to the bathing medium (3). What is probably of more relevance, however, is the calcium release that has been reported to be stimulated by high local concentrations of calcium externally and that is enhanced by protein kinase phosphorylation (14). Kirchberger and Wong (15) reasoned that this release was not the same as the pump reversal mentioned previously, since that reversal is inhibited by high external calcium concentration and by ATP. The release fostered by elevating calcium is postulated to be one mechanism by which the calcium entering the cell during the slow inward current of the action potential may trigger calcium egress from the sarcoplasmic reticulum. Calcium release has been studied in other ways, e.g., the report by Limas (16) that phosphotidate, a glycerol lipid intermediate, causes increased permeability of the sarcoplasmic reticulum to calcium, and inhibits calcium uptake and binding while it increases the ATPase activity and potentiates calcium release. This kind of alteration in calcium permeability of the sarcoplasmic reticulum might be a controlling factor in calcium release.

SARCOPLASMIC RETICULUM IN CARDIAC HYPERTROPHY

Page and McCallister (17) have shown that the area occupied by the sarcotubular membranes increases in proportion to the total cell volume in the presence of cardiac hypertrophy. It is possible that this biosynthesis of new membrane material might lead to altered membrane function.

Table 5 lists some of the reports on sarcoplasmic reticulum function in states of cardiac hypertrophy that have been produced by abnormal systolic or diastolic overload of the heart. Suko et al. (18) produced marked right ventricular hypertrophy and heart failure in the cat by pulmonary artery banding. This resulted in a significant depression in calcium uptake and calcium ATPase of sarcoplasmic reticulum from the right ventricle and also a tendency to lower values in left ventricular preparations. Sordahl et al. (19) studied rabbits with banding of the ascending aorta and found calcium binding of sarcoplasmic reticulum to be reduced in rabbits that had hypertrophy without cardiac failure; a further reduction was found in preparations from hearts with hypertrophy plus failure. Studying a less severe systolic overload, Lamers and Stinis (20) constricted the descending aorta of rabbits, causing significant left ventricular hypertrophy. They observed depressions in sarcoplasmic reticular calcium uptake and in the calcium uptake response to cAMP stimulation. Calcium ATPase activity was also found to be depressed in these studies. Limas and co-workers (21) have also studied sarcoplasmic reticular functions in preparations from rats with very mild left ventricular hypertrophy produced by abdominal aorta constriction. Their findings were unique in that increases in calcium uptake and calcium stimulated ATPase were observed; the phosphoenzyme intermediate was also found to be increased as was the rate of dephosphorylation. This is the first observation that in mild systolic overload the findings may not be the same as in severe and abrupt systolic overload.

TABLE 5. *Cardiac SR function in "pathologic" hypertrophy*

	Hypertrophy	Failure	Findings
A. Animal studies			
Calf: PA banding (18)	RV +(103%)	+	Ca uptake ↓18% ATPase ↓50% LV tended to be lower
Rabbit: Ascending	+	−	Ca binding ↓23%
Aortic banding (19)	+	+	Ca binding ↓30%
Rabbit: Descending aortic constriction, 1 month (20)	+59%		Ca^{2+} uptake ↓30% cAMP stimulation ↓26% Ca^{2+} ATPase ↓49%
Rat: abdominal aortic constriction (21)	+16–25%		Ca uptake ↑53% Ca^{2+} ATPase ↑31% ↑EP intermediate Kd ↑70% (rate of dephosphorylation)
Rat: Spontaneous hypertension (SHR) (22)	+		Ca uptake ↓35% Ca binding ↓34% Ca ATPase ↓27% cAMP phosphorylation ↓
Rabbit: AI			
2 weeks	+ mild	−	Ca uptake–NC
4–7 weeks	+ severe	−	Ca uptake ↓41%
4–7 weeks (23)	+	+	Ca uptake ↓56%
B. Human studies			
Human: ASHD with CHF (24,25)	?	+	Ca binding ↓
Human: MV disease and papillary muscle	+	+	Binding ↓56%; uptake ↓51% 50% less in LV with CHF than RV without CHF
Pulmonic stenosis, subvalvular muscle (26)	RV+	−	Ca ATPase ↓21% in both

Another kind of systolic overload that is found in spontaneous hypertensive rats was studied by Limas and Cohn (22). Significant reductions in several measures of sarcoplasmic reticular function were reported.

Diastolic overload has been studied less frequently, but Ito et al. (23) reported on rabbits in which aortic regurgitation had been created for varying periods of time. In animals with mild hypertrophy developing two weeks after creation of aortic regurgitation, no change was observed in calcium uptake of sarcoplasmic reticulum. In the animals with severe hypertrophy but no heart failure there was a 40% reduction of calcium uptake, whereas in those with hypertrophy the reduction was 66%.

Studies in tissues from humans have been limited, but Harigaya and Schwartz (24) and Lindenmayer et al. (25) studied hearts removed from patients at time of cardiac transplant. These patients mainly presented with atherosclerotic heart disease and congestive heart failure. The degree of hypertrophy in these hearts is unclear; the rates of calcium binding were depressed in comparison to preparations from rabbits and dogs. Lentz et al. (26) attempted to carry this study further in a more systematic fashion by analyzing preparations from the papillary muscles of patients with mitral valve disease, cardiac hypertrophy, and failure. Calcium binding and uptake were depressed in the sarcoplasmic reticular preparations. They further studied crista supraventricularis muscle from hearts of patients with pulmonic stenosis and right ventricular hypertrophy but no heart failure, and although calcium binding, uptake, and calcium ATPase were depressed, the depression was greater in patients with left ventricular failure than in those with right ventricular hypertrophy. Control studies in experimental animals had shown that sarcoplasmic reticulum binding and uptake was similar in the right and left ventricle of animals without hypertrophy.

Table 6 shows some studies of sarcoplasmic reticulum function from hearts of a different type of hypertrophy: that observed in the cardiomyopathic hamster. McCollum and colleagues (27) found that before hypertrophy developed calcium binding and uptake by sarcoplasmic reticulum were not abnormal, but that as heart failure developed, marked deficiencies were observed. Gertz et al. (28) demonstrated reductions in sarcoplasmic reticular calcium binding during the hypertrophic stage in these animals when failure was absent, but this became exaggerated when heart failure became manifest. In this study, like those in systolic overload and diastolic overload, it appears that an abnormality in the sarcoplasmic reticulum appears before the onset of congestive heart failure.

Hyperthyroidism, as opposed to severe systolic or diastolic overload or cardiomyopathy, is considered to be a form of "physiologic hypertrophy." Table 7 lists some of the studies on cardiac sarcoplasmic reticular function from animals subjected to various thyroid states. Suko (29) created hyperthyroidism in rabbits for several weeks and found increased sarcoplasmic reticulum calcium uptake and ATPase activity; these measurements were depressed when hypothyroidism was created. Nayler et al. (30) did a similar study in dogs and

TABLE 6. *Cardiac SR function and the myopathic hamster*

Ref.	No. of days	Hypertrophy	Findings
28	200	no CHF	Ca binding ↓23%
	320	no CHF	↓32%
	300	CHF	↓77%
27	60	no H	Ca binding NC
			Ca uptake NC
	216	+45% H and CHF	Ca binding ↓29%
			Ca uptake ↓22%
	262	+53% H and CHF	Ca binding ↓25%
			Ca uptake ↓19%

TABLE 7. *Cardiac SR function in abnormal thyroid states[a]*

(Ref.) study	Hypertrophy	Findings
(29) Rabbit: Thyroxine 25–100 µg/kg 3–4 weeks I[131] 4–5 mos	Not measured	Ca uptake ↑21% Ca ATPase ↑28% Ca uptake ↓38% Ca ATPase ↓44%
(30) Dog: 1 µg/kg 10 days		Ca binding ↑74% Ca uptake ↑60% Ca exchangeability +45% Total ATPase ↓ Ca ATPase NC
(31,32) Rat: Thyroxine 1 mg/kg 2× weeks	+26–37%	Ca uptake ↑39% ATPase ↑42% EP formation ↑ PL content ↑ cAMP effect ↑ Possible ↑ endogenous PK activity
(33) Dog: Dessicated thyroid 1 g/kg 55–177 days	+39% RV +15% LV	Ca content ↓48% Ca uptake ↓38%

[a] PL = phospholipid.

examined the animals after 10 days of treatment. They similarly found increases in sarcoplasmic reticulum calcium binding and uptake, but observed a decrease in the total ATPase and no change in the calcium ATPase activity. In two studies, Limas (31,32) treated rats with thyroxine for 2 weeks, and he reported an increased calcium uptake, ATPase activity, and phosphoenzyme formation even in the presence of hypertrophy. Limas also found an increase in phospholipid content of the sarcoplasmic reticulum and enhanced responsiveness of the cAMP dependent reaction. He postulated that hyperthyroidism was associated with increased endogenous protein kinase activity. Limas' studies demonstrate that increased sarcoplasmic reticulum function can coexist in the presence of thyroxine-induced cardiac hypertrophy. Conway et al. (33), on the other hand, produced cardiac hypertrophy by administering a large dose of dessicated thyroid to dogs for a longer period of time. In this study, calcium content of the sarcoplasmic reticulum was depressed, as was calcium uptake. Thus, the direct effect of thyroid hormone may be to increase function of sarcoplasmic reticulum, and this can exist with thyroid induced hypertrophy. But perhaps the duration and severity of the hypertrophic stimulus even in hyperthyroidism may govern whether SR function increases or decreases.

Another type of physiologic overload is that induced by physical training. Penpargkul and co-workers (34–36), in a series of papers from 1977 through 1981, have reported on cardiac sarcoplasmic reticulum function in preparation from hearts of rats chronically trained by swimming or running. Male swimmers and runners did not develop cardiac hypertrophy, but male swimmers demonstrated significant increases in calcium binding and uptake of sarcoplasmic reticulum; male runners developed lesser increases. Female swimmers developed significant cardiac hypertrophy and increased contractile performance, and preparations from their hearts demonstrate enhanced calcium binding and uptake but no change in calcium ATPase activity. Enhanced sarcoplasmic reticular function was associated with increased rates of ventricular relaxation. On the other hand, Sordahl et al. (37) found no change in sarcoplasmic reticulum extracted from hearts of dogs conditioned by running, but there was no hypertrophy in those animals.

In all of the above studies it is difficult to compare absolute values or percent changes in sarcoplasmic reticulum function reported from different laboratories because of variations in the way some of the assays are performed. For instance, certain groups use different temperatures and different substrate systems; some groups use ATP regenerating systems and others do not; some studies are performed with different ionic compositions and at different temperatures.

Although conclusions must be tentative from the studies that have been reviewed, one possible unifying thread may be that a mild or gradual onset of overload, such as observed in Limas' study with constricting the abdominal aorta of rats (21), in the hyperthyroid studies of several of the groups, and in the studies of physical training may cause sarcoplasmic reticulum function to be either normal or increased. On the other hand, in those states where the load is imposed abruptly, where it is severe and perhaps prolonged, hypertrophy is accompanied by depressed sarcoplasmic reticulum function. This is observed in most of the studies where there is systolic overload of the heart, and in the study in which hyperthyroidism was produced by administering a large dose of dessicated thyroid for a prolonged period of time (33). This possible conclusion is similar to that one can make from closely examining studies of actomyosin and myosin ATPase activity in various types of cardiac stress, where the ATPase activity tends to be increased in hyperthyroidism, physical training, and mild systolic overload, but is depressed when systolic or diastolic

TABLE 8. *Cardiac SR function with physical training*

(Ref.) study	Hypertrophy	Findings
(36) Rat: male swimmers	—	Ca binding ↑27% Ca uptake ↑33%
(35) Rat: male runners	—	Ca binding ↑10–20% Ca uptake NS
(34) Rat: female swimmers	+24%	Ca binding ↑17% Ca uptake ↑30% Ca ATPase NS
(37) Dog: running	—	Ca uptake NS

overload of a severe nature are imposed abruptly or for long periods of time (38,39).

PITFALLS IN STUDIES OF SARCOPLASMIC RETICULUM

Although the studies mentioned in the previous section appeared to be quite consistent, there are certain methodologic problems that should be mentioned.

Many of the workers studying preparations from rat heart may have performed the analyses under substrate limiting conditions. The total ATPase activity of rat heart is extremely high (40). Yet most of the studies in rat heart preparations have been performed without employing ATP regenerating systems. Penpargkul (41) emphasized the importance of using ATP regenerating systems when studying rat heart sarcoplasmic reticulum, finding that when 7 mM phosphoenolpyruvate was included in the incubation medium, the ATP concentration remained constant throughout the incubation period, whereas in the absence of phosphoenolpyruvate ATP concentrations fell remarkably. There was a reciprocal relationship between the amount of phosphoenolpyruvate present and calcium binding of sarcoplasmic reticulum. It is possible that studies under the substrate limiting conditions might minimize differences in calcium binding and uptake by sarcoplasmic reticulum and in some cases lead to false negative results.

A major problem in studies which compare extracts of different types of hearts relates to the impurities that may be found in sarcoplasmic reticulum. In a series of articles, Besch et al. explored the issue of the purity of the preparation (42,43). They have demonstrated that there is a marked contamination with sarcolemmal membranes in usual preparations of sarcoplasmic reticulum.

These kinds of careful analyses have not always been employed to compare preparations from experimental hearts and to determine the amount of contamination by other membrane systems.

Jones et al. (43) have developed new methods for isolating purer preparations of sarcolemma and sarcoplasmic reticulum. These very pure types of membrane preparations have not been employed in studies comparing vesicles from hearts in one physiologic or pathologic state to preparations from hearts of control animals.

SUMMARY

Sarcoplasmic reticular vesicles are made up of combinations of various proteins and lipids. Calcium binding and uptake are controlled by calcium concentration outside and inside the vesicle, ATP availability, the ATPase protein activity, and the concentrations of a variety of ions. The phosphorylation of the membrane protein by cAMP-dependent protein kinase and other protein kinases also appears to govern the rate of calcium movements.

In this chapter, a series of papers have been reviewed in which sarcoplasmic reticular function of a variety of models of cardiac hypertrophy have been examined. In general, with severe systolic and diastolic overload and myocardiopathy a depression in sarcoplasmic reticular function has been found. In very mild hypertrophy, sarcoplasmic reticular function may be enhanced, particularly in physiologic hypertrophy due to hyperthyroidism or physical training, but also in hypertrophy due to very mild systolic overload. It has been suggested that the function of the sarcoplasmic reticulum may be enhanced in mild hypertrophy of gradual onset and may be depressed in hypertrophy due to abrupt or prolonged imposition of a hemodynamic load.

The role of sarcoplasmic reticular dysfunction causing myocardial failure remains uncertain; a cause and effect relationship has not been established, and also reversibility of sarcoplasmic reticular abnormalities has not been explored.

Finally, methodologic problems have been mentioned. Some studies of sarcoplasmic reticulum function have been conducted under substrate limited conditions. It is clear that most of the comparative studies between control hearts and hearts subjected to various modes of overload have not paid rigorous attention to this problem of sarcolemmal contamination.

Nevertheless, the principles elucidated by the studies of hypertrophy are probably correct, but studies of sarcoplasmic reticulum must be expanded to investigate purer preparations, to define alterations in biochemical makeup of the vesicles, and to explore the factors that control sarcoplasmic reticular function in greater depth.

ACKNOWLEDGMENTS

Related work was supported by U. S. Public Health Service Grants HL 15498 and HL 21482. I wish to thank Ms. Janet Holwell for typing the manuscript, and Ms. Carol Gundlach for the editorial assistance.

REFERENCES

1. Fabiato, A., and Fabiato, F. (1979): *Ann. Rev. Physiol.*, 41:473–484.
2. MacLennan, D. H., and Holland, P. C. (1975): *Ann. Rev. Biophys. Bioeng.*, 4:377–404.
3. Tada, M., Yamamoto, T., and Tonomura, T. (1978): *Physiol. Rev.*, 58:1–79.
4. Jones, L. R., Besch, H. R., Jr., and Watanabe, A. M. (1978): *J. Biol. Chem.*, 263:1643–1653.
5. Katz, A. M. (1979): In: *Advances in Cyclic Nucleotide Research, Vol. 11,* edited by P. Greengard and G. A. Robinson, pp. 304–343. Raven Press, New York.
6. Barany, M., and Barany, K. (1981): *Am. J. Physiol.*, 241:H117–H128.
7. Tada, M., Ohmori, F., Yamada, M., and Abe, H. (1979): *J. Biol. Chem.*, 254:319–326.
8. LePeuch, C. J., Haiech, J., and Demaille, J. G. (1979): *Biochemistry*, 18:5150–5157.
9. Lopaschuk, G., Richter, B., and Katz, S. (1980): *Biochemistry*, 19:5603–5607.
10. Limas, C. J. (1980): *Biochem. Biophys. Res. Comm.*, 96:1378–1383.
11. Weller, M., and Laing, W. (1979): *Biochim. Biophys. Acta*, 555:406–419.
12. Fabiato, A., and Fabiato, F. (1977): *Circ. Res.*, 40:119–129.
13. Endo, M. (1977): *Physiol. Rev.*, 57:71–108.

14. Kirchberger, M. A., and Wong, D. (1978): *J. Biol. Chem.*, 253:6941–6945.
15. Kirchberger, M. A., and Wong, D. (1980): *Adv. Myocardial.*, 1:179–187.
16. Limas, C. J. (1980): *Biochem. Biophys. Res. Comm.*, 95:541–546.
17. Page, E., and McCallister, L. P. (1973): *Am. J. Cardiol.*, 31:172–181.
18. Suko, J., Vogel, J. H. K., and Chidsey, C. A. (1970): *Circ. Res.*, 27:235–247.
19. Sordahl, L. A., McCollum, W. B., Wood, W. G., and Schwartz, A. (1973): *Am. J. Physiol.*, 224:497–502.
20. Lamers, J. M. J., and Stinis, J. T. (1979): *Life Sci.*, 24:2313–2320.
21. Limas, C. J., Spier, S. S., and Kahlon, J. (1980): *J. Mol. Cell. Cardiol.*, 12:1103–1116.
22. Limas, C. J., and Cohn, J. N. (1977): *Circ. Res.*, 40:I62–I69.
23. Ito, Y., Sulo, J., and Chidsey, C. A. (1974): *J. Mol. Cell. Cardiol.*, 6:237–247.
24. Harigaya, S., and Schwartz, A. (1969): *Circ. Res.*, 25:781–794.
25. Lindenmayer, G. E., Sordahl, L. P., Harigaya, S., Allen, J. C., Besch, H. R., Jr., and Schwartz, A. (1971): *Am. J. Cardiol.*, 27:277–283.
26. Lentz, R. W., Harrison, C. E., Jr., Dewey, J. D., Barnhorst, D. A., Danielson, G. K., and Pluth, J. R. (1978): *J. Mol. Cell. Cardiol.*, 10:3–30.
27. McCollum, W. B., Crow, C., Harigaya, S., Bajusz, E., and Schwartz, A. (1970): *J. Mol. Cell. Cardiol.*, 1:445–457.
28. Gertz, E. W., Stam, A. C., Jr., and Sonnenblick, E. H. (1970): *Biochem. Biophys. Res. Comm.*, 40:746–753.
29. Suko, J. (1971): *Biochim. Biophys. Acta*, 252:324–327.
30. Nayler, W. G., Merrillees, N. C. R., Chipperfield, D., and Kurtz, J. B. (1971): *Cardiovasc. Res.*, 5:469–482.
31. Limas, C. J. (1978): *Am. J. Physiol.*, 235:H745–H751.
32. Limas, C. J. (1978): *Am. J. Physiol.*, 234:H426–H431.
33. Conway, G., Heazlitt, R. A., Fowler, N. O., Gabel, M., and Green, S. (1976): *J. Mol. Cell. Cardiol.*, 8:39–51.
34. Malhotra, A., Penpargkul, S., Schaible, T., and Scheuer, J. (1981): *Am. J. Physiol.*, 241:H263–H267.
35. Penpargkul, S., Malhotra, A., Schaible, T., and Scheuer, J. (1980): *J. Appl. Physiol.*, 48:409–413.
36. Penpargkul, S., Repke, D. I., Katz, A. M., and Scheuer, J. (1977): *Circ. Res.*, 40:134–138.
37. Sordahl, L. A., Asimakis, G. K., Dowell, R. T., and Stone, H. L. (1977): *J. Appl. Physiol.*, 42:426–431.
38. Scheuer, J., and Bhan, A. (1979): *Circ. Res.*, 45:1–12.
39. Wikman-Coffelt, J., Parmley, W. W., and Mason, D. T. (1979): *Circ. Res.*, 45:697–707.
40. Nayler, W. G., Dunnett, J., and Berry, D. (1975): *J. Mol. Cell. Cardiol.*, 7:275–288.
41. Penpargkul, S. (1979): *Cardiovasc. Res.*, 13:243–253.
42. Besch, H. R., Jr., and Jones, L. R. (1980): *Adv. Myocardiol.*, 1:123–138.
43. Jones, L. R., Besch, H. R., Jr., Fleming, J. W., McConnaughey, M. M., and Watanabe, A. M. (1979): *J. Biol. Chem.*, 254:530–539.

Perspectives in Cardiovascular
Research, Vol. 8,
edited by R. C. Tarazi and J. B. Dunbar.
Raven Press, New York © 1983.

Model Dependence of Contractile and Energetic Function of Hypertrophied Myocardium

George Cooper, IV

*Departments of Medicine and Physiology, Temple University School of Medicine,
Philadelphia, Pennsylvania 19140*

The response of the organism to hemodynamic overloading includes a variety of compensatory adaptations, the most obvious and basic of which is myocardial hypertrophy. The appearance of congestive heart failure after a period of functional compensation for a fixed hemodynamic overload implies a loss of one or more of these adaptive responses. Hypertrophy contributes to compensation of ventricular pump function by increasing the number of contractile elements, albeit at the cost of enhanced myocardial energy utilization. Hypertrophy, then, while allowing functional compensation of the stressed ventricle as a whole, is necessarily associated with basic changes in myocardial structure and energetics. It is possible that, at a time when the increased myocardial mass permits normal pump function, particularly in the resting organism, abnormalities of the contractile or energetic behavior of each unit of this tissue might appear, initially masked by the increased muscle mass and other adaptive responses to the hemodynamic overload. However, if either or both of these possible abnormalities were progressive, pump decompensation and the congestive heart failure state would be expected to ensue. In this sense, the quantitative adaptation of increased cardiac mass would eventually become maladaptive on the basis of the associated qualitative, functional changes.

The study of tissue removed from non-failing ventricles, in terms of intrinsic contractile and energetic properties per unit mass of hypertrophied myocardium, should allow the detection of relatively early changes that might have etiological significance for the later appearance of congestive heart failure. The data presented in this chapter will be confined to such studies of hemodynamic overloads of the right ventricle. In order to limit the scope of this material, only hemodynamic causes of hypertrophy have been selected. The right ventricle is discussed because of simplicity of experimental design and interpretation: For this chamber, it is possible to alter the myocardial loading conditions without a concomitant alteration in the hemodynamics of the perfusing vascular supply. Data presented are from studies of three distinct models of hemodynamic overloads of the cat right ventricle. Because all of these data were gathered from the same species in the same laboratory using identical techniques, the major variable responsible for any differing experimental results in these three models should be the nature of the hemodynamic overload. Data on the *in vivo* pump level are included to document that each model produced hypertrophy without associated congestive heart failure. Data on the *in vitro* muscle level will be presented more fully to characterize the intrinsic contractile and energetic properties of the myocardium apart from neurohumoral support mechanisms available in the intact animal.

METHODS

Experimental Models

The right ventricle of the cat was used to produce hypertrophy in response to a hemodynamic overload in each case (1–5). This is the only species that I have found both to tolerate extensive operative procedures and to provide a right ventricular papillary muscle of a size suitable for prolonged support by superfusion in the majority of the animals.

Volume Overload

A substantial volume overload of the right ventricle was produced surgically by resecting the atrial septum. For this procedure, the cats were anesthetized with sodium pentobarbital (25 mg/kg, i.p.), intubated, and placed on a respirator. Following a right thoracotomy, the azygos vein was ligated, and during inflow occlusion of the venae cavae, a large atrial septal defect was created through a right atriotomy. The atriotomy was then repaired, the lungs expanded, and the chest closed. A control group of adult cats had a sham operation consisting of a thoractomy and pericardiotomy.

Acute Reversible Pressure Overload

A major pressure overload of the right ventricle was produced by placing a biologically inert band around the proximal pulmonary artery; this band could be removed at a second operation to reverse the pressure overload. For either procedure, the cats were anesthetized with sodium pentobarbital (25 mg/kg, i.p.), intubated, and placed on a respirator. A left posterior thoracotomy was made in the fourth intercostal space, and the base of the aorta and the pulmonary artery were separated. The band, with an internal diameter of 3.5 mm when closed, was placed around the pulmonary artery, and its ends were apposed. The lungs were then expanded, and the chest was closed. The control group of adult cats was sham-operated. Pressure-overload reversal consisted of a similar operation in which the band was removed.

Chronic Progressive Pressure Overload

A pressure overload of similar eventual degree to that in the previous acute group, but of gradual onset, was produced by placing the same band on the proximal pulmonary artery of 7- to 8-week-old kittens. Small solid-state pressure transducers chronically implanted in the right ventricle showed that right ventricular pressure was normal initially and reached a stable, elevated level at 16 weeks after operation. The sham operation for another group of kittens consisted of pericardiotomy and dissection of the pulmonary artery from the base of the aorta.

Experimental Measurements

The techniques used for these measurements were similar for each of the three hemodynamic models employed; they are described in detail in the original reports (1–5). Each experimental model was assessed as follows: (a) hemodynamically, in terms of the type and the extent of the stimulus to hypertrophy and the pump function of the intact heart; (b) morphologically, in terms of the degree of ventricular and cellular hypertrophy; (c) mechanically, in terms of the contractile function of isolated right ventricular papillary muscles; and (d) energetically, in terms of the oxygen consumption of the isolated hypertrophied myocardium.

Hemodynamics

In the volume-overload model, cardiac catherization was performed in anesthetized cats to measure the left-to-right shunt by dye dilution techniques. Cardiac output and right ventricular and venous pressures were also measured at this time. In the acute pressure-overload and reversal models, the cardiac output and pressure were measured in the same way. In the chronic progressive pressure-overload model, these hemodynamic measurements in the anesthetized animal were supplemented by measuring the radioistopically determined right ventricular ejection fraction in the lightly sedated cat.

Morphology

The extent of right ventricular hypertrophy was quantitated in each model as the ratio of the weight of the right ventricular free wall to the weight of the cat. The extent of cellular hypertrophy and the participation of the papillary muscle in overall ventricular hypertrophy were quantitated as myocyte cross-sectional area in each tissue specimen.

Mechanics

Papillary muscles were studied in the flow respirometer shown in Fig. 1 and described in its legend. The measurements consisted of the force-velocity and

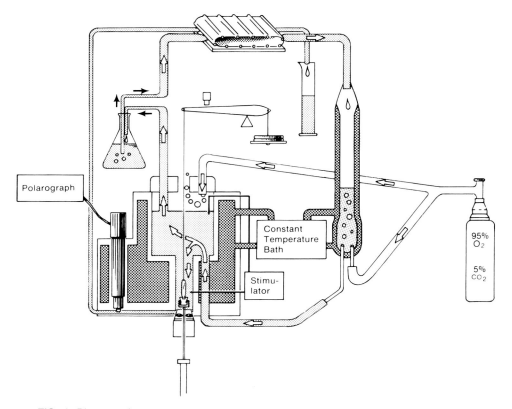

FIG. 1. Diagram of the polarographic myograph used for the simultaneous determination of myocardial contractile and energetic function. The superfusate is passed by a proportioning pump from a 1-liter Erlenmeyer flask to the column to the right of the myograph. There it is equilibrated with 95% O_2 and 5% CO_2 and brought to the desired temperature. From there, it passes by gravity to a chamber above the muscle in which back-diffusion is prevented by a second gas line. Most of the superfusate is recirculated to the flask, but a smaller quantity is drawn past the muscle and then past an oxygen cathode attached to a polarograph. The muscle is shown affixed to a rigid clip on the bottom, which in turn passes through a mercury seal and is affixed to an isotonic lever. Oxygen consumption is determined from the flow rate of the superfusate past the cathode, the solubility of oxygen at that temperature, and a calibration curve of pO_2 versus cathode current.

length-tension relationships for each muscle. All results were normalized to muscle dimensions to facilitate comparisons.

Energetics

The energetics of the quiescent and contracting papillary muscles were measured as myocardial oxygen consumption (MVO_2) at the same time that the force-velocity and length-tension relationships were being defined, as described in the legend of Fig. 1. In the volume overload and acute pressure-overload and reversal models, subcellular energetics were determined as indexes of oxidative phosphorylation of mitochondria isolated from the same right ventricles from which the papillary muscles were removed.

RESULTS

Volume Overload

Hemodynamics

These animals and the sham-operated controls were studied at two times after the atrial septal resection: 4 to 8 weeks and 15 to 16 weeks. The right ventricular systolic pressure had increased in the long-term group, when compared to control, from 23 ± 2 mm Hg to 31 ± 1 mm Hg, whereas in the earlier group, this value did not differ from that of the control group. The results were otherwise identical for the short-term and long-term groups in each of the other aspects of this study and will be reported together.

The atrial septal defect produced a major volume-overload of the right ventricle. The ratio of pulmonary blood flow to systemic blood flow increased from 1.04 ± 0.01 in the controls, to 3.30 ± 0.28 in the cats with atrial septal defects.

There was no evidence of congestive heart failure in these cats: Cardiac output and venous and right ventricular end diastolic pressures did not differ from control, the ratio of liver weight to body weight was not increased, and neither ascites nor plural effusion were found in any cat at the time of study.

Morphology

Selective hypertrophy of the right ventricle was demonstrated by an increase in the ratio of right ventricular weight to body weight from 0.59 ± 0.03 g/kg to 0.97 ± 0.03 g/kg in the volume-overloaded cats, while the ratio of left ventricular weight to body weight did not vary from control. Cellular hypertrophy was shown by a 125% increase in right ventricular myocyte cross-sectional area in the hypertrophied ventricles; the extent of cellular hypertrophy was the same in the papillary muscles and the right ventricular free wall.

Mechanics

Contractile performance during isotonic contractions is shown in the upper panel of Fig. 2. The top panel shows that the velocity of shortening at each load was the same for the control and hypertrophied muscles. The middle panel shows that the extent of shortening at each load was the same for the two groups. External work and the maximum isotonic load were also the same for the two groups.

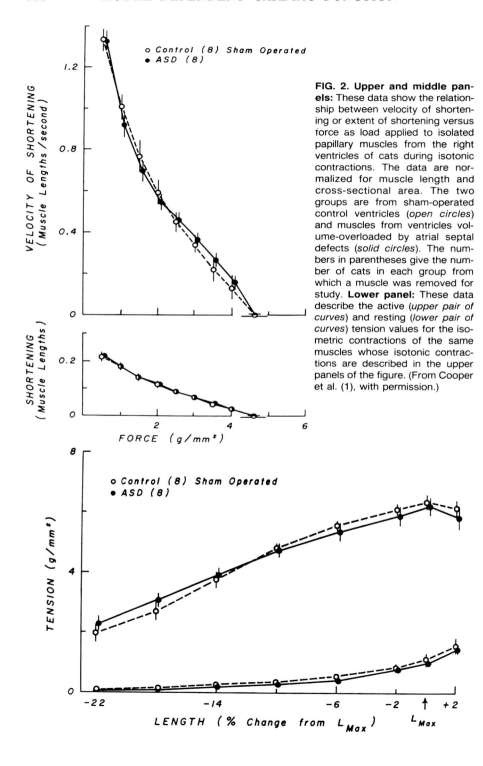

FIG. 2. **Upper and middle panels:** These data show the relationship between velocity of shortening or extent of shortening versus force as load applied to isolated papillary muscles from the right ventricles of cats during isotonic contractions. The data are normalized for muscle length and cross-sectional area. The two groups are from sham-operated control ventricles (*open circles*) and muscles from ventricles volume-overloaded by atrial septal defects (*solid circles*). The numbers in parentheses give the number of cats in each group from which a muscle was removed for study. **Lower panel:** These data describe the active (*upper pair of curves*) and resting (*lower pair of curves*) tension values for the isometric contractions of the same muscles whose isotonic contractions are described in the upper panels of the figure. (From Cooper et al. (1), with permission.)

Isometric contractile performance for the two groups is shown in the bottom panel of Fig. 2. Neither active tension, the upper pair of curves, nor resting tension, the lower pair of curves, differed in the volume overloaded (ASD) and control muscles. Other contractile indexes at L_{max}, that isometric muscle length at which developed tension is greatest, were also the same in the two groups. The maximum rate of tension development was 344 ± 20 mN/mm^2/sec control and 309 ± 23 mN/mm^2/sec for ASD; time to peak tension was 317 ± 6 msec control and 320 ± 11 msec for the ASD group.

Energetics

The oxygen consumption of the quiescent papillary muscles was the same in the two groups: 2.55 ± 0.26 μL/mg/hr control and 2.57 ± 0.15 μL/mg/hr ASD. The oxygen consumption for the contractions defining the force-velocity and force-shortening relationships of Fig. 2 are shown in the upper panel of Fig. 3: MVO$_2$ did not differ in the two groups over the entire range of loads examined.

The oxygen consumption for the control and volume-overload muscles at each of the points used to define the isometric active length-tension relationship of Fig. 2 is shown in the bottom panel of Fig. 3. There was no significant difference in either the slopes or the intercepts of the ordinate for these two sets of linear regression data.

The respiration of mitochondria isolated from the same right ventricles from which the papillary muscles had been removed was entirely comparable in the two groups. Mitochondrial oxygen consumption during adenosine diphosphate (ADP) phosphorylation was 236 ± 38 n atoms/mg/min control and 273 ± 39 n atoms/mg/min for ASD; the rate of mitochondrial oxygen consumption after ADP phosphorylation was complete was 15.8 ± 2.1 n atoms/mg/min control and 19.1 ± 2.2 n atoms/mg/min for ASD.

Acute Reversible Pressure Overload

Hemodynamics

These animals were studied at three times: The first group was studied with the pulmonary artery band in place, 4 to 6 weeks after the banding procedure; the second group was studied following pressure-overload reversal, 4 to 6 weeks after the unbanding procedure; the third group was studied 5 to 7 weeks after reversal of a more prolonged, 15 to 16 week, period of pressure overload. All data for the last two groups were similar and will be reported together as the unbanded group.

The pulmonary artery band produced a significant pressure overload of the right ventricle. The right ventricular systolic pressure increased from a control value of 23 ± 2 mm Hg to 58 ± 2 mm Hg in the banded group; unbanding immediately returned the right ventricular systolic pressure to normal, and this normal pressure was maintained at the time of subsequent study.

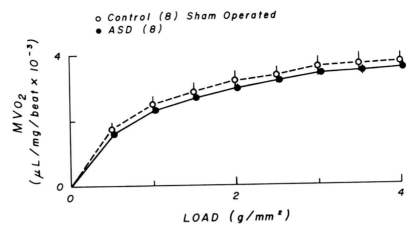

FIG. 3. Upper panel: Isotonic oxygen consumption data for the same muscles whose isotonic contractile performance is shown in Fig. 2. The MVO_2 values are shown for the same loads used in the force-velocity and force-shortening diagrams.

Neither the banded nor the unbanded groups showed evidence of congestive heart failure: Cardiac output and venous and right ventricular end diastolic pressures did not differ from control, the ratio of liver weight to body weight was not increased, and neither ascites nor pleural effusion were found in any cat at the time of study.

Morphology

Selective hypertrophy of the right ventricle was shown by an increase for the banded group in the ratio of right ventricular weight to body weight from 0.58 ± 0.03 g/kg control to 1.05 ± 0.06 g/kg in the banded group; the ratio of left ventricular weight to body weight did not vary from control. The unbanded group showed a return of right ventricular mass to normal at 0.56 ± 0.02 g/kg.

Cellular hypertrophy in the banded group was shown by a 135% increase in right ventricular myocyte cross-sectional area in the hypertrophied ventricles; this returned to the control value after unbanding. Changes in papillary muscle myocyte size paralleled those in the right ventricular free wall in each case.

Mechanics

Contractile performance during isotonic contractions for the control and experimental groups is shown in the upper panel of Fig. 4. The entire force-velocity and force-shortening relationships for the banded group were depressed, with decreases in both velocity and extent of shortening at all loads.

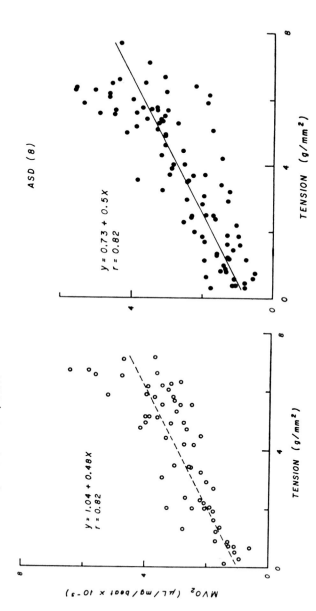

FIG. 3. *(Cont'd).* **Lower panels:** Each of these panels defines the relationship between isometric active tension and myocardial oxygen consumption during the contractions used to produce the length-tension diagrams in Fig. 2. The **left panel** gives the data for the control group, and the **right panel** for the volume-overloaded group. (From Cooper et al. (1), with permission.)

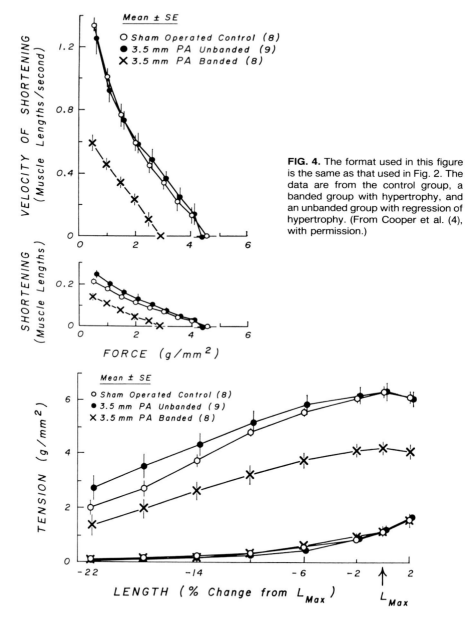

FIG. 4. The format used in this figure is the same as that used in Fig. 2. The data are from the control group, a banded group with hypertrophy, and an unbanded group with regression of hypertrophy. (From Cooper et al. (4), with permission.)

Thus, external work and the maximum isotonic load were also depressed for the banded group. For the unbanded group, each of these isotonic contractile defects returned to the control level with hypertrophy reversal.

Isometric contractile performance for these groups is shown in the bottom panel of Fig. 4. While the lower triad of curves shows that resting tension was the same in each group at all muscle lengths, the upper set of curves shows that there was a depression in developed tension in the muscles from the banded cats that was reversed with band removal. The maximum rate of tension generation at L_{max} was reduced from 344 ± 20 mN/mm²/sec control to 147 ± 13 mN/mm²/sec in the banded group and returned to 322 ± 9 mN/mm²/sec in the unbanded group. Time to peak tension at L_{max} increased from 317 ± 6 msec control to 411 ± 18 msec in the banded group and returned to 313 ± 5 msec in the unbanded group.

Energetics

The oxygen consumption of the quiescent papillary muscles was increased from the control value of 2.55 ± 0.26 μL/mg/hr to 3.40 ± 0.15 μL/mg/hr for the banded group and returned to 2.70 ± 0.09 μL/mg/hr for the unbanded group. The oxygen consumption for the contractions used to obtain the isotonic data in Fig. 4 is shown in the upper panel of Fig. 5. Despite the marked reduction in contractile state found for the pressure hypertrophied muscles, the MVO_2 was slightly increased rather than reduced when compared to the control group. The isotonic oxygen consumption of the muscles from unbanded cats was entirely normal.

The oxygen consumption for each group during isometric contractions is summarized in the bottom panel of Fig. 5. For the banded group, as reflected in the slope of its linear regression line, there was a marked increase when compared to control in the oxygen cost of tension development, despite its reduced contractile state. For the unbanded group, this relationship had returned to normal.

The respiration of mitochondria isolated from the right ventricles of the banded cats showed an abnormality of nonphosphorylating respiration which is illustrated in Fig. 6. The left columns of this figure show that the initial rate of nonphosphorylating respiration, measured after ADP phosphorylation was complete, was increased in the mitochondria isolated from the pressure-hypertrophied right ventricles; no other aspect of mitochondrial metabolism was found to be abnormal. When oligomycin was added to block oxidative phosphorylation, the abnormal respiration persisted; when ruthenium red, an inhibitor of energy-dependent mitochondrial calcium uptake, was added to the medium, the abnormality was abolished. It was further found that the extent of the increase in whole muscle respiration paralleled that of the increase in mitochondrial nonphosphorylating respiration in the same right ventricles. I concluded that both defects might be based on disordered sarcoplasmic reticulum calcium kinetics, with abnormal contractile behavior and enhanced whole muscle and mitochondrial respiration resulting from a diminished ability of the sarcoplasmic reticulum to accumulate ionized calcium. No abnormality of mitochondrial respiration was found in the unbanded, hypertrophy reversal right ventricles.

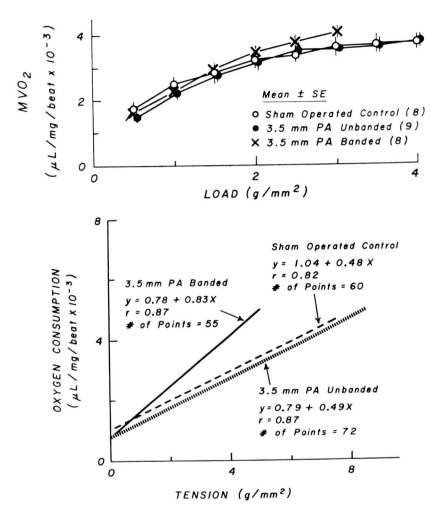

FIG. 5. Upper panel: The format used for this figure is the same as that used in Fig. 3. The data are from the control group, a banded group with hypertrophy, and an unbanded group with regression of hypertrophy. These are the isotonic oxygen consumption data accompanying the isotonic contractile data shown in Fig. 4. **Lower panel:** These data summarize the relationship between isometric active tension development and myocardial oxygen consumption for the same contractions characterized in Fig. 4. The format is the same as that used in Fig. 3. (From Cooper et al. (4), with permission.)

Chronic Progressive Pressure Overload

Hemodynamics

These animals and their respective sham-operated control groups were studied at two times: Group I was studied 25 weeks after banding, which was

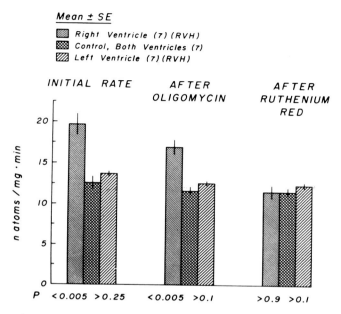

FIG. 6. These data describe the nonphosphorylating respiration of mitochondria isolated from control cats and the banded group with the band in place. **Left,** the rate of oxygen uptake in the absence of ADP; **middle,** the rate after the addition of enough oligomycin to block ADP phosphorylation; **right,** the rate after the addition of enough ruthenium red to block calcium uptake. (Mean ± SE.) (From Cooper et al. (2), with permission.)

approximately 10 weeks after the pressure overload had become maximal; group II was studied 60 weeks after banding, which was approximately 45 weeks after the pressure overload had become maximal.

The pulmonary artery band produced a pressure overload of the right ventricle that was comparable in the two experimental groups. The right ventricular systolic pressure increased from a mean control value of 25 ± 2 mm Hg to 51 ± 4 mm Hg for group I and 50 ± 1 mm Hg for group II.

No group showed evidence of abnormal ventricular pump function or of congestive heart failure. Cardiac output was identical at 0.18 L/kg/min for each control and experimental group; the right ventricular ejection fraction was the same in each group; venous and right ventricular end diastolic pressures were the same in each group; the ratio of liver weight to body weight was not increased; and neither ascites nor pleural effusion were found in any animal at the time of study.

Morphology

Selective hypertrophy of the right ventricle was shown by an increase in the ratio of right ventricular weight to body weight from 0.54 ± 0.03 g/kg to

0.82 ± 0.04 g/kg for group I, and from 0.50 ± 0.03 g/kg to 0.72 ± 0.03 g/kg for group II. The ratio of left ventricular weight to body weight did not differ from control in either group.

Cellular hypertrophy in both groups was shown by an increase in right ventricular free wall myocyte cross-sectional area from 186 ± 8 μm^2 for control to 267 ± 18 μm^2 for the banded cats; for the right ventricular papillary muscle, this increase was from 182 ± 6 μm^2 to 266 ± 11 μm^2. Mean diastolic sarcomere length did not differ from control with hypertrophy. Of note, only myocyte hypertrophy rather than hyperplasia was found by autoradiography in the hypertrophying myocardium, although progressive connective tissue proliferation was suggested by an increase in hydroxyproline content in group I from 3.48 ± 0.36 $\mu g/mg$ to 5.09 ± 0.14 $\mu g/mg$, and in group II from 3.35 ± 0.40 $\mu g/mg$ to 6.02 ± 0.69 $\mu g/mg$ of myocardium.

Mechanics

Contractile performance during isotonic contractions for each control and experimental group is shown in Fig. 7. The entire force-velocity and force-shortening relationships for each banded group were depressed, with a somewhat greater depression in the longer term group II muscles. External work and the maximum isotonic load were also depressed for both hypertrophied groups.

Isometric contractile performance for these groups is shown in Fig. 8. Active tension during contraction was depressed at all muscle lengths for the group I muscles, while resting tension did not differ significantly from control. Active tension was further depressed for the group II muscles, and there was an increase in the resting tension that was more pronounced at longer muscle lengths. The maximum rate of tension generation decreased from a control value of 302 ± 35 mN/mm^2/sec to 149 ± 18 mN/mm^2/sec for group I, and from a control value of 272 ± 28 mN/mm^2/sec to 120 ± 16 mN/mm^2/sec for group II. Time to peak tension increased to a comparable extent in each hypertrophy group.

Energetics

The oxygen consumption of the quiescent papillary muscles did not differ from control in either hypertrophied group. The oxygen consumption for the contractions used to obtain the isotonic data of Fig. 7 is shown in the left panels of Fig. 9. In parallel with the depressed velocity and extent of shortening at each load, there was a progressive reduction with time after banding in the associated oxygen cost of these contractions.

The oxygen consumption for each hypertrophy group and its control for the isometric contractions characterized in Fig. 8 are shown in the right panels of Fig. 9. The time integral of active tension during contraction ($\int$ active

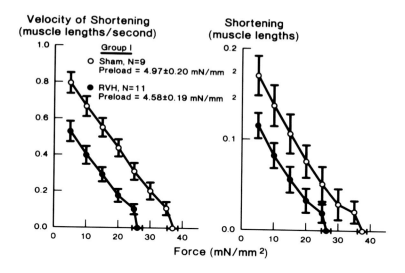

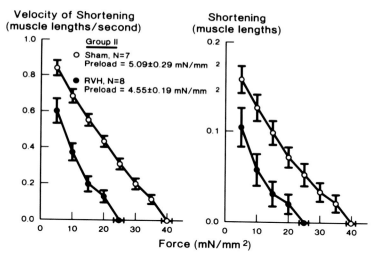

FIG. 7. Upper panels: The force-velocity and force-shortening data for the group I animals and their controls, studied at a relatively early time after initiation of a chronic progressive pressure overload. **Lower panels:** The same relationships for the longer-term group II animals and their controls. The format in each case is the same as that used in Fig. 2. (From Cooper et al. (5), with permission.)

tension) was markedly reduced in the hypertrophy groups, and this reduction was progressive with time: $\int$ active tension at L_{max} was 26.43 ± 3.91 mN/mm^2 × sec control, versus 15.27 ± 2.68 mN/mm^2 × sec for hypertrophy in group I, and was 24.04 ± 3.29 mN/mm^2 × sec control, versus 11.69 ± 2.08 mN/mm^2 × sec for hypertrophy in group II. Figure 9 demonstrates a reduction

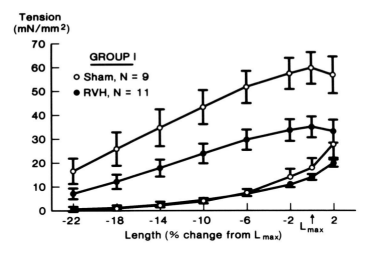

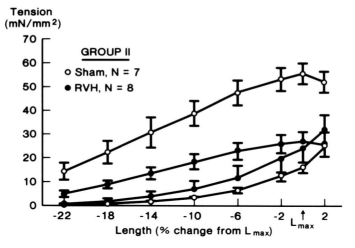

FIG. 8. Top: Length-tension data for the short-term group I animals; **bottom:** Same data for the long-term group II animals. The format is the same in each case as that used in Fig. 2. (From Cooper et al. (5), with permission.)

in the oxygen cost of this important mechanical determinant of myocardial energetics in parallel with the reduced isometric contractile state.

DISCUSSION

The major findings of these studies on the hypertrophied cat right ventricle can be summarized briefly. (a) In hypertrophy induced by a volume overload, there are no abnormalities of contractile or energetic function either with

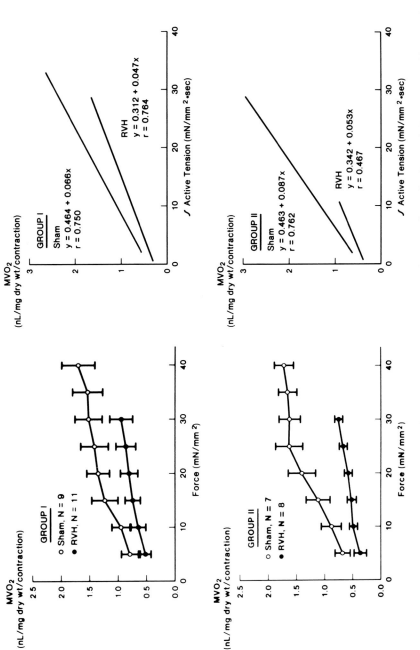

FIG. 9. **Left panels:** Isotonic oxygen consumption for the group I muscles (**top**) and the group II muscles (**bottom**). **Right panels:** Upper and lower panels show the isometric oxygen consumption for the group I muscles (**top**) and the group II muscles (**bottom**). The *abscissa* is the time integral of active tension during contraction. (From Cooper et al. (5), with permission.)

relatively short-term or long-term hypertrophy; (b) in hypertrophy of a similar degree and duration induced by a pressure overload applied acutely in the adult, there are marked abnormalities of both contractile and energetic function that are fully reversible at either relatively short or relatively long times after the hypertrophy is induced; (c) in hypertrophy of a similar degree induced by a chronic progressive pressure overload applied initially in the juvenile animal, there are marked contractile but not energetic abnormalities which worsen with time as the pressure overload persists in the adult. In none of these studies was abnormal pump function of the right ventricle in the intact animal apparent. This very wide range of differing results obtained in the same ventricle of the same species by a single investigator using the same techniques demonstrates that it is the nature of the inducing hemodynamic stress rather than the hypertrophy process itself that must be responsible for these model dependent functional abnormalities. Thus, the catholic view that the particular set of findings characteristic of any specific model of hemodynamic cardiac hypertrophy has broad implications for the behavior of hypertrophied myocardium in general is not warranted.

From this perspective, the disparity of recent conclusions regarding hemodynamically induced cardiac hypertrophy, based as they are on variable degrees of hypertrophy of the left or right ventricle in response to differing stresses in several species, is more to be expected than it is surprising. A précis of only a few of these studies, even with the emphasis limited to the question of contractile dysfunction, will substantiate this point. These can be separated into first, *in vitro* studies of muscle function, and second, *in vivo* studies of ventricular function. The first type of study is simpler to interpret, since these studies are not complicated by continuous changes in cardiac pump function in relation to neurohumoral factors and the systemic circulation. These *in vitro* studies provide the background which other factors may modulate in the intact animal.

A potentially important study (6) published in 1974 reported that the contractile defect produced by abrupt pulmonary artery banding in the adult cat was only transient. This suggested that in this model the contractile abnormality might be a self-limited defect produced by the acute hemodynamic stress rather than a fixed or progressive defect characteristic of myocardium with significant hypertrophy in response to a pressure overload. Unfortunately, there are two serious flaws in this study. The first is that the dimensions of the superfused muscles not only differed in the control and hypertrophy groups but were also too large to allow adequate metabolic support (5). The second is that, while absolute mass data were not provided, it appears that the long-term group had substantially less hypertrophy than the short-term group. Further, it was not clear why the results were so much at variance with those of the other studies (7–9) of contractile function following abrupt pressure overloading; in these studies the contractile defect was persistent after its initial appearance following acute pressure overloading.

Another study (10) published in 1975 also reported an early but largely transitory contractile defect following acute pressure overloading of the rat left ventricle. This study, too, has several serious limitations. The first is that the pattern of hypertrophy observed was singularly unusual, with the heart weight first increasing and then decreasing with time despite the same degree of aortic constriction said to be present throughout. Second, there was a modest and variable degree of hypertrophy, with the greatest contractile deficit associated not only with the earlier stages of hypertrophy but also with the greater degrees of hypertrophy; therefore, no realistic correlation of contractile defects with hypertrophy duration alone can be made. Third, mechanical data for all groups, including controls, were distinctly depressed and exhibited abnormal force-frequence behavior when compared to other data from this preparation in which adequate metabolic support was assured (11).

Despite the serious limitations to the conclusions that can be drawn from them, these studies, together with an anatomical study describing structural injury following acute but not gradual pressure overloading (12), did make the valuable point that acute, fixed afterload increments in the adult are not pathophysiologically appropriate models for pressure overload in the clinical setting. This has served as an impetus for the development of models employing gradually progressive afterload increments. I have reviewed the findings of one of these studies (5) here, and another (13) has recently confirmed the existence of a more restricted but progressive contractile defect in another, very different model of gradual afterload increase.

Turning to studies of ventricular function in the intact organism, and with the clear proviso that one is characterizing here not simply intrinsic contractile capabilities but instead the interaction of the ventricle with the rest of the organism, there have been several recent studies of interest. In two (14,15), the left ventricular function of conscious dogs was assessed after supracoronary aortic constriction. The first of these demonstrated a very early contractile defect that returned to normal two weeks after the afterload increment and was found in the second study to remain normal at a slightly later time. These two studies suggest that for the very modest degree and short duration of hypertrophy studied, the heart in the intact dog resumes normal function after the basic compensation of hypertrophy has occurred in response to an acutely applied pressure overload. However, this does not imply that the same degree of compensation occurs in the gradual onset of left ventricular pressure overload encountered clinically, since in patients with clinically apparent hypertrophy but not failure, the left ventricular mass typically doubles (16) rather than undergoing the 20 to 35% hypertrophy found in these two experimental studies. Indeed, in our studies (1–5) of *in vitro* myocardial function, our models each produced a doubling of right ventricular mass, intrinsic contractile abnormalities with each pressure overload, and yet normal *in vivo* ventricular pump function. The finding in another study (17) utilizing subcoronary aortic constriction to produce a progressive pressure overload of the left ventricle of puppies that ventricular function in the anesthetized animal is normal is therefore not surprising; the mean aortic pressure gradient was 25 mm Hg, and the extent of hypertrophy was approximately 35%.

Another model of hypertrophy without failure, in which a more substantial progressive pressure overload is associated with an eventual doubling of left ventricle weight, is the spontaneously hypertensive rat (SHR). It has been found here (18) that stressed ventricular performance is normal in the earlier phases and abnormal in the later phases of hypertrophy, perhaps reflecting a deterioration of intrinsic muscle function which ultimately results in compromised pump function. However, the dissociation of pressure overload from hypertrophy which can be produced pharmacologically (19) or by sympathectomy (20) in this model suggests that there are one or more genetic alterations that result in some form of hypertrophic cardiomyopathy not having a necessary, causal relationship to the usually accompanying hypertension. Thus, the SHR is not an appropriate model for myocardial hypertrophy induced solely by a pressure overload.

Considering very briefly the question of possible energetic as opposed to contractile dysfunction of hypertrophied myocardium, there is no greater unanimity of findings here. While there is general agreement that energy production and energy stores are both normal in hypertrophied but nonfailing myocardium, my findings (2) that the oxygen consumption of acutely pressure overloaded cat myocardium is increased is in distinct contrast to data showing reduced heat output from a similar model of hypertrophied myocardium in the rabbit (20). While no basis for this disparity other than species difference is apparent, the fact that this energetic abnormality was absent in chronic, progressive pressure overload suggests that, at least in my hands, a transient injury accompanying the acute pressure overload may have been responsible for the energetic abnormality.

In summary, it appears to me that there are two reasons for most of the conflicting views regarding the contractile and energetic behavior of myocardium hypertrophying in response to hemodynamic overloads: First, general conclusions have frequently been drawn from very specific and often very limited models; second, very real differences do exist in the biological responses to differing mechanical stresses, of which hypertrophy is only a single common factor. Given the increasing complexity and difficulty of current efforts to unravel the pathophysiology of myocardial hypertrophy and failure, it would therefore seem reasonable to devote an increasing share of our effort to the selection and thorough definition of pathophysiologically appropriate hemodynamic models.

ACKNOWLEDGMENT

This work was supported in part by grant HL21570 from the National Institutes of Health.

REFERENCES

1. Cooper, G., Puga, F. J., Zujko, K. J., Harrison, C. E., and Coleman, H. N. (1973): *Circ. Res.*, 32:140–148.
2. Cooper, G., Satava, R. M., Harrison, C. E., and Coleman, H. N. (1973): *Circ. Res.*, 33:213–223.
3. Cooper, G., and Satava, R. M. (1974): *J. Appl. Physiol.*, 37:762–764.
4. Cooper, G., Satava, R. M., Harrison, C. E., and Coleman, H. N. (1974): *Am. J. Physiol.*, 226:1158–1165.
5. Cooper, G., Tomanek, R. J., Ehrhardt, J. C., and Marcus, M. L. (1981): *Circ. Res.*, 48:488–497.
6. Williams, J. F., and Potter, R. D. (1974): *J. Clin. Invest.*, 54:1266–1272.
7. Bassett, A. L., and Gelband, H. (1973): *Circ. Res.*, 32:15–26.
8. Meerson, F. Z., and Kapelko, V. I. (1972): *Cardiology*, 57:183–199.
9. Hamrell, B. B., and Alpert, N. R. (1977): *Circ. Res.*, 40:20–25.
10. Jouannot, P., and Hatt, P. Y. (1975): *Am. J. Physiol.*, 229:355–364.
11. Henry, P. D. (1975): *Am. J. Physiol.*, 228:360–364.
12. Bishop, S. P., and Melsen, L. R. (1976): *Circ. Res.*, 39:238–245.
13. Capasso, J. M., Strobeck, J. E., and Sonnenblick, E. H. (1981): *Am. J. Physiol.*, 241:H435–H441.
14. Sasayama, S., Ross, J., Franklin, D., Bloor, C. M., Bishop, S., and Dilley, R. B. (1976): *Circ. Res.*, 38:172–178.
15. Sasayama, S., Franklin, D., and Ross, J. (1977): *Am. J. Physiol.*, 232:H418–H425.
16. Fulton, R. M., Hutchinson, E. C., and Jones, A. M. (1952): *Brit. Heart J.*, 14:413–420.
17. Carabello, B. A., Mee, R., Collins, J. J., Kloner, R. A., Levin, O., and Grossman, W. (1981): *Am. J. Physiol.*, 240:H80–H86.
18. Pfeffer, M. A., Pfeffer, J. M., and Frolich, E. D. (1976): *Circ. Res.*, 38:423–429.
19. Sen, S., Tarazi, R. C., Khairallah, P. A., and Bumpus, F. M. (1974): *Circ. Res.*, 35:755–781.
20. Cutiletta, A. F., Erinoff, L., Heller, A., Low, J., and Oparil, S. (1977): *Circ. Res.*, 40:428–434.
21. Alpert, N. R., and Mulieri, L. A. (1977): *Basic Res. Cardiol.*, 72:153–159.

*Perspectives in Cardiovascular
Research, Vol. 8,*
edited by R. C. Tarazi and J. B. Dunbar.
Raven Press, New York © 1983.

Changes in Creatine Kinase System During the Transition from Compensated to Uncompensated Hypertrophy in the Spontaneously Hypertensive Rat

Joanne S. Ingwall

*Departments of Medicine, Brigham and Women's Hospital, and Harvard Medical
School, Boston, Massachusetts 02115*

The heart adapts to increased work load by increasing its mass. The severity and duration of the increased work load, the nature of the stimulus (volume or pressure), and its rate of onset all contribute to the increase in myocardial mass and changes in contractility. These factors determine the rate of increase of myocardial mass and the time course of progression through the various stages of hypertrophy: (a) developing hypertrophy, (b) compensated stable hypertrophy, and (c) hypertrophy with failure. Many cellular and biochemical characteristics of the increase in cardiac mass and attendant changes in nucleic acid and protein composition are well documented (1–4).

In spite of a large body of work defining biochemical characteristics of the hypertrophied heart, many aspects of the metabolic machinery that controls the synthesis and utilization of high-energy phosphate-containing compounds in normal and hypertrophying heart remain to be defined fully. It seems possible that one characteristic of the uncompensated hypertrophied heart is a derangement in an enzyme system(s) involved with maintaining normal adenosine triphosphate (ATP) and creatine phosphate (CrP) contents. The research reported here addresses two goals: First, to test the hypothesis that changes in the concentration and distribution of certain proteins involved in maintaining the balance between ATP and CrP synthesis and utilization, namely the creatine kinase (CK) isozymes [ATP, creatine (Cr) N-phosphotransferase, EC 2.7.3.2.], are important characteristics of cardiac hypertrophy. The second goal is to determine the significance of these changes on the dynamics of energy metabolism in the hypertrophied heart. Evidence will be presented supporting this hypothesis and suggesting that a derangement in energy metabolism occurs during the transition from compensated to uncompensated hypertrophy in hearts of the spontaneously hypertensive rat (SHR).

THE CK SYSTEM

Creatine kinase catalyzes the following reaction:

$$MgATP + creatine \rightleftharpoons creatine\ phosphate + MgADP$$

Four CK isozymes have been identified and characterized: creatine kinase 1 or BB-creatine kinase, creatine kinase 2 or MB-creatine kinase, creatine kinase 3 or MM-creatine kinase, and creatine kinase 4 or mitochondrial creatine kinase. (The isozymes can be separated electrophoretically, and the designations, creatine kinases 1 through 4, refer to the relative migration of the proteins.) The double letter designations define the composition in terms of polypeptide chains characteristic of brain (B) or muscle (M). The B- and M-chains are synthesized on different genes and are chemically different (5–7). Experiments using techniques such as immunofluorescence and cell fractionation have defined the intracellular localization of several creatine kinase isozymes. Eppenberger and colleagues (8) identified one of the components of the M-line in the sarcomere as MM-CK. Scholte (9) and Saks et al. (10) have shown that, in heart, as much as one-half of the total cellular MM-CK is associated with the myofibril (this value is much lower in skeletal muscle). The mitochondrial creatine kinase is, as its name suggests, associated with the mitochondria, and is located on the outside of the inner membrane (11–13). Depending on the species, as much as one-third of the total cellular CK is the mitochondrial isozyme.

Figure 1 shows a diagrammatic representation of the energy transport system of the myocardial cell: The mitochondria with its CK isozyme, and the myofibrils and ion transport sites with MM-CK. It can be seen that if creatine phosphate is indeed a product of oxidative metabolism, then CrP and Cr [not ATP and adenosine diphosphate (ADP)] may constitute the energy shuttle between the site of production and sites of utilization of energy in the cell. This may not be an all-or-none phenomenon, but evidence from our laboratory suggesting that the localized mass action ratio favors the net synthesis of CrP in the environment of the mitochondrial CK isozyme makes this an attractive hypothesis (14). If CrP is produced as the ultimate end product of oxidative phosphorylation, it can diffuse to the myofibril and to various cellular membranes to be converted into ATP by the MM-CK isozyme localized in these organelles. Diffusion of CrP/Cr instead of ATP/ADP would be a more rapid process due to their smaller size, thus improving the efficiency of cellular energy transport. Much of the evidence describing the creatine kinase system has been previously reviewed (15).

Changes in the concentration, localization, or type of CK isozymes synthesized in the hypertrophied muscle cell could have important physiological consequences. Reduced tissue contents of MM- and mitochondrial-CK isozymes, the two isozymes characteristic of differentiated muscle, could limit not only the transfer of high-energy phosphate from ATP to CrP at the mi-

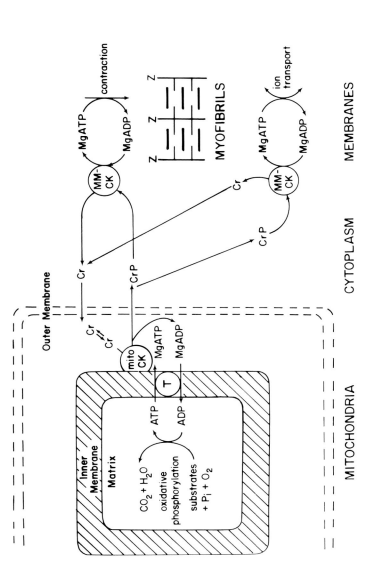

FIG. 1. Scheme of energy transport processes in the myocyte. The mitochondrial creatine kinase (mito CK) and MM-creatine kinase (MM-CK) isozymes are shown on various organelles. Creatine (Cr) and creatine phosphate (CrP) energy shuttle is illustrated.

tochondria, but also, if the energy transport system were compromised, limit the rate of rephosphorylation of ADP to ATP at the myofibril and sites of ion transport. Such changes may be the basis for decreased efficiency of energy transport and could contribute to depressed mechanical performance. In addition to changes in the CK isozymes, changes in the concentrations of the substrates for the reaction could also be important in regulating ATP and creatine phosphate turnover and transport in hypertrophied myocardium.

To assess these possibilities, this laboratory has used a combination of biochemical and biophysical techniques, first, to define changes in the steady state myocardial contents of the CK isozymes and its substrates, and second, to assess the significance of these changes on the rate of high-energy phosphate transfer between Cr and ADP, using saturation transfer phosphorous-31 nuclear magnetic resonance (P-31 NMR). The preparation used for the studies reported here is the hypertrophied heart of the SHR. Between 12 and 18 months of age, hearts of these animals exhibit signs of pump failure: specifically, dilation and reduced cardiac output (16). Such hearts are undergoing the transition from compensated to uncompensated hypertrophy. This preparation is well suited for both biochemical and biophysical measurements. Rat hearts can be isolated easily and perfused in the working heart mode (17). Even the largest rat heart can be easily accommodated in a 20-mm NMR tube for measurements of ATP and CrP contents and rates of phosphate transfer catalyzed by the CK reaction. The opportunity to assess the significance—whether causal or coincident—of changes in the distribution of these enzymes and in its substrate pools using NMR in this way may be unique and illustrates the power of applying these biochemical and biophysical techniques to an important problem in physiology.

METHODS

Twelve- and eighteen-month-old male SHR (Okamato-Aoki strain) and age-matched rats from two normotensive rat (NTR) strains (Wistar-Kyoto and American-Wistar) were obtained for the study (the Pfeffer colony at Brigham and Women's Hospital, Boston, MA).

Biochemical Analyses

Ten to thirty mg heart biopsy samples were homogenized in 0.1 M phosphate buffer, pH 7.4, with 1 mM EGTA and 1 mM β-mercaptoethanol and 0.1% triton at 0°C (final concentration 5 mg/ml). Aliquots were taken for protein determination (18) prior to the addition of triton and for total creatine kinase activity and isozyme composition. Total CK activity was measured using the coupled enzyme scheme of Rosalki (19) measuring the rate of appearance of reduced nicotinamide-adenine dinucleotide phosphate (NADPH). The relative proportion of CK isozymes was determined using cellulose acetate strip electrophoresis coupled with scanning fluorometry (Fig. 2) (20). To obtain quantitative results, 1 mM dithiothreitol was added to the electrophoresis buffer to prevent oxidation of the B-chain. In addition, any interfering fluorescence generated by the adenylate kinase reaction was determined by measuring only CrP-dependent fluorescence. This is accomplished by cutting each strip in half length-wise and soaking one-half in complete reaction mixture and the other half in reaction mixture lacking CrP; non-CrP-dependent fluorescence was subtracted. By adding diadenosine pentaphosphate ($\sim 10^{-5}$ M) to the electrophoresis buffer, most of the adenylate kinase activity was inhibited. Non-CrP-dependent activity usually constituted <5% of total activity. This method combines speed and convenience with sensitivity and precision, and permits measurement of the relative population of all four creatine kinase isozymes in one analysis.

Biophysical Analyses

NMR experiments were carried out in a Nicolet wide-bore NT 360 pulsed Fourier transform spectrometer equipped with fully broad-banded electronics, a dedicated 80k 1180 mini-computer, a Diablo dual moving head disc system

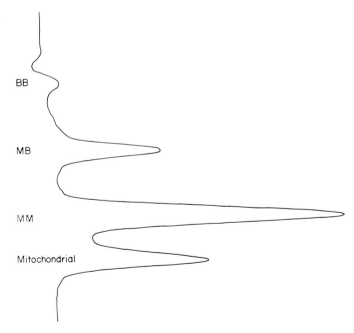

FIG. 2. Cellulose acetate strip electrophoretogram of creatine kinase isozymes of left ventricular tissue of 12-month-old SHR. The four isozymes, BB, MB, MM, and mitochondrial, are shown. Details of the method used are given in text.

and 89 mm bore 82.5 kG superconducting magnet. The spectrometer operates at 145.74 MHz for P-31. Experiments on perfused hearts were carried out in 20 mm OD sample tubes in a fixed frequency probe as previously described (21). The spectrometer was operated with 8 kHz spectral width and 30-, 45-, or 90-degree radio-frequency pulses repeated every 1 to 10 sec. Data were automatically stored as the free-induction decay on discs and were retrieved following the completion of the experiment for complete analysis. Details regarding quantitation of ATP and CrP contents have been described (21). The principles of saturation transfer NMR spectroscopy are described below.

RESULTS AND DISCUSSION

Between 12 and 18 months of age, when hearts begin to show signs of pump failure (16), hearts of the SHR undergo an increase in heart size (1.68 ± 0.04 to 1.96 ± 0.08 g) with no change in body weight ($\sim$420 g). The ratio of left ventricular weight to body weight increases from 3.00 ± 0.10 to 3.53 ± 0.12 mg/g. Compared to both NTR strains, this elevated ratio of left ventricular weight to body weight is nearly doubled (3.53 ± 0.12 mg/g for SHR versus 1.85 ± 0.10 mg/g for normotensive rats). These results not only show that hearts of the 18-month-old SHR are hypertrophied compared to the age-matched NTR, but also that a significant increase in heart size occurs between 12 and 18 months in the SHR. Accordingly, hearts from 12- and 18-month-old normotensive and hypertensive rats were analyzed for comparison of creatine kinase activity and isozyme distribution.

Biochemical Analyses

Values for total CK activities of left ventricular tissue for the 12- and 18-month-old SHR and NTR are shown in Table 1. Compared to the younger SHR and the age-matched NTR, the total CK activity of hearts of the 18-month-old SHR was 25 to 30% lower. This is the case whether results are expressed as activity per unit wet weight (data shown), dry weight, or total

TABLE 1. *Creatine kinase activity (IU/mg wet weight) in left ventricular tissue of normotensive and spontaneously hypertensive rat hearts*

	Age	
Strain	12 months	18 months
Normotensive	1.23 ± 0.07^a	1.20 ± 0.08^c
Hypertensive	1.19 ± 0.08^b	0.87 ± 0.07^d

[a] $N = 16$.
[b] $N = 8$.
[c] $N = 6$.
[d] $N = 10$.

cardiac protein (data not shown). Analysis of the distribution of CK isozymes also shows that significant changes occur only for hearts of the 18-month-old SHR. Approximately 50 to 60% of the total CK activity in adult rat myocardium of all ages in all strains is the MM isozyme, and 30 to 36% is the mitochondrial isozyme. (The remaining activity is MB; changes in its distribution will not be discussed here.) In the ventricles of 18-month-old SHR, however, the distribution of these two enzymes is $56 \pm 4\%$ MM and $19 \pm 2\%$ mitochondrial CK. Multiplication of the percentage distribution by the specific activity of total CK provides an estimate of the specific activity or tissue concentration of each isozyme. Performing this calculation for the hearts of the four groups of animals studied shows that the tissue content of the MM isozyme for 12-month-old animals of all strains and for the 18-month-old NTR is 0.66 ± 0.06 IU/mg wet weight, while the value for this isozyme for the 18-month-old SHR was reduced 25%, to 0.49 IU/mg wet weight. The change in the tissue content of the mitochondrial creatine kinase isozyme is more profound. Left ventricular tissue of all 12-month-old animals studied and 18-month-old normotensive animals contain 0.39 IU mitochondrial isozyme/mg wet weight, whereas left ventricular tissue of the 18-month-old SHR contains only ~ 0.16 IU/mg wet weight ($\sim 60\%$ reduction).

Thus, analysis of total CK activity and isozyme distribution of left ventricular tissue from the 12- and 18-month-old SHR and NTR shows that in hearts exhibiting impaired ventricular performance—from the 18-month-old SHR—the total CK and MM-CK activities per unit myocardial mass are reduced $\sim 30\%$, while the activity of the mitochondrial CK isozyme is reduced $\sim 60\%$. In order to assess whether changes in the tissue content of these isozymes have any impact on energy metabolism in the hypertrophied heart, hearts were isolated and perfused as Neely-Morgan working hearts for measurement of steady state ATP and CrP contents and transfer of high-energy phosphate between Cr and ADP using P-31 NMR spectroscopy.

Biophysical Analyses

P-31 NMR is being used to study the metabolism of ATP, creatine phosphate, and inorganic phosphate in isolated, intact functioning organs. Using this technique, dynamic aspects of the metabolism of these compounds can now be defined quantitatively, non-destructively, and repetitively in the intact organ while normal physiological function is maintained.

Information contained in the P-31 NMR spectrum of heart, such as that shown in Fig. 3, includes identifying the composition and quantitating the amount of phosphorus-containing metabolites present in relatively high concentration (>0.6 mM), in this case ATP and CrP. Since the position of the resonance corresponding to the phosphate moiety is sensitive to the chemical environment of that group, it is also possible to obtain information about the structure, motion, binding sites and pH of the molecule. Using saturation

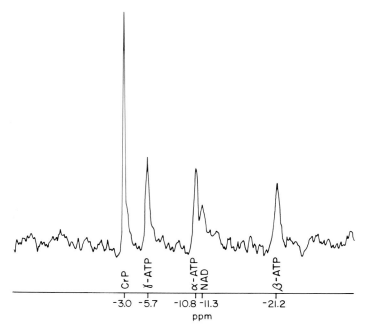

FIG. 3. P-31 NMR spectrum of a perfused working normotensive rat heart. The heart was perfused with Krebs-Henseleit buffer, pH 7.4, without glucose or phosphate, but with 10 mM pyruvate. Peak aortic pressure was ~140 mm Hg. The major resonances are labeled. To obtain this spectrum, 256 acquisitions were signal averaged. The flip angle was 45° and the repetition rate 1.2 msec; under these conditions, the CrP resonance is saturated ~40% and the γ-phosphate resonance is saturated ~15%.

transfer techniques and reaction rates, fluxes and lifetimes of reactants for enzymes such as CK can be measured directly in the intact heart. Most important, it is possible to obtain this information while normal physiological function is maintained. Thus, using NMR, it is possible to assess molecular bioenergetics and mechanical and electrical events simultaneously.

One relatively simple application of P-31 NMR spectroscopy to studies of energy metabolism in the hypertrophied heart is to quantitate the size of the unbound ATP and CrP pools in normotensive and hypertensive rat hearts. Preliminary experiments suggest that in the uncompensated heart of the 18-month-old hypertensive rat, the CrP pool is slightly smaller than in hearts of younger animals and in age-matched normotensive animals, but that the ATP pool is the same. Several other laboratories have also reported decreases in ATP and CrP pools in failing hearts (22,23).

Thus, in the uncompensated hypertrophied heart, changes occur in total CK activity, in the distribution of CK isozymes, and in the concentration of the CrP pool. Although it is attractive to speculate that these changes in the accumulation of certain organellar-bound proteins and one of their substrates signal a derangement in energy metabolism (and perhaps mechanical performance), such steady state measurements cannot prove that a derangement actually occurs. P-31 saturation transfer NMR offers the possibility of directly testing whether these changes are associated with (and perhaps causal to) changes in the rate of high-energy phosphate transfer between ADP and Cr in the beating heart.

Saturation transfer NMR can be used to measure unidirectional reaction rates with a time resolution in the order of 1 sec under steady state or equilibrium conditions. The method was developed by Forsen and Hoffman (24) in 1963 to measure exchange rates and lifetimes of chemical reactants of base-catalyzed proton exchanges. In 1977, Brown and Ogawa (25) used P-31 double resonance techniques to measure unidirectional reaction rates of adenylate kinase and lifetimes of some of its reactants. Several groups have now used this technique to study directly the chemical transfer of inorganic phosphate between CrP and ATP in muscle, i.e., to study the whole organ enzymology of the CK reaction (26–28). The CK reaction is fast enough to be measured using this technique, and muscle is an ideal system for such measurements because the primary reactants, CrP and ATP, are the dominant species observed in the spectrum.

The technique is based on the following principle: It is possible to selectively irradiate the CrP resonance (for one example) and make the phosphate of creatine phosphate NMR-invisible. Over time, the high-energy phosphate group is transferred from CrP to ADP via the chemistry of the creatine kinase reaction. Since this phosphate "remembers" that it is saturated or NMR-invisible, there is a transfer of saturated phosphate to the γ-ATP resonance (hence the name "saturation transfer"). Experimentally, the transfer is observed as a decrease in the intensity of the γ-ATP resonance. From measurement of the change in γ-ATP intensity and its relaxation properties over time, the apparent unidirectional rate constant for the transfer of phosphate from γ-ATP position to Cr can be calculated. Similarly, the γ-ATP resonance can be selectively irradiated and the unidirectional rate constant for transfer of phosphate from CrP to the γ-phosphate position of ATP can be calculated. Other information that can be obtained from this experiment includes (a) the lifetime of the species, (b) unidirectional fluxes, and (c) the net flux.

Preliminary experiments suggest that flux through the CK reaction in hearts of 18-month-old hypertensive rats is threefold lower than fluxes in hearts of younger hypertensive animals and age-matched normotensive animals (29). Decreased flux through the CK reaction is consistent with the observed decrease in the CrP pool. Since the ATP pool is unchanged in the uncompensated heart, these results also suggest that flux through other ATP-producing reactions must be increased to compensate for decreased phosphate transfer from CrP to ADP. Although tentative, these results show that P-31 NMR spectroscopy offers the opportunity to quantitate several features of the CK enzymology in the intact beating heart. This represents a unique opportunity to use a biophysical tool to assess the significance of a change in CK composition and distribution on the metabolism of its substrates.

The hypothesis that control of high-energy phosphate metabolism may play a role in determining ventricular performance of the hypertrophying myocardium has long been recognized. The possibility that changes in energy metabolism may constitute the trigger for hypertrophy has been suggested. In 1974, Meerson (30) proposed that a deficiency in high-energy phosphate levels, characterized by an increase in the phosphorylation potential, (ADP)(Pi)/ (ATP), may be the initial stimulus to hypertrophy. He reasoned that early on in work overload, ATP utilization increases, and the resulting increase in phosphorylation potential signals the need for increased capacity for ATP synthesis. Similar arguments can be made for the CrP/Cr ratio. Support for this hypothesis comes from observations that early in pressure overload hypertrophy, there is an increase in the volume of mitochondria relative to cell volume (31– 33), presumably increasing the capacity of the myocardium to synthesize ATP and CrP.

The results presented here, although preliminary in many respects, suggest that changes in the content and distribution of creatine kinase isozymes— particularly the mitochondrial isozyme—in the uncompensated hypertrophied heart of the 18-month-old SHR have a profound effect on the transfer of high-energy phosphate between creatine and ADP. It seems likely that such changes could compromise the efficiency of transport, synthesis, and utilization of high-energy phosphate during the transition from compensated to uncompensated hypertrophy and could presage pump failure.

ACKNOWLEDGMENTS

This work was supported by NIH grant HL 20552. Dr. Ingwall is an Established Investigator of the American Heart Association.

REFERENCES

1. Fanberg, B. (1974): In: *The Mammalian Myocardium*, edited by G. A. Langer and A. J. Brady, pp. 283–306. Wiley, New York.
2. Rabinowitz, M., and Zak, R. (1972): *Ann. Rev. Med.*, 23:245–262.
3. Morkin, E. (1974): *Circ. Res. (Suppl.)*, II:37–48.
4. Zak, R., and Rabinowitz, M. (1979): *Ann. Rev. Physiol.*, 41:539–552.
5. Eppenberger, H. M., Dawson, D. M., and Kaplan, N. O. (1967): *J. Biol. Chem.*, 242:204–209.
6. Dawson, D. M., Eppenberger, H. M., and Kaplan, N. O. (1967): *J. Biol. Chem.*, 242:210–217.
7. Watts, D. C. (1973): In: *The Enzymes, Vol. 8*, edited by P. D. Boyer, pp. 383–455. Academic Press, New York.
8. Turner, D. C., Wallimann, T., and Eppenberger, E. M. (1973): *Proc. Natl. Acad. Sci. USA*, 70:702–705.
9. Scholte, H. R. (1966): *Biochem. Biophys. Res. Comm.*, 22:597–602.
10. Saks, V. A., Chernousova, G. B., Vorronkon, Y. I., Smirnov, V. W., and Chazov, E. I. (1974): *Circ. Res.*, 34, III:138–149.

11. Jacobs, H., Heldt, H. W., and Klingenberg, M. (1964): *Biochem. Biophys. Res. Comm.*, 16:516–521.
12. Bessman, S. P., and Fanyo, A. (1966): *Biochem. Biophys. Res. Comm.*, 22:597–602.
13. Jacobus, W. E., and Lehninger, A. L. (1973): *J. Biol. Chem.*, 248:4803–4810.
14. DeFuria, R., Ingwall, J. S., Fossel, E. T., and Dygert, M. K. (1980): In: *Heart Creatine Kinase*, edited by W. E. Jacobus and J. S. Ingwall, pp. 135–139. Williams and Wilkins, Baltimore.
15. Jacobus, W. E., and Ingwall, J. S. (1980): *Heart Creatine Kinase*. Williams and Wilkins, Baltimore.
16. Pfeffer, J. M., Pfeffer, M. A., Fishbein, M. C., and Frohlich, E. D. (1979): *Am. J. Physiol.*, 237:H461–H468.
17. Neely, J. R., and Rovetto, M. J. (1973): *Methods in Enzymology*, 34:45–63.
18. Lowry, O. H., Rosebrough, N. J., Farr, A. L., and Randall, R. J. (1953): *J. Biol. Chem.*, 193:265–275.
19. Rosalki, S. P. (1967): *J. Lab. Clin. Med.*, 69:696–705.
20. Hall, N. F., and DeLuca, M. (1976): *Anal. Biochem.*, 76:561–567.
21. Fossel, E. T., Morgan, H. E., and Ingwall, J. S. (1980): *Proc. Natl. Acad. Sci. USA*, 77:3654–3658.
22. Fox, A. (1971): In: *Cardiac Hypertrophy*, edited by N. R. Alpert, pp. 203–212. Academic Press, New York.
23. Pool, P. E., Spann, J. R., Buccino, R. A., Sonnenblick, E. H., and Braunwald, E. (1967): *Circ. Res.*, 21:365.
24. Forsen, S., and Hoffman, R. (1963): *J. Chem. Phys.*, 39:2892–2901.
25. Brown, T. R., and Ogawa, S. (1977): *Proc. Natl. Acad. Sci. USA*, 74:3627–3631.
26. Ackerman, J. J. H., Bore, P. J., Gadian, D. G., Grove, T. H., and Radda, G. K. (1980): *Phil. Trans. R. Soc. (Lond.)*, B289:425–436.
27. Brown, T. R., Gadian, D. G., Garlick, P. B., Radda, G. K., Seeley, P. J., and Styles, P. (1978): In: *Frontiers of Biological Energetics, Vol. II*, edited by P. L. Dutton, J. S. Leigh, and A. Scarpa, pp. 1341–1349. Academic Press, New York.
28. Nunnally, R. L., and Hollis, D. P. (1979): *Biochemistry*, 18:3642–3646.
29. Ingwall, J. S., and Fossel, E. T. (1980): *Circulation (abstract)*, 62:III-19.
30. Meerson, F. V. (1974): *Circ. Res. (Suppl.)*, I:58–63.
31. Anversa, P., Loud, A. V., and Vitali-Massa, L. (1976): *Lab. Invest.*, 35:475–483.
32. Astorri, E., Bolognesi, R., Colla, B., Chizzola, A., and Visioli, O. (1977): *J. Molec. Cell. Cardiol.*, 9:763–775.
33. Rabinowitz, M., and Zak, R. (1975): *Circ. Res.*, 36:367–376.

*Perspectives in Cardiovascular
Research, Vol. 8,*
edited by R. C. Tarazi and J. B. Dunbar.
Raven Press, New York © 1983.

Myocardial Myosin Isoenzymes and Thermomechanical Economy

Norman R. Alpert and Louis A. Mulieri

*Department of Physiology and Biophysics, University of Vermont
College of Medicine, Burlington, Vermont 05405*

The relationship of energy utilization to contractile performance in the hypertrophied heart has been difficult to assess for the following reasons. First, energy utilization involves the contractile, mitochondrial, and excitation contraction coupling systems as well as the processes concerned with maintaining the constancy of the internal milieu and the structure of the intracellular organelles. Second, the development of the hypertrophied heart is not a monolithic event. Each of the systems and processes may be restructured in a manner determined by the nature, intensity, and duration of the stress as well as the age and species under investigation. The contractile protein, myosin, participates in the stress-induced reorganization of the heart by increasing in quantity and changing its specific adenosine triphosphatase (ATPase) activity (1). The change in specific ATPase activity is now believed to result from alterations in the relative content of the myocardial myosin isoenzymes. Three isoenzymes of myosin were reported (2–8). These were distinguished by electrophoretic mobility (2,3,5–8), and heavy chain peptide differences (5,9–12). In pressure overload, myocardial hypertrophy in the rabbit, V_3, with low ATPase activity predominates (5). Thyroxine-induced hypertrophy in the rabbit results in a high proportion of V_1 which has a high ATPase activity (5,7). This chapter is a review of our work on the contribution of V_1 and V_3 isoenzymes of myosin to the thermomechanical economy of hypertrophied rabbit hearts (13–22).

METHODS

Animal Models

Young rabbits (1.9 kg) were subjected to two types of hypertrophic stress in order to produce hearts containing primarily the V_3 or the V_1 isoenzyme of myosin. Pressure-overload hypertrophy was produced by twisting a spiral monel metal spring around the pulmonary artery reducing its diameter 67% (19,23). The animals were used 21 to 48 days after surgery. Thyrotoxic hypertrophy was produced by 14 daily intramuscular injections of 0.2 mg/kg of L-thyroxine (5,24,25). Injections were suspended on the days when body weight fell below 80% of the value at the start of the experiment. The relative concentrations of the V_3 (slow electrophoretic motility) and V_1 (fast electrophoretic motility) isoenzymes of myosin were assessed from the densitometer tracing of polyacrylamide gels of myosin prepared from each of the hearts (Fig. 1) (5). The ratio of V_1 to V_3 in the P and T hearts was <0.05 and 0.90, respectively.

Systolic and Diastolic Pressure Measurements

Right ventricular systolic and diastolic pressures were measured in lightly anesthetized (methoxyfluorane), closed-chest animals using an 18-gauge, 2-inch needle connected to an Ailtech (MS10-D) pressure transducer and recorded on a Beckman Type R Dynagraph (18,20,26).

Papillary Muscle Preparation and Force Measurements

Excised hearts from rabbits, stunned by a blow to the base of the skull, were washed out in a Kreb's-Ringer's bathing solution at 37°C and then transferred to a dissection chamber at room temperature (18). The right ventricle was

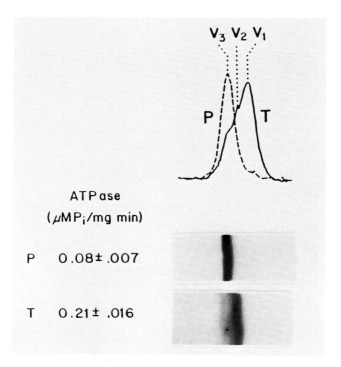

FIG. 1. The densitometer tracing (**upper right**) of pyrophosphate gels (**lower right**) of myosin from pressure overload (P) and thyrotoxic (T) hypertrophied hearts. **Lower left:** The steady state actin-activated myosin ATPase activity is tabulated. (From ref. 5, with permission.)

then opened and the thinnest available papillary muscle dissected free and mounted on the thermopile as previously described (18,27). The planar thermopile was made of vacuum deposited bismuth and antimony (27). The cut end of the papillary muscle was attached to a glass rod which extended through the thermopile frame and fastened to the capacitance force transducer (28). The tendinous end of the muscle was tied to a stationary hook below the thermopile, while a tether was used to guarantee close contact between the whole length of the muscle and the active junctions of the thermopile. The stimulating electrodes ($25\text{-}\mu$-diameter platinum wires) were threaded through the braided silk ties at each end of the muscle and kept in contact with the muscle by the ties. The muscles were stimulated with 10% supramaximal square wave pulses at a frequency of 0.2 Hz (18). After mounting the muscle on the thermopile, the assembly was placed in an incubating chamber containing Krebs solution with continuous oxygenation. The chamber was then submerged in a 70-liter constant temperature water bath where equilibration was carried out for 2 hr at 21°C. At the end of the equilibration period, the muscle was stretched in small increments (0.10–0.05 mm) until optimum length was reached. Muscles are discarded if active-to-passive force ratio was less than four and if the force and heat production were not steady throughout the experiment. The cool-off time constant and heat capacity of the muscle and adhering solution were then determined for each set of measurements made in the experiment by a modification (27) of the Kretzschmar and Wilkie (29) method.

Initial and Tension-Dependent Heat Measurements

The increase above ambient temperature of a repetitively stimulated muscle is a function of resting, initial, and recovery heat production and the cool-off characteristics of the muscle and system (27). Initial heat is a reflection of the ATP hydrolyzed as a result of Ca^{++} cycling and actomyosin crossbridge cycling during contraction and relaxation (Fig. 2, lower left). The initial heat can be calculated from the steady state temperature oscillation that occurs in phase with the contraction relaxation cycle (Fig. 2, upper left). The temperature change associated with the initial heat, θ_{i1}, is multiplied by the heat loss coefficient and the effective thermal capacity of the muscle (17,19,27,30). The initial heat consists of the tension dependent heat, TDH, and the tension independent heat, TIH (Fig. 2, left upper and lower diagram). The strategy for obtaining the TDH involves the measurement of the initial heat portion of TIH by measuring the triggerable heat output when tension is eliminated by incubating the muscle in 2.5 times normal hyperosmotic mannitol Krebs solution (Fig. 2, right upper and lower diagrams). The temperature change associated with the initial portion of the TIH, θ_{i2}, is obtained by the extrapolation procedure previously described. The temperature change associated with TDH is $\theta_{i1}\text{-}\theta_{i2}$. TDH is obtained by multiplying $\theta_{i1}\text{-}\theta_{i2}$ by the heat loss coefficient and

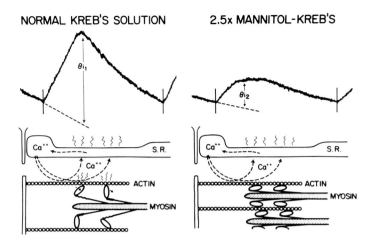

FIG. 2. The temperature oscillation of a repetitively stimulated (0.2 Hz) papillary muscle in normal (**upper left**) and 2.5 × hyperosmotic mannitol (**upper right**) Krebs-Ringer solution. The *dashed line* is obtained by taking the cool-off curve occurring when the stimulus is terminated and transposing that to the previous temperature oscillation. The source of initial heat (**lower left**) is presumed to be ATP hydrolized in conjunction with myosin crossbridge head cycling and Ca^{++} cycling. θ_{i1} is the temperature change of the papillary muscles associated with initial heat (**upper left**). **Upper right:** The source of TIH is presumed to be ATP hydrolyzed in conjunction with Ca^{++} cycling. θ_{i2} is the temperature change of the papillary muscle associated with TIH. (From ref. 17, with permission.)

the thermal capacity of the muscle and adhering Ringer's solution (14,16, 19,27,30).

In using 2.5 times normal hyperosmotic mannitol treatment to eliminate tension and partition the measurement of initial heat, we have assumed that the mannitol does not alter the amount and economy of Ca^{++} released and removed in each contraction relaxation cycle. We tested this assumption by using the natural twitch tension treppe that occurs when a 1-hr rest period is followed by the imposition of a steady 0.2-Hz pacing regimen (19). The tension treppe results from the presence of varying amounts of free intracellular Ca^{++}, and thus varying amounts of activation. Presumably, this would mean a changing number of functioning crossbridges in direct proportion to the force developed. The muscle is then subjected to the same pattern of rest and activity after blocking force development with 2.5 × hyperosmotic mannitol. The TIH for each individual stimulus in the train of sitmuli is subtracted from the appropriate initial heat obtained in normal solution to give the TDH for each contraction in the treppe. When the TDH is plotted against force, a linear relationship implies that each recruited crossbridge is identical with all others. This result is similar to that found in frog skeletal muscle using stretch above L_o to reduce active crossbridge number (31,32). The zero intercept of the twitch tension TDH curve suggests that mannitol does not markedly affect the amount of Ca^{++} release or the heat lost in removing it (19).

RESULTS

General

Peak right ventricular systolic and diastolic pressures were 17 and 1.2 mm Hg in the control animals. Systolic pressures were increased to 38 and 31 mm Hg in the P and T preparations, respectively (21). Diastolic pressures were elevated to 2.2 mm Hg in the P and unchanged in the T hearts (21). Right ventricular heart-weight-to-body-weight ratios increased from 0.31 g/kg in the normal animal to 0.66 g/kg ($p < 0.002$) in the P, and 0.61 g/kg ($p < 0.002$) in the T preparations (20). The cross-sectional area of the right ventricular papillary muscles was 0.59 mm². This was significantly increased in the P hearts (1.05 mm²; $p < 0.001$) and unchanged in the T preparations (20).

Isometric Force

Isometric peak force was 5.8 g/mm² and was attained in 630 msec in normal muscle. In the P hearts, the force was 4.93 g/mm², a value not significantly different from normal, and rose to its peak level in 806 msec ($p < 0.01$) (20). The T hearts developed an isometric force of 4.2 g/mm² ($p < 0.05$) and reached their peak value in 334 msec ($p < 0.01$) (20).

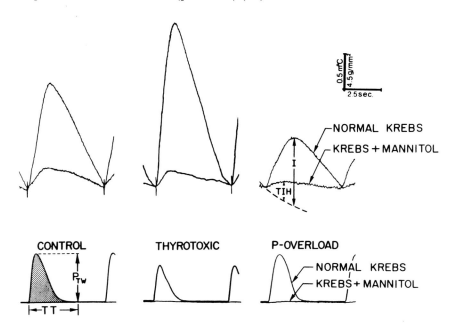

FIG. 3. Records of right ventricular papillary muscle heat production (**above**) and isometric force (**below**) for control, thyrotoxic, and pressure-overload hearts. For both the heat production and force records, the upper trace was obtained in normal Krebs-Ringer solution and the lower trace in 2.5 × hyperosmotic mannitol Krebs-Ringer solution. TT, twitch time; P_{TW} is the isometric force.

Initial Heat Measurements

Records of force (below) and heat production (above) are presented for the N, P, and T preparations in Fig. 3 (19). The initial heat production for the normal muscle was 1.66 mcal/g (18). In the P and T preparations it was 1.05 and 2.01 mcal/g, respectively (15). The ratio of initial heat produced to tension development for the normal muscle was 2.91 μcal/g cm (18). In the P and T preparations these values were 2.04 and 4.66 μcal/g cm, respectively (19). From the heat and force records it is clear that the economy of force development (force production ÷ initial heat) is greater than normal in the P muscles and less than normal in the T muscles.

TDH Measurements

The TDH is the difference between the initial heat and the TIH. The TIH records in 2.5 × hyperosmotic mannitol for N, P, and T preparations (smaller heat records) are shown in Fig. 3. The TDH in the normal hearts was 1.21 mcal/g; in the P and T hearts, the TDH was 0.74 and 1.52 mcal/g, respectively. When the TDH was normalized for peak tension, the values for the N, P, and T hearts were 2.08, 1.50, and 3.64 μcal/g cm, respectively (19).

DISCUSSION

Our plan was to examine the energy cost of force development in two types of hypertrophy in which the relative proportion of the V_1 and V_3 isoenzymes of myosin are changed (Fig. 1). The pressure-overload hypertrophy resulting from banding the pulmonary artery is relatively stable (4–11 weeks) and involves alterations in the following functional parameters: (a) decrease in maximum velocity of unloaded shortening (23,33); (b) a decrease in actin activated myosin ATPase activity (4,34–36); and (c) an increase in the *a* to *Po* ratio[1] (23,26). Hearts hypertrophied secondary to daily injection of L-thyroxine exhibit changes in the opposite direction (9–11,13,16,24,25,37–41,44–46). In each of these preparations, the hypertrophy is produced without hemodynamic evidence of failure. The slight increase in diastolic pressure of the P hearts is not sufficient to be an index of congestion (21,23).

From the initial heat measurements, it is clear that the economy of isometric force development is greater in the P than in the T preparations. This alteration in economy may be attributable to the contractile or to the excitation–contraction coupling processes. Partitioning the initial heat enables us to assess the contribution of alterations in the contractile proteins to the change in economy.

---

[1] In the ratio *a/Po*, *a* is constant and *Po* is the isometric force at optimum length used in the standard force velocity equation $(P + a)(V + b) = (Po + a)$. As *a/Po* increases, the curvature of the force velocity decreases.

The values of TDH per unit tension indicate that the increased V_1 isoenzyme content in the T preparation is associated with a 43% decrease in economy of isometric force production, while the increased V_3 content in the P preparation is associated with a 39% increase in economy.

The P hearts consist mainly of the V_3 isoenzyme of myosin, while the T hearts are made up primarily of V_1 isoenzyme (Fig. 1) (5). The ratio of the actin-activated myosin ATPase of the V_1 (T) to V_3 (P) preparations is 2.6, while the ratio of TDH is 2:1. The view that TDH is directly related to myosin crossbridge cycling is supported by the linear correlation that exists between TDH and actin-activated myosin ATPase activity over the broad range from pressure overload to thyrotoxic hypertrophy (19,20). Thus, the TDH measurements can be used in conjunction with currently acceptable kinetic schemes of actomyosin interaction to explain the altered economy (16,17, 19,20,47).

According to the scheme shown in Fig. 4, top, force is developed when the crossbridge heads of the myosin molecule are connected to actin and rotate from the 90° position to the 45° position (Fig. 4, step 5). In the complete cycle (steps 1–6), one ATP is hydrolyzed and two distinct states exist: the "on" force producing state (steps 4–6), where actin and myosin are associated and the "off" dissociated state (steps 1–4). A possible additional pathway (step 7) involving a noncycling "on" step is not considered for the purpose of this analysis. The steady state force seen at the tendons is the summation of the force impulses of the randomly attached and rotating myosin crossbridge heads as they stretch the compliant portion of the myosin molecule. The force developed is a function of the unitary strength of the crossbridge, the rate of crossbridge cycling, and the duration of the "on" time in the force generating configuration. The TDH is a measure of the number of moles of ATP split by the cycling crossbridge heads during a contraction–relaxation cycle (48). The cycling rates of P and T preparations relative to normal are determined by comparing the ratios of the TDH to twitch time for the experimental and normal hearts. The crossbridges of the P muscles cycle 35% slower than normal, while those from the T muscles cycle 56% faster (Fig. 4, bottom). The time in the force producing configuration, the "on" time, is determined by comparing ratios of tension–time integral to TDH for normal and experimental preparations (assuming each crossbridge from each preparation develops identical unitary force). In P and T preparations, the "on" time is 54% longer than normal in P preparations and 53% shorter than normal in T preparations (Fig. 4, bottom).

SUMMARY

The increased economy of force generation at the crossbridge level reflects the functioning of the V_3 isoenzyme of myosin, which is characterized by a slower "cycling rate" and a longer "on" time. The decrease in economy of the T preparations is consistent with the presence of the V_1 isoenzyme of myosin

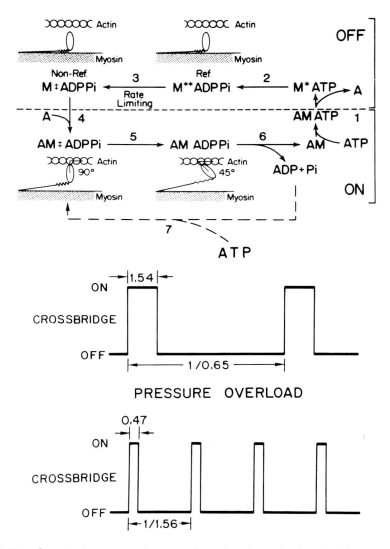

FIG. 4. Top: Steps in the actomyosin contraction–relaxation cycle. A, actin; M, myosin; ATP, adenosine triphosphate; ADP, adenosine diphosphate; P, inorganic phosphate; *, **, ‡, different conformational states of myosin. **Bottom:** Force development in terms of crossbridge "cycling rate" and "on" time. The height of each pulse is the force exerted by the crossbridge (assumed to be unity for all preparations). The "on" time or period of crossbridge force generation is indicated by the width of the pulse. The cycling rate is indicated by the frequency at which the pulses occur. (From ref. 19, with permission.)

characterized by faster "cycling rate" and a shorter "on" time. The P hearts with the slower, more economical contractile system are adapted for the maintenance of persistent high pressure. Where the demand in the T hearts is to move the blood at high velocity, the adaptation produces a fast muscle, which is less economical. The adaptations involve the redistribution of specific myosin isoenzymes which uniquely prepare the muscle for the stress at hand.

ACKNOWLEDGMENT

The authors are grateful for the technical assistance of Robert P. Goulette. This work was supported in part by PHS R01 17592-05 and P01 HL28001.

REFERENCES

1. Scheuer, J., and Bhan, A. K. (1979): *Circ. Res.*, 45:1–12.
2. Dillman, W. (1980): *Diabetes*, 29:579–582.
3. Hoh, J. F. Y., McGrath, P. A., and Hale, P. T. (1977): *J. Mol. Cell. Cardiol.*, 10:1053–1076.
4. Leger, J. J., Berson, G., Delcayre, C., Klotz, C., Schwartz, K., Leger, J., Stephens, M., and Swynghedauw, B. (1975): *Biochimie*, 57:1247–1273.
5. Litten, R. Z., Martin, B. J., Low, R. B., and Alpert, N. R. (1982): *Circ. Res.* 50:856–864.
6. Lompre, A. M., Schwartz, K., d'Albis, A., Lacombe, G., Thiem, N. V., and Swynghedauw, B. (1979): *Nature* (Lond.), 282:105–107.
7. Martin, A. F., Pagani, E. D., and Solaro, R. J. (1982): *Circ. Res.*, 50:117–124.
8. Mercadier, J. J., Lompre, A. M., Wisnewsky, C., Samuel, J. L., Bercovici, J., Swynghedauw, D., and Schwartz, K. (1981): *Circ. Res.*, 49:525–532.
9. Flink, I. L., and Morkin, E. (1977); *FEBS Lett.*, 81:391–394.
10. Flink, I. L., Morkin, E., and Elzinga, M. (1977): *FEBS Lett.*, 84:261–265.
11. Flink, I. L., Rader, J. H., and Morkin, E. (1979): *J. Biol. Chem.*, 254:3105–3110.
12. Hoh, J. F. Y., Yeoh, G. P. S., Thomas, M. A. W., and Higgenbottom, L. (1979): *FEBS Lett.*, 97:330–334.
13. Alpert, N. R., Litten, R. Z., and Mulieri, L. A. (1978): *The Physiologist*, 21:2.
14. Alpert, N. R., and Mulieri, L. A. (1977): *Basic Res. Cardiol.*, 72:153–159.
15. Alpert, N. R., and Mulieri, L. A. (1980): *J. Mol. Cell. Cardiol.*, 12:5.
16. Alpert, N. R., and Mulieri, L. A. (1980): *Basic Res. Cardiol.*, 75:179–184.
17. Alpert, N. R., and Mulieri, L. A. (1981): In *The Heart in Hypertension*, edited by B. E. Strauer, pp. 153–163. Springer Verlag, Berlin.
18. Alpert, N. R., and Mulieri, L. A. (1982): *Circ. Res.* 50:491–500.
19. Alpert, N. R., and Mulieri, L. A. (1982): *Fed. Proc.*, 41:192–198.
20. Alpert, N. R., Mulieri, L. A., and Litten, R. Z. (1979): *Am. J. Cardiol.*, 44:947–953.
21. Alpert, N. R., Mulieri, L. A., Litten, R. Z., Goulette, R., and Schine, L. (1979): *Circ. Res.*, 60:II–224.
22. Alpert, N. R., and Mulieri, L. A. (1982): In: *Myocardial Hypertrophy and Failure*, edited by N. R. Alpert. Raven Press, New York.
23. Hamrell, B. B., and Alpert, N. R. (1977): *Circ. Res.*, 40:20–25.
24. Banerjee, S. K., Flink, I. L., and Morkin, E. (1976): *Circ. Res.*, 34:319–326.
25. Banerjee, S. K. and Morkin, E. (1977): *Circ. Res.*, 41:630–634.
26. Schine, L. (1982): Masters Thesis, University of Vermont.
27. Mulieri, L. A., Luhr, R., Trefry, J., and Alpert, N. R. (1977): *Am. J. Physiol.*, 233:146–156.
28. Hamrell, B. B., Panaanan, R., Trono, J., and Alpert, N. R. (1974): *J. Appl. Physiol.*, 38:190–193.
29. Kretzschmar, K. M., and Wilkie, D. R. (1972): *J. Physiol*, 224:18P–20P.
30. Mulieri, L. A., and Alpert, N. R. (1982): *Can. J. Physiol. Pharmacol. (in press)*.
31. Homsher, E., Mommaerts, W. F. H. M., Ricchiutti, N. W., and Wallner, A. (1972): *J. Physiol.*, 220:601–625.
32. Smith, I. C. H. (1972): *J. Physiol.*, 220:583–599.

33. Maughan, D., Low, E., Litten, R., Brayden, J., and Alpert, N. R. (1979): *Circ. Res.*, 44:279–287.
34. Litten, R. Z., Brayden, J. E., and Alpert, N. R. (1978): *Biochem. Biophys. Acta*, 523:377–384.
35. Shiverick, K. T., Hamrell, B. B., and Alpert, N. R. (1976): *J. Mol. Cell. Cardiol.*, 8:837–851.
36. Thomas, L. L., and Alpert, N. R. (1977): *Biochem. Biophys. Acta*, 481:680–688.
37. Buccino, R. A., Spann, J. F., Pool, P. E., Sonnenblick, E. H., and Braunwald, E. (1967): *J. Clin. Invest.*, 46:1669–1682.
38. Conway, G., Heazlitt, R. A., Fowler, N. O., Gabel, M., and Green, S. (1976): *J. Mol. Cell. Cardiol.*, 8:39–51.
39. Goodkind, M. J., Dambach, G. E., Thyrum, P. T., and Juchi, R. J. (1974): *Am. J. Physiol.*, 226:66–72.
40. Gunning, J. F., Harrison, C. E., Jr., and Coleman, H. N., III (1974): *Am. J. Physiol.*, 226:116.
41. Marayama, M., and Goodkind, M. J. (1968): *Circ. Res.*, 23:743–751.
42. Skelton, C. L., and Sonnenblick, E. H. (1974): *Circ. Res.*, 34:II-83.
43. Strauer, B. E., and Scherpe, A. (1975): *Res. Cardiol.*, 70:115.
44. Katz, A. (1970): *Physiol. Rev.* 50:63–158.
45. Taylor, R. R., Covell, J. W., and Ross, J., Jr. (1969): *J. Clin. Invest.*, 48:775–784.
46. Yazaki, Y., and Raben, M. S. (1975): *Circ. Res.*, 36:208–215.

Perspectives in Cardiovascular Research, Vol. 8,
edited by R. C. Tarazi and J. B. Dunbar.
Raven Press, New York © 1983.

Myocardial Mechanics in Two Models of Pressure Overload Hypertrophy

Oscar H. L. Bing, Wesley W. Brooks, and Allen W. Wiegner

Thorndike Laboratory and Department of Medicine, Harvard Medical School, and Department of Medicine, Boston Veterans Administration Medical Center, Boston, Massachusetts 02130

Hypertrophy is a fundamental adaptive response of the myocardium, by which the increased muscle mass normalizes an increased load. A major question regarding hypertrophy is whether the process contains pathological elements that eventually lead to hemodynamic compromise. Changes described with hypertrophy include those that involve myocardial passive properties (such as fibrosis) and those affecting active properties (such as changes described with pressure overload hypertrophy). At this point, it is not clear as to whether or not these changes are the result of hypertrophy, and, in addition, whether or not they represent an adaptive response, or result in hemodynamic impairment in the intact animal.

Before comparing findings in two models of pressure overload hypertrophy, an overview of isolated muscle mechanics in cardiac hypertrophy will be presented. No attempt is made to be exhaustive in reporting; rather, an update of some concepts based on isolated muscle findings is presented.

PASSIVE PROPERTIES OF ISOLATED CARDIAC MUSCLE IN HYPERTROPHY

Attention has focused recently on the connective tissue response, which is associated in some cases with hypertrophy. It has been considered that abrupt loading is associated with connective tissue proliferation. Likewise, long-standing hypertrophy appears to be associated with increased myocardial collagen. The role of the connective tissue response on the active and passive mechanical performance of cardiac muscle has been considered; however, the literature in this area is inconclusive. There are studies of stiffness in hypertrophy without measurements of tissue collagen, and studies of collagen without measurement of mechanical properties. It is not clear that hypertrophy is necessarily associated with increased connective tissue or that connective tissue elements are responsible for changes in stiffness.

Differing methods of estimating stiffness have led to differing conclusions regarding the presence of altered stiffness in cardiac hypertrophy. For example, Spann et al. (1), measuring resting length–tension relations in papillary muscles, concluded there was no change in passive stiffness in their model of the pulmonary artery banded cat. However, Mirsky et al. (2) evaluated Spann's data and concluded that they indicated the presence of increased passive stiffness.

In recent years, an increasing number of studies have reported an increase in passive stiffness in association with hypertrophy (3–8). It should be emphasized, however, that all forms of hypertrophy need not be associated with changes in stiffness, and it is also possible that increased stiffness not present in the hypertrophied heart of a young animal may appear over the course of time. For example, we have found no change in active or passive stiffness of muscle preparations from the spontaneously hypertensive rat (SHR) studied at 6 and 12 months of age, while stiffness was found to increase in the SHR at 18 months (9).

In a study to further elucidate the role of connective tissue on the passive and active properties of cardiac muscle, β-amino proprionitrile (BAPN), an inhibitor of collagen cross-linking, was administered to rats at the time of aortic banding (5). Hypertrophy that developed after aortic banding was not associated with increased left ventricular hydroxyproline content, as was the case in animals not fed BAPN. It was found that an index of passive stiffness did not increase in banded rats fed BAPN, while passive stiffness increased in similarly banded rats not fed BAPN. Changes in myocardial active properties were similar to those reported in an earlier study (4) and were not affected by dietary BAPN. These studies suggest that (a) the change in the passive properties of cardiac muscle in association with hypertrophy appears to be due to the connective tissue response, and (b) changes in connective tissue are not responsible for the changes in active mechanical properties seen with aortic banding in the rat. Additional studies must be carried out to confirm these findings in other models of cardiac hypertrophy.

ACTIVE PROPERTIES OF ISOLATED CARDIAC MUSCLE IN CARDIAC HYPERTROPHY

In general, isolated muscle findings in cardiac hypertrophy may be outlined as follows: Hypertrophy that occurs with hyperthyroidism is associated with an increase in contractile activity (10). While volume loading does not appear to alter the mechanical responses of isolated muscle preparations, considerable variability in findings has been observed with pressure overload hypertrophy. Findings of increased (11), unchanged (12), and depressed (3–5,7,13–15) contractile activity have been reported. In other studies, contractile state has been observed to vary with time, being associated with early depression followed by later recovery (16).

To clarify a seemingly confused picture, it may be useful to reduce variables and carefully examine findings in a relatively well studied preparation such as the left ventricle (LV) of the rat subject to pressure overload. Models of hypertrophy in this subgroup include aortic banding (AC) (4,5,14), renal hypertension (6,7,17), DOCA treatment (18), and the SHR (18,19). All of these studies have been carried out in animals with hypertrophy without evidence of hemodynamic impairment. In examining data from this subgroup, one sees that despite differences in these models, findings have been generally similar. Force–velocity relationships reveal minor depression or no change. Active tension development is unchanged and time-to-peak tension (TPT) is usually prolonged.

COMPARISON OF ACTIVE MECHANICAL ACTIVITY IN TWO MODELS OF CARDIAC HYPERTROPHY

In this chapter, we compare findings in two models of pressure-overload hypertrophy studied in our laboratory: The aorta banded rat and the SHR. While it would be optimal if the effects of abrupt and gradual loading were the only variables compared, one must be quick to point out that these studies were carried in our laboratories at differing times and with different strains of rats at differing ages.

METHODS

SHR aged 6, 12, and 18 months used in the present study were from the colony of Okamoto-Aoki rats (20) at Peter Bent Brigham Hospital. Normotensive Wistar and Wistar-Kyoto rats were combined, as insufficient numbers were present in either group to provide a sufficiently large normotensive population of animals. Aorta-banded animals were from a strain of Charles River rats subjected to aortic constriction (4). Animals were studied at approximately 3 months of age, 4 weeks after acute banding of the ascending aorta.

Hearts of freshly decapitated rats were quickly removed and placed in oxygenated Krebs-Henseleit (21) solution at 28°C. The anterior papillary muscle of the left ventricle was dissected free, placed between two spring clips, and mounted vertically in a 100-ml plexiglas chamber containing Krebs-Henseleit solution at 28°C and gassed with 95% O_2 and 5% CO_2.

Muscles were stimulated 12/min by parallel platinum electrodes delivering 5-msec pulses at voltages 10% greater than the minimum necessary to produce a maximum mechanical response. For studies with SHR preparations, the apparatus is as described below; for studies with aorta-banded rats, the apparatus is as described previously (4). The spring clip on the tendon end of the muscle was connected to the lever arm of a low-inertia DC motor; the lower clip was attached to a semiconductor strain gauge transducer immersed in the bath.

Either the length or tension of the preparation could be controlled by means of an electronic servosystem controlled by a digital computer (22). Muscle contractions were recorded by sampling length and force at a rate of 1 kHz. Quantitation error was less than 5 μm for length and 20 mg for force.

After each experiment, muscles were removed from the spring clips, blotted, and weighed. Cross-sectional areas were calculated by assuming cylindrical uniformity and a density of 1.00 g/cm^3. Preparations with cross-sectional areas <0.5 or >1.5 mm^2 were not included in the data base used for this study. All data were normalized for muscle length and cross-sectional area. Data were evaluated statistically using 2-way analysis of variance with replication and by unpaired t-test where appropriate.

RESULTS

In comparing animal and heart weight (Fig. 1), it can be noted that aorta-banded animals were considerably smaller. This is because aortic banding was carried out in 200-g rats when they were approximately 8 weeks of age. Significant left ventricular hypertrophy is present in the SHR at all three ages, with a considerable increase seen at 18 months. Hypertrophy in the aorta-banded rat, as measured by the LV/BW (body weight) ratio, appears intermediate in degree between the 6- and 18-month SHR.

Isometric performance parameters normalized for papillary muscle cross-sectional area are compared to the appropriate control groups in Fig. 2. In the SHR, an increase in active tension and tension development (dT/dt) is seen in both 6- and 18-month animals, while these parameters did not change in the aortic-banded animal. TPT is significantly prolonged in the 18-month SHR and the aortic banded rat, but not the 6- or 12-month SHR.

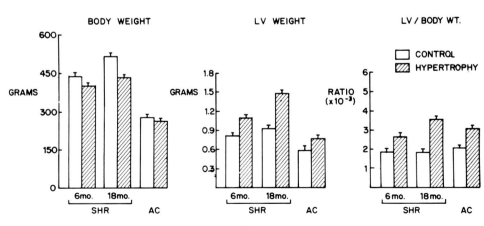

FIG. 1. Body weights, LV weights, and LV/BW ratios in SHR and normotensive rats (control) at 6 and 18 months, and rats subjected to AC with appropriate control animals. Data are mean + SEM.

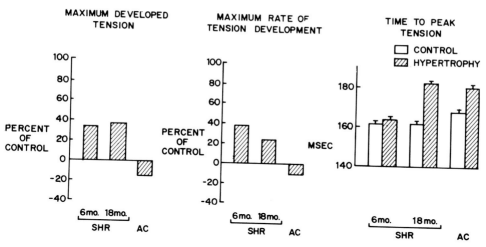

FIG. 2. Isometric performance parameters: Maximum developed tension (T), maximum rate of tension development (dT/dt), and time-to-peak tension (TPT) in muscle preparations from SHR at 6 and 18 months and rats with aortic banding (AC) (all with appropriate controls). T and dT/dt normalized for papillary muscle cross-sectional area.

In SHR, force–velocity relations were plotted from quick release data (Fig. 3A). Velocities were measured 17 msec after release, which was the earliest time a uniformly stable velocity could be measured. Releases were performed at 25, 50, 75, and 100% of TPT. While overlap between data from SHR and normotensive preparations is present at light loads, a separation between SHR and normotensive data is seen at increasing loads. Thus, force–velocity relations in the SHR at all ages studied seem to be characterized by small changes in maximum velocity and a relatively larger increase in maximum force developed.

In the AC rat, force–velocity relations were plotted from afterloaded–isotonic contraction data (Fig. 3B). These relations reveal a small depression of maximum shortening velocity with no change in peak force.

Using a point counting technique, the constituents of papillary muscle preparations of SHR rats were estimated. Muscle content was simply divided into 4 components: mitochondria, myofibrils, other (intracellular), and other (extracellular) (Fig. 4A). If papillary muscle contents are extrapolated to total the left ventricle, one finds that the increase in left ventricular mass seen in the 6- and 12-month SHR is almost totally due to an increase in myofibrils (Fig. 4B). Changes in mitochondria and other elements are small. In the 18-month SHR, a further increase in myofibrils is seen; the increase in mitochondria in this age group does not quite achieve statistical significance.

Since the contractile unit of the myocardium is the myofibril, it may be reasonable to normalize mechanical performance for myofibrillar cross-sec-

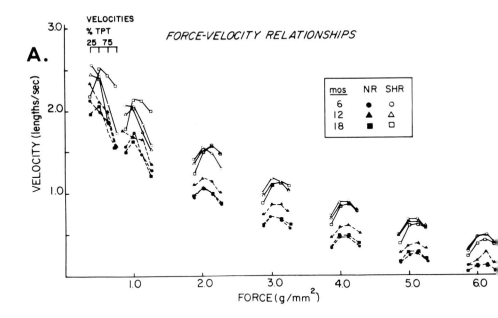

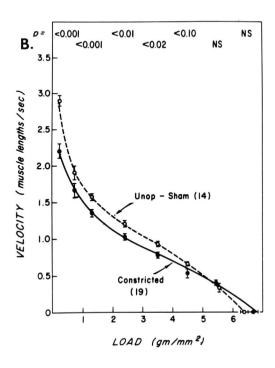

FIG. 3. A: Quick release force–velocity relations in muscle preparations from SHR and normotensive rats, age 6, 12, and 18 months, measured at 25, 50, 75, and 100% TPT. **B:** Force–velocity relations in preparations from aorta banded rats and controls measured from afterloaded isotonic contractions.

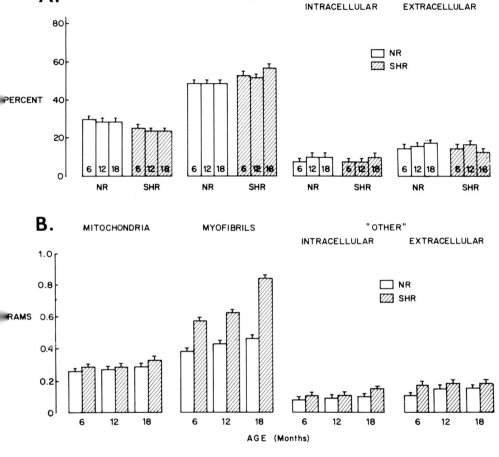

FIG. 4. A: Papillary muscle constituents in preparations from SHR and normotensive rats, measured by a point-counting technique. Constituents were divided into 4 groups: mitochondria, myofibrils, other (intracellular), and other (extracellular). **B:** Papillary muscle constituents multiplied by LV weight (g). This calculation assumes left ventricular constituents to be similar to that of the papillary muscle.

tional area (Fig. 5). If this is done, increases in AT and dT/dt in data normalized for papillary muscle cross-sectional area in the SHR are no longer statistically significant. Although we have not carried out point-counting studies in the aorta banded rat, if we assume a change in myofibrillar concentration proportional to that of the SHR with a similar degree of hypertrophy estimated from the LV/BW ratio, we find that tension (T) and dT/dt are somewhat depressed in the aorta-banded rat.

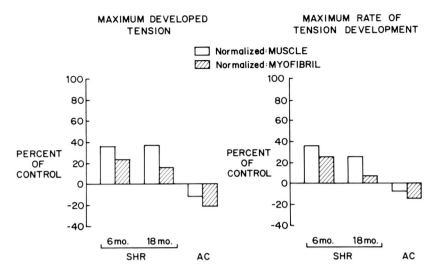

FIG. 5. Isometric performance parameters in preparations from SHR and AC rats normalized for papillary muscle cross-sectional area (as in Fig. 2) compared with data normalized for myofibrillar cross-sectional area. Myofibrillar cross-sectional areas calculated from point-counting data. AC data calculated assuming a change in myofibrillar concentration proportional to that of the SHR with a similar degree of hypertrophy as estimated from the LV/BW (see text).

DISCUSSION

Before discussing the effects of hypertrophy on mechanical performance, it may be useful to consider some of the difficulties with and attributes of the isolated muscle preparation relevant to studies of cardiac hypertrophy.

These preparations are removed from the right ventricle of most larger animals such as cat, rabbit, and dog, but left ventricular preparations can be utilized in the rat. Preparations must be carefully dissected to avoid damage and they must be thin—usually less than 1 mm in cross-sectional area. To prevent problems associated with diffusion, studies must be carried out with high bath P_{O_2}, low temperature, and low stimulation rate. Such experimental conditions raise questions of the relevance of findings in isolated muscle studies to events occurring in the intact animal.

On the other hand, much useful information has been gained from appropriately designed experiments using this preparation. Inotropic effects, such as those of hypoxia and isoproterenol, for example, are clearly demonstrable when each preparation serves as its own control. The more difficult studies are those comparing two or more groups of animals, such as in studies of hypertrophy. Technique must be expert as one should not discard preparations; even then, it may be well to consider that many workers in cardiac muscle mechanics discard many hearts before finding an "adequate" preparation. In studies such as the present one, one must, for the most part, accept every preparation, and technical errors should not take place, since it is subsequently unclear whether a poorly performing preparation is the result of an alteration in intrinsic muscle properties or technical difficulties.

With this in mind, it is perhaps less surprising to find an incomplete concensus among investigators with respect to the effects of hypertrophy on isolated cardiac muscle mechanics. Technical problems, species differences, type of hypertrophy, rate of hypertrophy development, degree of loading, and chamber involved may all be reasons for the variability in findings between laboratories.

The present studies are interpreted as indicating that two models of pressure-overload hypertrophy demonstrate relatively minor differences in active muscle performance. Force–velocity relations in the SHR, measured by the quick release technique, demonstrate minor changes in maximum shortening velocity. These relations measured from afterloaded isotonic contractions in the aorta banded rat reveal a slight depression of maximum velocity. If one examines afterloaded isotonic force–velocity relations in the same rats as quick release studies were recorded, one finds that in the 18-month SHR, a depression of maximum shortening velocity is apparent (Fig. 6), where, in quick release data, such depression is not evident (compare with Fig. 3A).

What is the explanation? In studies utilizing afterloaded isotonic contractions, velocity of shortening at increasing loads is measured at progressively later times in the contraction. As indicated by quick release velocity profiles, the onset of activity is delayed or slowed in the 18-month SHR (5) and possibly, also, the aorta banded rat where a prolongation in TPT is clearly evident. It is suspected that the previously described depression of maximum shortening velocity in pressure overload hypertrophy may be due, in part, to the slow onset of mechanical activity.

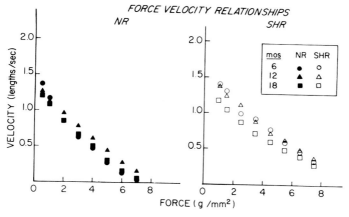

FIG. 6. Force–velocity relations in preparations from 6-, 12-, and 18-month SHR and normotensive rats recorded from afterloaded isotonic contractions.

Neither depression of maximum shortening velocity (measured from after-loaded isotonic contractions) nor prolongation of mechanical activity are seen in 6- and 12-month SHRs, but are only seen in the 18-month SHR and rats with acute aortic banding. It is interesting that after a period of stable hyper-trophy at 6 and 12 months, as indicated by the LV/BW ratio, a further increase in hypertrophy is seen in 18-month SHRs. In both the 18-month SHR and the rat subjected to acute banding, an increase in LV/BW ratio above a pre-vious stable value appears to be associated with prolonged mechanical activity. This raises the question of whether changes in the active properties are related to hypertrophy per se or to a relatively abrupt change in loading conditions.

Using a point-counting technique (23), papillary muscle constituents were calculated. Mechanical data were then renormalized for myofibrillar cross-sectional area. Findings based on this data suggest that peak isometric force or force–velocity relations at heavy loads may be no different from controls. Thus, increases in T and dT/dt in data normalized for papillary muscle cross-sectional area appear to be due, at least in part, to an increased concentration of contractile units in parallel: in other words, more dense packing of myo-fibrillar material. If one assumes a similar change in contractile unit density for the aorta banded rat, it might be concluded that peak force and rate of force development are unchanged or slightly depressed.

It is in the aged SHR that evidence for impaired ventricular function is seen (24). We have been particularly interested in defining the isolated muscle cor-relates of impaired hemodynamic performance. Although current data are only preliminary, some interesting trends may be developing. If hypertrophy as indicated by LV/BW ratio is plotted against mitochondria–myofibrillar ratio, one sees that as hypertrophy increases in 6- and 12-month SHRs, the mito-chondria/myofibrillar (M/MF) ratio falls, reflecting an increase in myofibrillar mass and a relatively unchanged mitochondrial population (see Fig. 4). In the 18-month SHR, there is a considerable increase in the LV/BW with little additional change in the M/MF ratio, suggesting that with further hypertrophy, some increase in mitochondria must be taking place. In looking more closely at the 18-month SHRs, one might anticipate that those hearts with the largest increase in LV/BW would have the smallest M/MF or the greatest numbers of myofibrils relative to mitochondria. It was surprising to find, however, that the opposite trend appeared to be the case. The least hypertrophied ventricles had the smallest M/MF ratio. This suggested to us the possibility that, in the course of hypertrophy, after a point, further myofibrillar hypertrophy may be linked to an increase in mitochondrial mass.

It was further surprising to note that those preparations associated with the least hypertrophy and the smallest M/MF ratios tended to have the poorest performance, as measured by lightly loaded shortening velocity. Although, at present, these data do not quite reach statistical significance, the trend suggests that hypertrophy associated with decreased cardiac performance may reflect a failure of the mitochondrial mass to increase.

It seems that the adaptive process associated with hypertrophy is at first associated with increased myofibrils without an increase in mitochondria. At a critical point, mitochondria must increase in relative proportion to the myofibrils. If a late increase in mitochondrial volume does not occur, depression of myocardial performance is seen. These preliminary data raise the possibility that hemodynamic impairment in the aging SHR may be related to a defect at the mitochondrial level.

ACKNOWLEDGMENTS

This work was supported in part by Grants HL-20552 and HL-18338 from the National Heart, Lung, and Blood Institute, National Institutes of Health. O.H.L. Bing is the recipient of NIH Career Development Award HL-00072.

The authors wish to thank Susan Miness-Farber, Karen B. Weinstein, and Kathleen Robinson for expert technical assistance, Patricia O'Shea for assistance with electron microscopic studies, and Deborah Marbut-Blaustein for assistance in the preparation of this manuscript.

REFERENCES

1. Spann, J. F., Jr., Buccino, R. A., Sonnenblick, E. H., and Braunwald, F. (1967): *Circ. Res.*, 21:341–354.
2. Mirsky, I., and Parmley, W. W. (1973): *Circ. Res.*, 33:233–242.
3. Alpert, N. R., Hamrell, B. B., and Halpern, W. (1974): *Circ. Res.*, 34:71–82.
4. Bing, O. H. L., Matsushita, S., Fanburg, B. L., and Levine, H. J. (1971): *Circ. Res.*, 28:234–245.
5. Bing, O. H. L., and Wiegner, A. W. (1983): In: *Cardiac Hypertrophy and Failure*, edited by N. Alpert. Raven Press, New York (*in press*).
6. Holubarsch, C. H. (1981): *Basic Res. Cardiol.*, 75:244–252.
7. Kämmereit, A., and Jacob, R. (1979): *Basic. Res. Cardiol.*, 74:389–405.
8. Williams, J. F., Jr., and Potter, R. D. (1981): *Circ. Res.*, 49:211–215.
9. Wiegner, A. W., Weinstein, K. B., and Bing, O. H. L. (1980): *Circulation*, 62(III):12.
10. Skelton, L., and Sonnenblick, E. H. (1974): *Circ. Res. (Suppl.)*, 34 & 35:83–96.
11. Kerr, A., Jr., Winterberger, A. R., and Giambattista, M. (1961): *Circ. Res.*, 9:103–105.
12. Grimm, A. F., Kubota, R., and Whitehorn, W. V. (1963): *Circ. Res.*, 12:118–124.
13. Grenning, F. J., and Coleman, H. N. (1972): In: *Myocardiology, Vol 1*, edited by E. Bajusz, G. Rona, pp. 190–199. University Park Press, Baltimore.
14. Jouannot, P., and Hatt, P. Y. (1975): *Am. J. Physiol.*, 229:355–364.
15. Kaufman, R. L., Homburger, H., and Wirth, H. (1971): *Circ. Res.*, 28:346–357.
16. Williams, J. F., Jr., and Potter, R. D. (1974): *J. Clin. Invest.*, 54:1266–1272.
17. Capasso, J. M., Fein, F., Kornstein, L. B., Strobeck, J. E., and Sonnenblick, E. H. (1980): *Am. J. Cardiol.*, 45:434.
18. Heller, L. J. (1978): *Am. J. Physiol.*, 235:H82–H86.
19. Perkins, F. M., Hamrell, B. B., and Alpert, N. R. (1975): *Fed. Proc.*, 34:365.
20. Okamoto, K., and Aoki, K. (1963): *Jpn. Circ. J.*, 27:282–293.
21. Krebs, H. A., and Henseleit, K. (1932): *Z. Physiol. Chem.*, 210:33–36.
22. Sulman, D. L., Bing, O. H. L., Mark, R. G., and Burns, S. K. (1974): *Biochem. Biophys. Res. Comm*, 56:947–951.
23. Page, E., and McCallister, L. P. (1973): *Am. J. Cardiol.*, 31:172–181.
24. Pfeffer, M. A., Pfeffer, J. M., and Frohlich, E. D. (1976): *Circ. Res.*, 38:423–429.

Perspectives in Cardiovascular Research, Vol. 8,
edited by R. C. Tarazi and J. B. Dunbar.
Raven Press, New York © 1983.

Myocardial Contractile Alterations Induced by Hypertensive Hypertrophy and Its Reversal

John E. Strobeck, Joseph M. Capasso, Ashwani Malhotra, and Edmund H. Sonnenblick

Cardiovascular Research Laboratories, Division of Cardiology, Albert Einstein College of Medicine, Bronx, New York 10461

Myocardial hypertrophy is a fundamental compensatory mechanism that allows the heart to maintain normal pump function in the face of abnormal hemodynamics (28,34). Although many models of myocardial hypertrophy have been utilized to assess alterations in contractile performance (1,14,32,34), results have been inconsistent due to variations in the severity and duration of the inciting stimulus (18,26,40).

Utilizing the isolated left ventricular papillary muscle to assess myocardial contractile performance, we have previously examined the effects of a gradually applied pressure overload (i.e., renovascular hypertension) over a 30-week period. These studies have shown that force development is maintained at the expense of prolongation of isometric and isotonic timing parameters, while there is a progressive decay in the speed of muscle shortening (11). In the present study, we have examined the possibility of reversing these abnormalities after lowering the blood pressure by unilateral nephrectomy.

METHODS

Experimental Model

Female Wistar rats (Charles River) weighing 175 to 200 g were divided into three experimental groups: control rats (C); animals made hypertensive for 10 weeks (H); and animals made hypertensive for 10 weeks followed by reversal of hypertension (by unilateral nephrectomy) for an additional 10 weeks (R).

Animals were made hypertensive by placing a silver clip with a 0.25-mm aperture around the left renal artery. The contralateral kidney was left untouched. Using the tail cuff method (41), systolic blood pressure was measured under light ether anesthesia before clipping and at 1-week intervals thereafter. Rats were considered hypertensive when systolic arterial pressure increased to 150 mm Hg within 3 to 5 weeks after clipping, and remained at or above this level until the time of study.

Ten weeks after the onset of hypertension, a group of hypertensive animals were randomly selected for removal of the ischemic kidney. Normotension resulted in these animals within 24 hr and blood pressure remained below 150 mm Hg until the time of study ten weeks later.

Mechanical Recordings

Animals were anesthetized with ether. The heart was rapidly excised and placed in oxygenated Tyrode's solution. Left ventricular papillary muscles were removed and suspended horizontally in a continuous perfusion myograph. Care was taken to select muscles of relatively cylindrical uniformity, whose cross-sectional area was less than 1.2 mm^2, to ensure adequate oxygenation of central fibers. The muscles were superfused with Tyrode's solution of the following composition in mM/liters: Na^+ 151.3, Ca^{2+} 2.4, K^+ 4.0, Mg^{2+} 0.5, Cl^- 147.3, $H_2PO_4^-$ 1.8, HCO_3^- 12.0, and dextrose 5.5. This solution was maintained at 30°C and gassed with 95% O_2, 5% CO_2. The nontendinous end of the papillary muscle was inserted into a spring-loaded stainless steel clip, which was mounted to the end of a micrometer assembly used to adjust external muscle length. The tendinous end was tied to a light steel wire with a short length of wet Ethicon 3-0 braided silk. The wire inserted into a 2-cm stainless steel lever that was connected in turn to a servo-controlled galvanometer. Control circuitry permitted operation in either afterloaded isotonic or isometric modes. The position of the lever was measured by a variable capacitor positioned at the rear of the galvonometer's moving iron core. Force at the tip of the lever was determined by scaling and amplifying the error signal produced in the position-servo section of the control circuitry during the contraction. Force and length measurements were both obtained from the galvanometer, eliminating the need for a separate force transducer. Velocity of shortening was determined by electronic differentiation of the muscle length signal (lever position). The rate of tension change was derived by differentiation of the force signal.

Studies of Contractile Proteins

In some studies, hearts were immediately prepared for extraction of contractile proteins. Other hearts were stored at -80°C in 50% glycerol containing 50 mM KCl and 10 mM KPO_4^- at pH 7.0 prior to preparing the extracts. In all cases, the hearts that were examined for calcium activated adenosine triphosphatase (ATPase) activity were the same hearts from which papillary muscles were removed and utilized for mechanical studies. There was no difference in values for ATPase activity when hearts were prepared immediately or after a period of storage. Hearts of experimental animals were always extracted and analyzed simultaneously with the hearts of controls using the same reagent and incubation conditions.

The methods for preparing and analyzing cardiac actomyosin from individual hearts (the same hearts from which papillary muscles are removed for additional study) have been detailed previously (5).

Study Design

One hundred and twenty female Wistar rats purchased at 6 weeks of age were housed in our animal facility. At 8 weeks of age, 70 animals underwent surgical clipping of the left renal artery. Hypertension (systolic arterial pressure ≥ 150 mm Hg) was produced in approximately 85% of all clipped animals 3 to 5 weeks after renal artery constriction. At 10 weeks after the onset of hypertension, a group of hypertensive animals were removed for mechanical study. Age-matched, unoperated, and sham-operated rats from the same initial group were used as controls. All hypertensive animals studied displayed significant left ventricular hypertrophy (≥40%) and for simplicity will be called hypertensives (H).

In addition, the mechanical effects of a reduction in systolic blood pressure were studied in this same group of rats. At 10 weeks after the onset of hypertension, approximately 10 hypertensive animals were removed for unilateral nephrectomy of the ischemic kidney. Blood pressure was monitored within 24 hr and then weekly for the following 10 weeks. All animals in which systolic blood pressure was decreased by nephrectomy also displayed a significant reduction in heart size and were considered to be hypertensive-reversal animals (R). At the completion of 10 weeks of normotension (systolic blood pressure < 150 mm Hg), R animals were sacrificed (along with appropriate age-matched controls), their left ventricular papillary muscles removed, and mechanical data collected. At this same time, both atria and the right ventricle were discarded and the remaining left ventricle was weighed and stored in 50% glycerol (see *Methods*) for analysis of contractile protein enzyme activity.

RESULTS

General features of the experimental model of renovascular hypertension and its regression are shown in Table 1. Results of body weight, heart weight, blood pressure, and bilateral kidney weight measurements are shown for C and H animals at 10 weeks after the development of hypertension, and in R animals, following the normalization of systolic blood pressure (<150 mm Hg) for an additional 10 weeks. No body weight differences were observed between any of the groups at either time of study. Blood pressure and heart weight values of hypertensive animals showed persistent elevations above controls throughout this study.

Since the left kidney was uniformly involved in the surgical renal artery stenosis, its weight progressively decreased during the course of hypertension

TABLE 1. General features of hypertensive, hypertensive-regression, and control animals

	10 weeks (N)			20 weeks (N)				
	C(8)	p	HT(8)	C(10)	p	HT(10)	p	R(10)
BW (g)	267 ± 5.3	NS	271 ± 4.6	285 ± 5.7	NS	280 ± 6.0	NS	286 ± 6.3
HW (g)	0.66 ± 0.03	≤0.01	0.98 ± 0.04	0.68 ± 0.02	≤0.01	0.96 ± 0.04	≤0.01	0.72 ± 0.02
HW/BW (mg/g)	2.47 ± 0.08	≤0.01	3.62 ± 0.09	2.39 ± 0.10	≤0.01	3.42 ± 0.10	≤0.01	2.51 ± 0.08
BP (mm Hg)	125 ± 5.0	≤0.01	186 ± 5.6	122 ± 5.3	≤0.01	193 ± 7.1	≤0.01	120 ± 6.7
RK (g)	0.93 ± 0.01	≤0.01	1.25 ± 0.07	1.00 ± 0.02	≤0.01	1.45 ± 0.05	≤0.01	2.13 ± 0.04[a]
LK (g)	0.95 ± 0.02	NS	0.91 ± 0.03	0.98 ± 0.04	≤0.01	0.81 ± 0.03	≤0.01	—

C = controls; HT = hypertensives; R = hypertensive-regression. BW = body weight; HW = heart weight; HW/BW = heart weight/body weight ratio; BP = systolic blood pressure; RK = right kidney; LK = left kidney.
Values are expressed as the mean ± SEM. NS = not significant ($p \geq 0.1$).
[a] Significantly different from control ($p \leq 0.01$).

while the contralateral kidney increased in weight significantly above the control level. Blood pressure and heart weight values of H animals dropped precipitously upon removal of the left kidney. Blood pressure decreased to control levels within 24 hr following nephrectomy, while heart weight decreased in a somewhat slower manner. At 20 weeks after the onset of hypertension, heart weights of R animals were virtually identical to those of C animals.

Myocardial Mechanics

Isometric contraction data obtained for all experimental groups are shown in Table 2. Also shown are average muscle length, muscle weight, and calculated cross-sectional area. Muscle weights in H animals were significantly greater than in C animals, although no differences in muscle lengths were observed. Therefore, H muscles displayed a significantly greater cross-sectional area. Calculated cross-sectional areas for all muscles were in the range of 0.85 ± 0.06 to 1.05 ± 0.07.

The time course of representative isometric contractions from C, H, and R muscles are depicted in Fig. 1A. This figure depicts, in addition, the method for measurement of various parameters of isometric force development and its rate of force development. Developed tension remained similar in all three groups throughout the 20-week study. Significant differences were noted in a peak rate of tension fall ($-T'$) between the groups throughout the 20-week period. The time to peak positive rate of force development (TPP) and time to peak negative rate of force decay (TPN) were significantly prolonged in H animals when compared to C or R muscles. R data was virtually identical to that of C.

Time to peak tension and time to ½ relaxation (T½R) increased in H muscles, while R animals showed values similar to those of C. Of note was the fact that TPT and T½R did not show progressive change between 10 and 20 weeks of hypertension.

Passive and active length tension relationships between the three experimental groups are shown in Fig. 2. No differences in resting length–tension relationships were observed at 10 or 20 weeks after the onset of hypertension between C, H, and R animals. Analysis of developed tension showed no significant differences between any of the groups studied.

Force–Velocity Relations

Data from isotonic contractions obtained at a Ca^{2+} concentration of 2.4 mM are shown in Table 3. No significant differences between H, C, and R muscles were observed in the amount of shortening from preload alone at L_{max}. Time to peak shortening (TPS), on the other hand, was significantly prolonged in muscles from H animals at both study points. Velocity of shortening (Vs) at a relative load of 50% was significantly depressed in muscles from

TABLE 2. *Isometric contraction data from hypertensive, hypertensive-regression, and control animals*

	10 weeks (N)			20 weeks (N)				
	C(8)	p	HT(8)	C(10)	p	HT(10)	p	R(10)
ML (mm)	6.0 ± 0.3	NS	6.1 ± 0.3	5.7 ± 0.3	NS	6.1 ± 0.3	NS	6.2 ± 0.3
MW (mg)	5.1 ± 0.3	≤ 0.05	6.4 ± 0.4	5.5 ± 0.4	≤ 0.05	6.6 ± 0.4	NS	6.0 ± 0.4
XS (mm^2)	0.85 ± 0.06	≤ 0.05	1.05 ± 0.07	0.96 ± 0.07	NS	1.08 ± 0.07	NS	0.97 ± 0.07
RT (g/mm^2)	1.94 ± 0.34	NS	2.01 ± 0.40	2.10 ± 0.24	NS	2.05 ± 0.30	NS	1.97 ± 0.31
DT (g/mm^2)	6.3 ± 0.56	NS	6.7 ± 0.51	7.30 ± 0.62	NS	7.89 ± 0.67	NS	7.21 ± 0.45
TPT (msec)	119 ± 1.8	≤ 0.01	153 ± 2.3	125 ± 2.1	≤ 0.01	155 ± 2.3	≤ 0.01	123 ± 1.8
T½R (msec)	143 ± 2.8	≤ 0.01	165 ± 3.0	146 ± 2.7	≤ 0.01	170 ± 2.4	≤ 0.01	144 ± 2.1
+T' (g/sec/mm^2)	101 ± 6.3	NS	96 ± 5.6	96 ± 6.4	NS	89 ± 5.7	NS	97 ± 5.6
−T' (g/sec/mm^2)	56 ± 2.0	NS	54 ± 2.4	53 ± 1.8	NS	51 ± 2.4	NS	55 ± 2.1
TPP (msec)	48 ± 0.3	≤ 0.01	68 ± 0.4	50 ± 0.5	≤ 0.01	71 ± 0.7	≤ 0.01	48 ± 0.4
TPN (msec)	123 ± 2.1	≤ 0.01	145 ± 3.1	126 ± 2.5	≤ 0.01	151 ± 3.4	≤ 0.01	123 ± 2.3

C = controls; HT = hypertensives; R = hypertensive-regression. ML = muscle length at L_{max}; MW = muscle weight; XS = muscle cross-sectional area; RT = resting tension; DT = developed tension; TPT = time to peak tension; T½R = time to ½ relaxation (50% DT); +T' = peak rate of tension rise; −T' = peak rate of tension fall; TPP = time from RT to peak rate of tension rise; TPN = time from peak tension to peak rate of tension fall. Values are expressed as mean ± SE. All values were obtained at a muscle length = L_{max}. NS = not significant ($p \geq 0.1$).

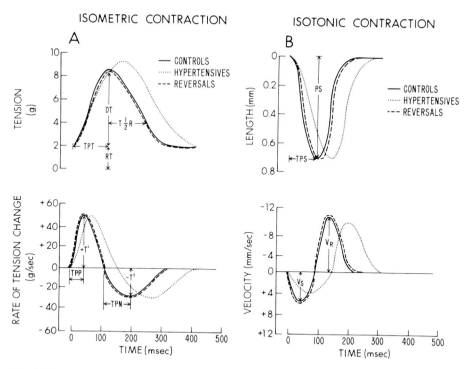

FIG. 1. Papillary muscle contraction at L_{max}. **A**: Isometric contractions from hypertensive, control, and reversal muscles. Tension (**upper panel**) and the rate of tension development (**lower panel**) are plotted against time. Mechanical parameters are indicated by arrows pointing to the control trace. RT = resting tension; DT = developed tension; TPT = time to peak tension; T½R = time to ½ relaxation (50% DT); +T′ = peak rate of tension rise; −T′ = peak rate of tension fall; TPP = time to peak rate of tension rise; TPN = time from peak tension to peak rate of tension fall. **B**: Isotonic contractions from hypertensive, control, and reversal muscles. Relative loads (total isotonic load/total isometric load × 100) were similar for hypertensive, control, and reversal. Muscle length (**upper panel**) and velocity (**lower panel**) are plotted against time. PS = peak shortening; TPS = time to peak shortening; Vs = peak velocity of shortening; Vr = peak velocity of relaxation.

H animals at 10 and 20 weeks after the onset of hypertension. TPS and Vs for R animals were virtually identical to age-matched C data.

Force–velocity relations expressed as a function of relative load for C, H, and R muscles are shown in Fig. 3. Representative isotonic contractions for muscles from C, H, and R animals, shown in Figure 1B, depict the general character of the C, H, and R isotonic contraction. They also illustrate the method by which measurements of shortening and shortening–velocity were measured. Force–velocity curves comparing H and C data at 10 and 20 weeks after the onset of hypertension were significantly depressed in the H muscles at all relative loads studied. Force–velocity curves of muscles from R animals were similar to controls at all relative loads.

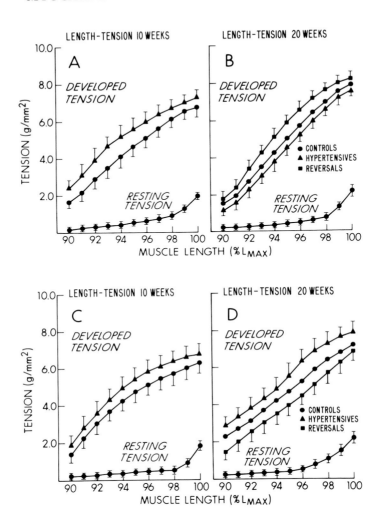

FIG. 2. Resting and development tensions are plotted as a function of muscle length in hypertensive, control, and reversal animals. Values are plotted as the mean ± SEM. Resting tension shown in **A** and **B** is from control animals; resting tension values from hypertensive and reversal groups were not significantly different ($p \geq 0.1$) from controls.

Contractile Protein Enzyme Activity

Table 4 shows actomyosin ATPase activity of preparations from the hearts of control and hypertensive animals. In addition, this table shows ATPase values for animals from this same group at 5 and 30 weeks after the onset of hypertension. Actomyosin ATPase activity was significantly depressed in preparations from hearts of all groups of hypertensive animals. Actomyosin ATPase activity in preparations from the hearts of animals hypertensive for 10 weeks

TABLE 3. *Isotonic contraction data from hypertensive, hypertensive-regression, and control animals*

	10 weeks (N)			20 weeks (N)				
	C(8)	p	HT(8)	C(10)	p	HT(10)	p	R(10)
PS (% ML)	5.8 ± 0.3	NS	5.6 ± 0.4	5.9 ± 0.3	NS	6.1 ± 0.4	NS	6.2 ± 0.3
TPS (msec)	121 ± 3.1	≤0.01	160 ± 5.0	124 ± 2.3	≤0.01	162 ± 5.6	≤0.01	127 ± 3.0
Vs (ML/s)	0.77 ± 0.02	≤0.01	0.61 ± 0.02	0.75 ± 0.02	≤0.01	0.59 ± 0.02	≤0.01	0.76 ± 0.02
Vr (ML/s)	0.98 ± 0.04	NS	0.95 ± 0.03	0.94 ± 0.03	NS	0.93 ± 0.03	NS	0.95 ± 0.03
TVs (msec)	67 ± 3.0	NS	72 ± 2.9	71 ± 2.8	NS	75 ± 2.5	NS	69 ± 2.5
TVr (msec)	48 ± 2.0	≤0.05	58 ± 1.0	52 ± 2.1	≤0.05	61 ± 2.3	≤0.05	50 ± 1.8

C = controls; HT = hypertensives; R = hypertensive-regression. PS = peak shortening; TPS = time to peak shortening; Vs = peak velocity of shortening divided by L_{max}; Vr = peak velocity of relaxation divided by L_{max}; TVs = time to peak velocity of shortening; TVr = time to peak velocity of relaxation; ML = muscle length.

Values are expressed as mean ± SE. Values were obtained at an initial muscle length = L_{max}, and at a relative load (total isotonic load/total isometric load × 100) of 50%. NS = not significant ($p \geq 0.1$).

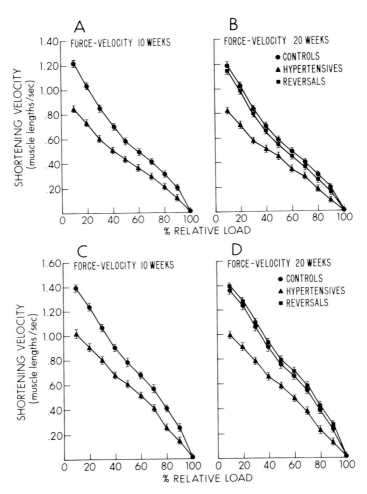

FIG. 3. Normalized force–velocity relations for a series of afterloaded isotonic contractions at an initial muscle length of L_{max}. Force is expressed as the percent relative load (total isotonic load/total isometric load × 100). Velocity is expressed as the number of muscle lengths per second, calculated as the peak velocity (in mm/sec) divided by L_{max}. Values are plotted as mean ± SEM. Significant differences were observed between control and hypertensive preparations at all loads studied; reversals were not significantly different from controls. **A**: Female hypertensive and control values at 10 weeks after the onset of hypertension. **B**: Female hypertensive, control, and reversal values at 20 weeks after the onset of hypertension.

and then normotensive for an additional 10 weeks (R) was not significantly depressed as compared to the actomyosin ATPase activity in preparations from control animals. The SDS gel electrophoretic bands for hypertensive, control, and hypertensive-reversal animals did not show any visible differences. Although actomyosin ATPase activity was significantly depressed at the end of

5 weeks of hypertension, it decreased further in the tenth week and then remained stable from the tenth to the thirtieth week after the onset of hypertension.

DISCUSSION

The precise delineation of the course and degree of contractile alterations in the pressure-overload hypertrophied heart is important in the critical evaluation and clinical treatment of hypertensive conditions. Use of a pertinent experimental model of pressure-overload hypertrophy, namely chronic renovascular hypertension in the rat, permits the detailed investigation of mechanical alterations in hypertrophied myocardium. In the present study, creation of a left renal artery stenosis resulted in the gradual application of a pressure overload. Ten weeks after the development of hypertension, normalization of systolic blood pressure was produced by unilateral nephrectomy of the ischemic kidney and experiments were conducted to determine the reversibility of the observed contractile abnormalities. This model of gradually applied pressure overload avoids the acute contractile failure of aortic or pulmonary artery banding (4) and the rapid increase in connective tissue that may result from an acute overload (10).

In examining the effects of pressure overload on heart function in dogs three days after bilateral renal artery constriction, Ferrario et al. (17) found that the relationship described by stroke volume and end-diastolic pressure was shifted downward and to the right. In the same study, dogs with severe hypertension had significantly greater left ventricular end-diastolic pressures (12 ± 2 mm Hg) as compared to animals with moderate hypertension (7 ± 3 mm Hg). Further, under conditions of fluid loading, hypertensive animals were unable to increase cardiac output to a similar degree as control animals.

TABLE 4. *Actomyosin ATPase activity in hearts of hypertensive, hypertensive-regression, and control animals*

Time after onset of hypertension	Control		Hypertensive		Hypertensive-regression
5 weeks	0.702 ± 0.007 (4)		0.652 ± 0.003 (4)		
p		≤ 0.01			
10 weeks	0.705 ± 0.006 (5)		0.523 ± 0.017 (4)		
p		≤ 0.01			
20 weeks	0.669 ± 0.008 (7)		0.560 ± 0.023 (12)		0.668 ± 0.017[a] (9)
p		≤ 0.01		≤ 0.05	
30 weeks	0.657 ± 0.008 (4)		0.499 ± 0.022 (5)		
p		≤ 0.01			

Results are shown as μmoles Pi/mg/min at 30°C. Values are expressed as mean $\pm$ SEM. Numbers of preparations used are shown in parentheses.

[a] Not significantly different from control value.

Utilizing bilateral renal artery constriction in rats, Ferrone et al. (16) found that renovascular hypertensive, spontaneous hypertensive, and control animals had similar cardiac outputs. Although these investigators studied the effects of hypertension only 14 days after the initiation of the pressure overload, they did find that total peripheral resistance was elevated significantly and to the same degree in either model of hypertension. Using a two-kidney, one-clip, Goldblatt hypertensive rat, Averill et al. (3) determined from cardiac function curves that chronic renovascular hypertension was associated with a depressed cardiac reserve, due either to diminished contractility or reduced ventricular compliance. Despite significant hypertrophy (44%) in this model, there was a twofold increase in myocardial connective tissue, which may account for the observed reduction in ventricular compliance. In addition, the rate of rise of blood pressure and the duration of hypertension prior to study was highly variable (6–22 weeks after the onset of hypertension), which prevents complete interpretation of their results due to poor control of these important factors.

Examining pressure-overload hypertrophy created by surgical constriction of the pulmonary artery in cats, Spann et al. (11) and Carey et al. (12) have shown, using isolated right ventricular papillary muscles, that contractility is depressed, while Natarajan and co-workers (30) concluded that this depression may, in part, be due to an increase in the stiffness of hypertrophied muscles. However, using the lathyrogen b-amino propriontrile, which inhibits the cross-linking of both collagen and elastin, Bing et al. (6) concluded that alterations associated with myocardial contractility occur independent of elevated connective tissue. Maughan et al. (27), studying chemically skinned right ventricular muscle bundles from hypertrophied rabbit hearts, correlated mechanical and biochemical changes. They found a 34% reduction in velocity of shortening (Vs) and a similar depression in the Ca^{2+} and actin-activated, myosin ATPase activity, showing a clear correlation between depressions of velocity of shortening and ATPase activity in hypertrophied muscle.

Measures of actomyosin ATPase activity as carried out in this study reflect the myosin ATPase activity of pure myosin (33). The present observations of depressed ATPase activity provide one explanation for the diminished contractile function from the hearts of hypertensive-hypertrophied rats. It is unlikely that the altered ATPase activity totally explains the mechanical abnormality. However, the decreased rates of relaxation observed in papillary muscles from hypertensive-hypertrophied hearts (9) suggest that there is some alteration at the level of the sarcoplasmic reticulum, as observed in other models of hypertrophy (35).

In the experiments described above, we have shown that hypertrophied myocardium taken from a stable, gradual-onset model of pressure overload is able to maintain normal levels of peak isometric tension despite depressions in the preloaded velocity of muscle shortening and myosin ATPase activity. This situation is possible only if the duration of contraction (TPT) is simultaneously prolonged—which was the observation made. The fact that reversal of hypertension (relief of the pressure load) returned all mechanical and biochemical alterations to control levels indicates that 10 weeks of hypertension in this experimental model does not result in irreversible myocardial damage. The mechanisms responsible for the reversible alterations in contractile behavior in 10-week hypertrophied myocardium are not clear, but the results suggest that viable myocardial fibers enlarge in response to a gradual pressure overload and initially develop disturbances of the excitation–contraction coupling sequence and probably the contractile protein interaction. The trigger elements, or the link between the pressure overload and the cellular enlargement of viable myocardial fibers, is still not clear. In addition, factors responsible for the observed reversibility of the contractile and biochemical alterations, as well as the longest duration of reversibility obtainable in this model, are important issues that are currently under study in longer term experiments.

ACKNOWLEDGMENT

This work was supported in part by NIH grants H1 21993-03, HL 07071-05, and HL 15498. The authors thank Renée M. Remily for her technical assistance.

REFERENCES

1. Alpert, N. R., Hamrell, B. B., and Halpern, W. (1974): *Circ. Res.*, 34:71–82.
2. Anderson, P. A. W., Manring, A., Arentzen, C. E., Rankin, J. S., and Johnson, E. A. (1976): *Circulation*, 53:II–33.
3. Averill, D. B., Ferrario, C. M., Tarazi, R. C., Sen, S., and Bajbus, R. (1976): *Circ. Res.*, 38:280–288.
4. Beznak, M., Korecky, B., and Thomas, G. (1969): *Can. J. Physiol. Pharmacol.*, 47:579–586.
5. Bham, A. K., and Scheuer, J. (1972): *Am. J. Physiol.*, 223:1486–1490.
6. Bing, O. H. L., Fanburg, B. L., Brooks, W. W., and Matsushita, S. (1978): *Circ. Res.*, 43(4):632–637.
7. Bing, O. H. L., Matsushita, S., Fanburg, B. L., and Levine, H. J. (1971): *Circ. Res.*, 28:234–245.
8. Bishop, S. P. (1972): In: *Comparative Pathophysiology of Circulatory Disturbances*, edited by C. M. Bloor, pp. 289–314. Plenum Press, New York.
9. Breisch, E. A., Bove, A. A., and Phillips, S. J. (1980): *Cardiovasc. Res.*, 14:161–168.
10. Buccino, R. H., Harris, E., Spann, J. F., and Sonnenblick, E. H. (1969): *Am. J. Physiol.*, 216:425–428.
11. Capasso, J. M., Strobeck, J. E., and Sonnenblick, E. H. (1981): *Am. J. Physiol.*, 241:H435–H441.
12. Carey, R. A., Bone, A. A., Coulson, R. L., and Spann, J. F. (1978): *Am. J. Physiol.*, 234:H711–H717.
13. Cooper, G., IV., Puga, F. J., Zujko, K. J., Harrison, C. E., and Coleman, H. N., III (1973): *Circ. Res.*, 32:140–148.
14. Cooper, G., IV, Satava, M., Jr., Harrison, C. E., and Coleman, H. N., III (1973): *Circ. Res.*, 33:213–233.
15. Coulson, R. L., Yazdanfar, S., Rubio, E., Bove, A. A., Lemole, G. M., and Spann, J. F. (1977): *Circ. Res.*, 40:41–49.
16. Dodge, H. T., Grimer, M., and Stewart, D. K. (1974): *Circ. Res.*, 34:122–127.
17. Ferrario, C. M., Kosoglov, A., Bajbus, R., and Madzan, G. R. (1976): *Clin. Sci. Mol. Med.*, 51:141s–143s.
18. Ferrone, R. A., Walsh, G. M., Tsuchiya, M., and Frohlich, E. D. (1979): *Am. J. Physiol.*, 236:H403–H408.

19. Fiske, C. H., and Subbarow, Y. (1925): *J. Biol. Chem.*, 66:375–400.
20. Graham, T. P., Jr., Jarmakani, J. M., Canent, R. U., Jr., and Anderson, P. A. W. (1971): *Circulation*, 44:1043–1052.
21. Grimm, A. F., Kubota, R., and Whitehorn, W. V. (1963): *Circ. Res.*, 12:118–124.
22. Hatt, P. Y., Jouannot, P., Moravec, J., Perennec, J., and Laplace, M. (1978): *Bas. Res. Cardiol.*, 73:405–421.
23. Hickson, R. C., Hammons, G. T., and Holloszy, J. O. (1979): *Am. J. Physiol.*, 236:H268–H272.
24. Jouannot, P., and Hatt, P. Y. (1975): *Am. J. Physiol.*, 299:355–364.
25. Kerr, A., Winterberger, A. R., and Giambattista, M. (1961): *Circ. Res.*, 9:103–105.
26. Lund, D. D., Twietmeyer, T. A., Schmild, P. G., and Tomanek, R. J. (1979): *Cardiovasc. Res.*, 13:39–44.
27. Maughan, D., Low, E., Litten, R., Brayden, J., and Alpert, N. (1979): *Circ. Res.*, 44:279–287.
28. Meerson, F. Z., and Kapelko, V. I. (1972): *Cardiology*, 57:183–199.
29. Mehmel, H. C., Mazzoni, S., and Krayenbuhl, H. D. (1975): *Am. Heart J.*, 90:236–240.
30. Natarajan, N., Bove, A. A., Coulson, R. L., Carey, R. A., and Spann, J. F. (1979): *Am. J. Physiol.*, 237:H676–H680.
31. Pool, P. E., Chandler, B. M., Sonnenblick, E. H., and Braunwald, E. (1978): *Circ. Res.*, 22:213–219.
32. Sasayama, S., Ross, J., Franklin, D., Bloor, C. M., Bishop, S., and Dilley, R. B. (1977): *Circ. Res.*, 38:172–178.
33. Scheuer, J., and Bhan, A. K. (1979): *Circ. Res.*, 45:1–12.
34. Spann, J. F., Jr., Covell, J. W., Eckberg, D. L., Sonnenblick, E. H., Ross, J., Jr., and Braunwald, E. (1972): *Am. J. Physiol.*, 233:1150–1157.
35. Spech, M. M., Ferrario, C. M., and Tarazi, R. C. (1980): *Hypertension*, 2:75–82.
36. Suko, J. (1971): *Biochem. Biophys. Acta*, 252:324–327.
37. Taylor, R. R., Covell, J. W., and Ross, J., Jr. (1968): *J. Clin. Invest.*, 47:1333–1342.
38. Turina, M., Bussmann, W. D., and Krayenbuhl, H. D. (1969): *Cardiovas. Res.*, 3:486–495.
39. Weber, K., and Osborn, M. (1969): *J. Biol. Chem.*, 224:4406–4412.
40. Weigman, D. L., Joshua, I. G., Morff, R. J., Harris, P. D., and Miller, F. N. (1979): *Am. J. Physiol.*, 236:H545–H548.
41. Williams, J. P., Jr., Harrison, T. R., Grollman, A. (1939): *J. Clin. Invest.*, 18:373–376.

*Perspectives in Cardiovascular
Research, Vol. 8,*
edited by R. C. Tarazi and J. B. Dunbar.
Raven Press, New York © 1983.

Cardiac Hypertrophy in the Spontaneously Hypertensive Rat: Adaptation or Primary Myopathy?

Marc A. Pfeffer and Janice M. Pfeffer

*Department of Medicine, Harvard Medical School, Brigham and
Women's Hospital, Boston, Massachusetts 02115*

The development of left ventricular hypertrophy in systemic hypertension is an adaptive response that permits the left ventricle to sustain the excessive pressure load. In fact, most individuals with systemic hypertension and left ventricular hypertrophy are asymptomatic and have normal ventricular volumes and contractile indices despite the elevated arterial pressures (1–3). However, other hypertensive individuals develop symptoms of left ventricular dysfunction, which may severely compromise the quality and duration of life. Indeed, in the Framingham cohort, hypertension was the most common precursor of the development of clinically detectable congestive heart failure (4).

The spontaneously hypertensive rat (SHR) was developed by the selective inbreeding of Wistar rats demonstrating elevations of systolic arterial pressure (5). Since 1963, the SHR has exhibited a 100% incidence of severe systemic hypertension and has been used as an animal model for studies of the genesis and consequences of systemic hypertension. These genetically hypertensive rats develop many of the cardiovascular lesions observed in hypertensive humans (6). Most significantly, the SHR have an attenuated lifespan that can be effectively prolonged by antihypertensive therapy (7,8).

Although it appears that the SHR provides an excellent experimental model for studies of the effects of sustained hypertension on left ventricular performance, the question has been raised as to whether or not these rats have a primary defect in myocardial contractility in addition to genetic hypertension (7,8). Indeed, a few studies have shown that the stroke volume of even the young SHR is reduced compared to that of normotensive rats and thus cardiac performance is depressed at an early age (7–9). This has lead to the speculation that the SHR has a cardiomyopathy with an intrinsic defect in cardiac function that is not the result of sustained hypertension. On the other hand, ours and other studies on left ventricular performance in the SHR indicated that the SHR demonstrates a stable phase of adaptive ventricular hypertrophy (10–14). Although we have demonstrated ventricular dysfunction in the SHR, it occurred only at an advanced age and with severe left ventricular hypertrophy

(12,13,15–17). Furthermore, antihypertensive therapy has been effective in preventing the development of ventricular dysfunction (12), suggesting that the dysfunction is a consequence of the level and duration of hypertension and not the result of an intrinsic genetic defect in the myocardium. The focus of this chapter is to address the controversy concerning cardiac performance of the SHR: Does hypertrophy of the left ventricle of the SHR represent an adaptive response that permits the heart to sustain elevated workloads, or is the increase in left ventricular mass the result of an intrinsic defect in ventricular performance that is not produced by systemic hypertension?

CARDIAC PERFORMANCE

Papillary Muscle

Several laboratories have examined the mechanical properties of papillary muscles isolated from the left ventricles of normotensive Wistar rats and SHR and found that the muscles from SHR functioned as well as those from normotensive rats (10,18,19). In no instance was the force–velocity relationship of the papillary muscle from the SHR depressed. Indeed, the length–active tension relationship demonstrated that the papillary muscles from SHR have an augmented ability to develop force when compared to papillary muscles from normotensive rats at similar muscle lengths. Therefore, the finding of normal or supranormal mechanical function of papillary muscles from SHR supports the concept of an adaptive hypertrophy and provides evidence against the hypothesis of a primary cardiomyopathy in the SHR.

Isolated Heart

Although the papillary muscle from hypertrophied left ventricles of SHR demonstrated adaptive hyperfunction, overall ventricular performance could still be impaired as a result of an altered ventricular geometry or compliance. Noresson et al. (20) developed an isolated working left ventricle preparation in which Frank-Starling curves were generated by varying preload. These curves (stroke volume versus filling pressure) were determined over a wide range of arterial pressures. When arterial pressure was maintained at normotensive levels, the left ventricles of SHR ejected stroke volumes similar to those of control rats over the entire range of filling pressures. However, as the pressure against which the left ventricle ejected was elevated, the stroke volume of the normotensive hearts was reduced to a greater extent than that of the SHR. Therefore, at higher arterial pressures the isolated left ventricle of the SHR pumped a considerably greater stroke volume than that of normotensive rats for any given filling pressure (Fig. 1). As in the papillary muscle studies, the performance of the isolated left ventricle of SHR was similar to that of normotensive rats and, in fact, demonstrated an augmented capacity to eject blood at higher workloads.

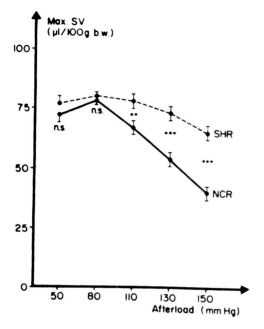

FIG. 1. The relationship between maximal stroke volume (max SV) and mean arterial pressure of hearts isolated from SHR and normotensive control (NCR) rats. **p < 0.01; ***p < 0.001. (From ref. 20, with permission.)

Intact Heart

We found that the alterations in stroke volume of the intact left ventricles of normotensive rats and SHR to elevations in systemic pressure were very similar to the observations in the isolated heart (21). The stroke volume of young adult SHR was similar to that of normotensive rats at mean arterial pressure levels between 120 to 140 mm Hg (Fig. 2). As arterial pressure was

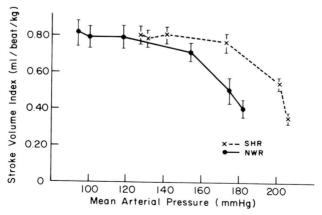

FIG. 2. Alterations in stroke volume index of the intact heart of SHR and normotensive Wistar rats (NWR) to acute elevations in mean arterial pressure during graded infusions of methoxamine.

elevated to levels between 160 to 175 mm Hg with increasing doses of meth-oxamine, the stroke volume of the normotensive rats progressively declined, whereas the stroke volume of the SHR was maintained, demonstrating that the hypertrophied left ventricle of the SHR is well adapted to sustain forward output against elevated pressure levels. Therefore, studies of papillary muscles and isolated and intact hearts provide strong evidence that the left ventricle of SHR undergoes an adaptive hypertrophic growth and does not support the concept of an intrinsic cardiomyopathy in the SHR.

SYSTEMIC HEMODYNAMICS

The suggestion of an intrinsic defect in left ventricular function in the SHR was based on the observation of Cutilletta and co-workers (7,8) that the stroke volume and cardiac output of young SHR anesthetized with pentobarbital were reduced compared to those of normotensive rats. Moreover, these investigators postulated that this ventricular dysfunction was an inherent trait of the SHR and was not related to the systemic hypertension. Spech, Ferrario, and Tarazi (9) reported that the stroke volume and cardiac indices of the SHR were less than those of normotensive rats under both basal and volume loaded conditions, and thus provided some support for this concept of left ventricular dysfunction early in SHR hypertension. However, these observations are at variance with a large number of studies in both anesthetized (6,10,11,13,22–27) and unanesthetized rats (26,28–32), which have demonstrated normal stroke volume and cardiac indices in SHR despite elevations in arterial pressure and peripheral resistance. Smith and Hutchins (29) made serial measurements of systemic hemodynamics in unanesthetized SHR and found that the cardiac index of SHR was equal to or greater than that of age-matched Wistar-Kyoto rats. Indeed, the external cardiac work of the SHR was consistently greater than that of normotensive rats.

The cardiac reserve capacity of young and mature SHR, as assessed by the peak stroke volume and cardiac indices attained with a rapid intravascular volume loading, was also comparable to that of normotensive rats (10,12,13). Comparisons of peak cardiac performance, using the intact heart preparation, are notoriously difficult because of the differences in loading conditions of the ventricle. Indeed, estimates of afterload based on left ventricular mass, volume, and systolic pressure confirmed that the SHR left ventricle operates against an increased afterload (33). However, as in the isolated heart (20), the intact left ventricle of the SHR is capable of sustaining normal baseline and stressed forward outputs despite the adverse load (21). These observations provide further evidence that ventricular hypertrophy is adaptive since the increased ventricular mass permits the SHR to maintain a normal forward output despite a marked elevation in arterial pressure.

RELATION OF VENTRICULAR DYSFUNCTION AND
ARTERIAL PRESSURE

Primary ventricular dysfunction is a central component in the scheme for the development of SHR hypertension proposed by Cutilletta and co-workers (7). According to their theory, a primary myocardial abnormality results in cardiac hypertrophy (which is not secondary to hypertension) and a reduced stroke volume. Sympathetic activity is increased secondarily in an attempt to maintain the cardiac output of the impaired left ventricle. The proponents of this theory claim that the increased sympathetic activity, in addition to providing extrinsic support for the genetically impaired ventricle, also elevates peripheral resistance and arterial pressure. This primary defect in ventricular contraction and the secondary augmentation of sympathetic activity thus result in the hemodynamic profile of a reduced cardiac output and an elevated arterial pressure in young SHR.

As already mentioned, this finding of a reduced cardiac output, which is central to the cardiomyopathy hypothesis, has not been substantiated by other investigators of the hemodynamic characteristics of either anesthetized or unanesthetized SHR. Moreover, there is little evidence to support the hypothesis that an impaired left ventricle may play a central role in the development of SHR hypertension. Indeed, we offer the opposite hypothesis: That a well adapted left ventricle is essential for the manifestation of SHR hypertension, and that an impairment in ventricular performance results in a reduction, not an elevation, of arterial pressure. This compensatory phase of cardiac hypertrophy in SHR is supported by the observations of papillary muscle, isolated left ventricle, and intact heart preparations described above. In each instance, the hypertrophied left ventricle of the SHR was capable of developing more force or of ejecting a normal stroke volume against higher arterial pressures than the nonhypertrophied left ventricle of normotensive rats.

Further support for the concept that a well adapted left ventricle is required for the expression of SHR hypertension has been provided by studies in which experimental myocardial infarctions produced graded degrees of left ventricular dysfunction in SHR and normotensive rats (34). Whether the rats were genetically normotensive or hypertensive, an impairment in left ventricular function was associated with a reduction in the level of arterial pressure. In both SHR and normotensive rats the magnitude of the reduction in pressure was directly proportional to the size of the myocardial infarction. Attempts to return the arterial pressure of the SHR with myocardial infarctions to levels comparable to those of SHR without infarctions underscored the importance of adaptive hypertrophy in the manifestation of SHR hypertension. Graded infusions of the alpha-adrenergic agonist, methoxamine, were used to increase the systemic vascular resistance of SHR with and without healed myocardial infarctions. The resistance level at each dose of methoxamine was similar in all groups of infarcted and noninfarcted SHR. However, both arterial pressure and cardiac output at each dose of methoxamine were considerably reduced in SHR with myocardial infarctions compared to noninfarcted SHR. Indeed, the relationship of either cardiac output or stroke volume to arterial pressure in SHR with myocardial infarctions was very similar to that of the noninfarcted normotensive rats (Fig. 2); that is to say, in the lower range of arterial pressures, normal flows were sustained, but in the higher range of arterial pressures, forward flows were reduced. Both the noninfarcted left ventricle of normotensive rats and the infarcted left ventricle of SHR were unable to sustain cardiac output at the elevated level of arterial pressure in which the noninfarcted ventricle of SHR functions normally. Contrary to the hypothesis that ventricular dysfunction leads to SHR hypertension, experimentally-induced dysfunction resulted in a reduction in arterial pressure. A well adapted, hypertrophied left ventricle is necessary for the SHR to maintain cardiac output against the elevated arterial pressure levels and thus manifest its genetic hypertension.

RELATION OF VENTRICULAR WEIGHT AND ARTERIAL PRESSURE

The lack of a strong direct correlation between terminal systolic pressure determinations and heart weight in the SHR has been used as suggestive evidence that the cardiac hypertrophy in these animals is not the result of their hypertension. Similarly, the apparent dissociation between the lowering of blood pressure by certain antihypertensive agents in the SHR and ventricular weight has contributed to the concept of a cardiomyopathy in these animals (35–37). Although these observations suggest that the heart weight of the SHR cannot be predicted by short-term arterial pressure determinations, they do not necessarily support the contention that the ventricular hypertrophy of the SHR is not produced or sustained by abnormal hemodynamic conditions. Heart weight should not be directly related simply to arterial pressure but, more appropriately, to afterload, in that other factors such as ventricular chamber volume and wall thickness are required to estimate the stresses against which the myocardium contracts. The duration of the hypertension must also be considered in any attempt to relate arterial pressure levels to cardiac mass. Clearly, the young person with new onset hypertension would not be expected to have the same degree of left ventricular hypertrophy as the older individual with comparable, but long-standing elevations of arterial pressure. Similarly, in the mature SHR, left ventricular weight increases despite the maintenance of relatively stable arterial pressure levels (12). Moreover, with advanced hypertensive heart disease and marked ventricular hypertrophy, arterial pressure levels may actually decline with the development of congestive heart failure (6,15). Therefore, the absence of a strong direct correlation between arterial pressure and heart weight does not imply that the two variables are unrelated.

The administration of antihypertensive drugs may variously affect neurohumoral and volume mechanisms that provide other stimuli for cardiac growth. The lack of regression of ventricular hypertrophy of the SHR following 6 weeks of effective antihypertensive therapy with vasodilators (hydralazine or minoxidil) does not indicate that the hypertrophy was unrelated to the hypertensive process (35,36). However, it is noteworthy that more chronic administration of hydralazine was effective in preventing the increase in ventricular weight that occurs in the aging SHR (17). Other antihypertensive agents have been even more effective in reducing the left ventricular mass of the SHR (17,38,39) and in returning the increased ratio of left ventricular mass to cavitary volume (concentric hypertrophy) toward normal (17). For the most part, effective antihypertensive therapy results in a reduction in ventricular weight in SHR.

SUMMARY

The SHR has been criticized as an animal model for hypertensive heart disease. A few studies have suggested that ventricular dysfunction and hypertrophy occur independently of the systemic hypertension in SHR. However, a large majority of hemodynamic studies have reported that ventricular performance is well maintained in SHR despite an augmented workload. Indeed, the mechanical properties of papillary muscles from these genetically hypertensive rats, as well as ejection characteristics of the isolated and intact left ventricles, have demonstrated that the SHR heart is capable of developing more force and of sustaining higher workloads than hearts from normotensive rats. Numerous hemodynamic studies have also shown that the SHR maintain normal systemic flows despite marked elevations in arterial pressure and moderate left ventricular hypertrophy. Therefore, we believe that the left ventricular hypertrophy of the SHR is an adaptive response to systemic hypertension and not a primary cardiomyopathy.

REFERENCES

1. Karliner, J. S., Williams, D., Gorwit, J., Crawford, M. H., and O'Rourke, R. A. (1977): *British Heart J.,* 29:1239–1245.
2. Savage, D. D., Drayer, J. I. M., Henry, W. L., Mathews, E. C., Ware, J. H., Gardin, J. M., Cohen, E. R., Epstein, S. E., and Laragh, J. H. (1979): *Circulation,* 59:623–632.
3. Takahashi, M., Sasayama, S., Kawai, C., and Kotoura, H. (1980): *Circulation,* 62:116–126.
4. Kannel, W. B. (1974): *Cardiovasc. Dis.,* 27:5–24.
5. Okamoto, K., and Aoki, K. (1963): *Jap. Circ. J.,* 27:282–293.
6. Nagaoka, A., Kawaji, H., Imai, Y., and Fukui, H. (1970): *Jap. J. Pharmacol.,* 20:509–516.
7. Cutilletta, A. F., Benjamin, M., Culpepper, W. S., and Oparil, S. (1978): *J. Molec. Cell. Cardiol.,* 10:689–703.
8. Cutilletta, A. F., Erinoff, L., Heller, A., Low, S., and Oparil, S. (1977): *Circ. Res.,* 40:428–437.
9. Spech, M. M., Ferrario, C. M., and Tarazi, R. C. (1980): *Hypertension,* 2:75–82.
10. Burger, S. B., and Strauer, B. E. (1981): In: *The Heart in Hypertension,* edited by B. E. Strauer, pp. 13–52. Springer-Verlag, Berlin.

11. Pfeffer, M. A., and Frohlich, E. D. (1973): *Circ. Res. (Suppl.)*, 32:I29–38.
11a. Pfeffer, M. A., Frohlich, E. D., Pfeffer, J. M., and Weiss, A. K. (1974): *Circ. Res.*, 34:235–244.
12. Pfeffer, J. M., Pfeffer, M. A., Fishbein, M. C. and Frohlich, E. D. (1979): *Am. J. Physiol.*, 237:H461–H468.
13. Pfeffer, M. A., Pfeffer, J. M., and Frohlich, E. D. (1976): *Circ. Res.*, 38:423–429.
14. Freis, E. D., and Ragan, D. (1975): *Proc. Soc. Exp. Biol. Med.*, 150:422–424.
15. Pfeffer, J. M., Pfeffer, M. A., and Braunwald, E. (1983): In: *Perspectives in Cardiovascular Research, Vol. 7,* edited by N. Alpert, pp. 73–84. Raven Press, New York.
16. Pfeffer, J., Pfeffer, M., Fletcher, P. and Braunwald, E. (1979): *Am. J. Cardiol.*, 44:994–998.
17. Pfeffer, J. M., Pfeffer, M. A., Fletcher, P. J., Fishbein, M. C. and Braunwald, E. (1982): *Am. J. Physiol.*, 242:H776-784.
18. Weiss, L. (1974): *Acta Physiol. Scand.*, 91:393–408.
19. Heller, L. J. (1978): *Am. J. Physiol.*, 235:H82–H86.
20. Noresson, E., Ricksten, S. E., Hallbäck-Nordlander, M., and Thorén, P. (1979): *Acta Phys. Scand.*, 107:1–8.
21. Pfeffer, M. A., and Frohlich, E. D. (1973): *Am. J. Physiol.*, 224:1066–1071.
22. Albrecht, I. (1974): *Japan. Circ. J.*, 38:991–996.
23. Hiley, C. R., and Yates, M. S. (1978): *Clin. Sci. Molec. Med.*, 55:317–320.
24. Iriuchijima, J. (1973): *Jap. Heart J.*, 14:267–272.
25. Iriuchijima, J., Numao, Y., and Suga, H. (1975): *Jap. Heart J.*, 16:257–264.
26. Tobia, A. J., Lee, J. Y., and Walsh, G. M. (1974): *Cardiovasc. Res.*, 8:758–762.
27. Tobia, A. J., Walsh, G. M., and Lee, J. Y. (1974): *Proc. Soc. Exp. Biol. Med.*, 146:670–673.
28. Ferrone, R. A., Walsh, G. M., Tsuchiya, M., and Frohlich, E. D. (1979): *Am. J. Physiol.*, 236:H403–H408.
29. Smith, T. L., and Hutchins, P. M. (1979): *Hypertension*, 1:508–517.
30. Tsuchiya, M., Walsh, G. M., and Frohlich, E. D. (1977): *Am. J. Physiol.*, 233:617–621.
31. Walsh, G. M., Baricos, W. H., and MacPhee, A. A. (1978): *Res. Comm. Chem. Pathol. Pharmacol.*, 22:135–143.
32. Walsh, G. M., Tsuchiya, M., Cox, A. C., Tobia, A. J., and Frohlich, E. D. (1978): *Am. J. Physiol.*, 234:H275–H279.
33. Mirsky, I., Pfeffer, J. M., and Pfeffer, M. A. (1983): In: *Perspectives in Cardiovascular Research, Vol. 7,* edited by N. Alpert, pp. 39–55. Raven Press, New York.
34. Fletcher, P. J., Pfeffer, J. M., Pfeffer, M. A., and Braunwald, E. (1980): *Clin. Sci.*, 59:385–387.
35. Sen, S., Tarazi, R. C., Khairallah, P. A., and Bumpus, F. M. (1974): *Circ. Res.*, 35:775–781.
36. Sen, S., Tarazi, R. C., and Bumpus, F. M. (1977): *Cardiovasc. Res.*, 11:427–433.
37. Tomanek, R. J. (1979): *Lab. Invest.*, 40:83–91.
38. Antonaccio, M. J., Rubin, B., Horovitz, Z. P., Laffan, R. J., Goldberg, M. E., High, J. P., Harris, D. N., and Zaidi, I. (1979): *Jap. J. Pharmacol.*, 29:285–294.
39. Sen, S., Tarazi, R. C., and Bumpus, F. M. (1980): *Hypertension*, 2:169–176.
40. Bing, O. H. L., Farber, S., and Wiegner, A. W. (1980): *Circulation (Suppl.)*, 62:13.
41. Tadepalli, A. S., Walsh, G. M., and Tobia, A. J. (1974): *Life Sci.*, 15:1103–1114.

*Perspectives in Cardiovascular
Research, Vol. 8,*
edited by R. C. Tarazi and J. B. Dunbar.
Raven Press, New York © 1983.

Mechanical and Structural Aspects of the Hypertrophied Human Myocardium

Karl T. Weber, Joseph S. Janicki, and Sanjeev Shroff

*Cardiovascular–Pulmonary Division, Department of Medicine,
University of Pennsylvania, Philadelphia, Pennsylvania 19104*

Structurally, the myocardium is composed of cardiac muscle fibers and a coronary vasculature, which are tethered within an extensive network of connective tissue (1). Functionally, the myocardium may be viewed as a muscular pump whose dynamic behavior is determined by the elastic properties, or stress–strain relation, of its muscular and connective tissue elements (2–3). Myocardial mass increases and cardiac muscle hypertrophies when the work requirements of the ventricle are elevated for any prolonged period of time. This applies to the physiological stress of exercise training and the excessive hemodynamic work that accompanies cardiac disease (4). The response in connective tissue to conditions of chronic overloading remains unclear, although there is evidence to suggest that collagen occupies a larger proportion of the hypertrophied, pressure-overloaded myocardium (5–7). An excessive formation of the collagenous matrix or endoskeleton of the myocardium would reduce its elasticity and compromise both the stretching and shortening of the cardiac muscle fibers. This structural remodeling of the myocardium would have significant implications as to the pathogenesis of cardiac pump failure. In this chapter we will examine how hypertrophy affects systolic wall stress and the functional architecture of the diseased human heart. We will also review our observations (7) on the increased collagen content of the hypertrophied human myocardium that accompanies the chronic left ventricular pressure overload of systemic hypertension.

STRESS AND STRAIN OF THE MYOCARDIUM

In considering the relationship between stress and strain of the myocardium, it is necessary to describe the force that exists across the myocardium in any given direction and the resulting deformation.

Wall Force

The force that exists across the myocardium in any given plane may be described as follows. Consider the heart to be filled with blood under a given pressure. If an imaginary horizontal plane divides the heart in half, as shown in Fig. 1, a force exists on either side of the plane, tending to pull the heart apart. This force in grams, which is equal to the product of chamber pressure and the cross-sectional area of chamber included in the plane, is counterbalanced by an equal and opposite force within the myocardium, which holds the heart together. Because this force runs perpendicular to the horizontal plane, it represents the net longitudinal force in the myocardium included in the plane. As can also be seen in Fig. 1, the cross-sectional area of the left ventricular (LV) chamber near the base of the heart is obviously greater than

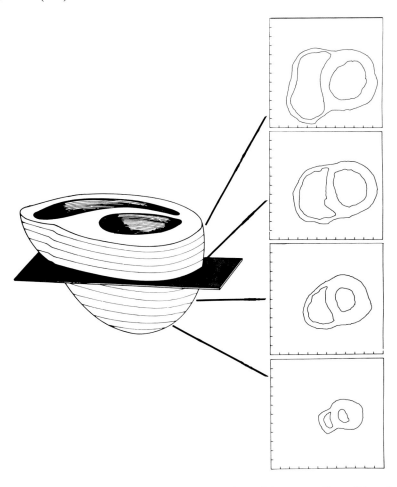

FIG. 1. The longitudinal force that exists in any given plane of the myocardium will be a function of ventricular pressure and the cross-sectional area of the ventricular chamber included in the plane. Because chamber area is greater at the base of the heart, longitudinal force will be greater there. Stress describes the distribution of wall force in any given plane over the corresponding cross-sectional area of myocardium.

that at the apex. The apex-to-base variation in transverse LV chamber area is shown in the left panel of Fig. 2. In accordance with this configuration, longitudinal force at the base of the LV will exceed that at the apex based on the difference in these cross-sectional chamber areas.

A circumferential force also exists in the myocardium, running perpendicular to any vertical plane passing through the long axis of the heart. Because this plane transcribes a larger cross-sectional area of the normally elliptical, human left ventricular chamber, circumferential force will exceed longitudinal force by the ratio of major-to-minor areas of the chamber. We have found this ratio to be 2:2. These concepts emphasize the central role of ventricular size and shape in establishing the two major components of net well force. Other components, such as radial and torsional forces (2), will not be discussed here.

Wall Stress

The distribution of the longitudinal and circumferential forces over their corresponding cross-sectional areas of myocardium represents longitudinal and circumferential wall stress (g/cm^2), respectively. Therefore, stress is inversely proportional to the area or thickness of myocardium. In the right panel of Fig. 2, the distribution of cross-sectional muscle area is shown as a function of the length of the LV chamber. The linear ($r = 0.84$) relationship between the cross-sectional area of LV myocardium and LV chamber area in the horizontal plane is shown in Fig. 3. This relationship indicates that, except for the apical region, longitudinal wall stress is uniformly distributed (*vide infra*). These findings are in agreement with the view of Woods (8) and Burton (9) that wall thickness is proportional to wall tension (g force per unit length of myocardium). The homogenous distribution of stress favors a uniform deformation of the myocardium during both diastole and systole. If this were not the case,

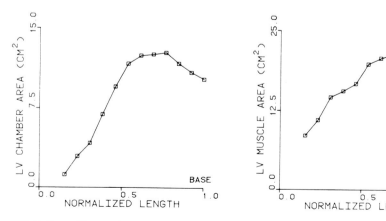

FIG. 2. Normal human heart. **Left:** LV chamber area, and **right:** muscle area versus normalized length.

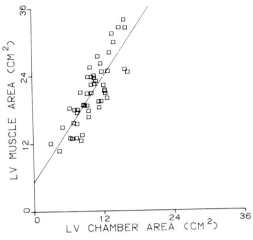

FIG. 3. The linear relation between LV muscle area and chamber area for 8 normal human hearts.

as may be true of patients with coronary artery disease, abnormal segmental wall motion would exist in regions of high wall stress.

During systole, the magnitude of longitudinal and circumferential stress will be determined by wall thickening and resultant increase in myocardial cross-sectional area, although muscle mass itself remains constant. The shortening of muscle fibers in the longitudinal and circumferential directions will determine wall thickening. Because the majority of muscle fibers of the normal human heart are located in the circumferential direction (7), the larger circumferential stress is supported by the shortening and corresponding thickening of these fibers. The lesser number of oblique fibers shorten in the longitudinal direction against the lesser longitudinal stress. Systolic stress normally peaks shortly after aortic valve opening. Thereafter, and because the cross-sectional area of the chamber declines while the wall thickens, systolic stress falls throughout the remainder of ejection. This fall in stress during systole allows the contracting myocardium to partially unload itself.

Systolic Stress and Strain

The relative deformation of the myocardium from its unstressed state is called strain. There are many strains that occur during the cardiac cycle. These strains, which vary according to their direction and their site of origin, include longitudinal, circumferential and radial strains as well as interfascicular strains and torsion (2). Because the myocardium is an anisotropic material, i.e., the elastic properties of the myocardium vary according to the direction of the applied stress, elongating strains are accompanied by shearing strains. Hence, the complete description of myocardial deformation requires the measurement of all strains. For our purposes, a simple expression of myocardial strain has been adopted based on the change in length (ΔL) of a theoretical midwall circumferential muscle fiber expressed with respect to its unstressed length (L_o) (10). During diastole, there is a positive strain on stretching of the fiber, while in systole there exists a negative strain or contraction of the fiber.

From the systolic stress–strain relationship, obtained for an isolated canine heart, it is apparent that fiber shortening, or strain, is an inverse function of systolic stress. Hence, the greater the systolic stress, the less the shortening. In our example, we have taken peak systolic stress to depict this relation (10). We have also reported that this relationship holds true when one considers instantaneous or mean systolic stress (11). As the contractile state of the myocardium is raised with catecholamines, one creates a more elastic system. The stress–strain relation is displaced to the right so that a greater deformation occurs for any given stress. Alternatively, depressing the heart by β-adrenergic receptor blockade makes it less elastic. In the failing heart as well, we find a less elastic system (10,12,13).

The Diseased Human Heart

Each of a variety of cardiovascular diseases imposes an excessive hemodynamic workload on the myocardium. This overloading may be expressed in terms of an augmented pressure or volume work. As a result, the systolic wall force and stress sustained by the myocardium are increased. In order for muscle fiber shortening to remain normal under these conditions, systolic wall stress must be returned to its normal value. Hence, the cross-sectional area of myocardium must increase. We consider the resultant increase in myocardial mass to represent myocardial hypertrophy. The link between these mechanical events and the chemical processes surrounding hypertrophy remains unclear. Whether or not the increment in myocardial mass is appropriate to normalize systolic force determines whether or not it is adequate. An elevated myocardial mass that is not associated with an appropriate increase in cross-sectional area of myocardium represents inadequate hypertrophy.

To explore the patterns of myocardial growth and chamber configuration that occur under various pathological conditions, we obtained both normal and diseased human hearts from the autopsy service of our hospital. The hearts were fixed in 10% formalin under normal or abnormal levels of distension; the level of elevated filling pressure was determined from antemortem cardiac catheterization data. After fixation and the preservation of shape, the hearts were then cast in gelatin, sectioned, traced, and digitized according to the technique developed by Janicki et al. (14).

Two groups of diseased hearts were compared to the normal human heart (2 males, 6 females; mean age 58 years, age range 36–78 years) without history or anatomical evidence of cardiac disease. One group (2 males, 4 females; mean age 59 years, age range 30–72 years) represented the chronic LV pressure overload of systemic hypertension without coronary artery disease, while the other group (5 males, 1 female; mean age 47 years, age range 36–58 years) had idiopathic congestive cardiomyopathy. Two of the patients with hypertension had an acute decompensation in their clinical status, while all patients with cardiomyopathy had severe heart failure. LV mass (free wall and septum) was significantly ($p < 0.001$) increased above the normal value of 102 ± 6.6 g in all patients with cardiac disease, as can be seen in Fig. 4. The degree of LV hypertrophy was graded as moderate (i.e., SD = 3 as compared to normal) or marked (i.e., SD = 6 as compared to normal). In the patients with compensated LV pressure overload, the predominant remodeling of the myocardium occurred between the minor axis and apex of the heart (Fig. 5), where the thickness-to-radius (h/r) and mass-to-volume (M/V) ratios were greater than those in the normal heart. Above the normalized length value of 0.6 the discrepancy in mass and wall thickness were less, h/r and M/V ratios resembling those of the normal heart. The transition from compensated to decompensated hypertrophy in two patients with systemic hypertension was reflected in a shape change of the LV chamber. The dominant chamber enlargement occurred in the lower half of the ventricle as indicated in Fig. 5. Hence, there are regional changes in myocardial mass and chamber configuration that occur during the natural course of LV pressure overload and that serve to reflect the transition from the compensated to the decompensated state.

As indicated in Fig. 5, the hypertrophy was adequate in the compensated patients with LV pressure overload. Here the ratios of thickness-to-chamber-radius and LV-mass-to-volume were normal at the base and greater than normal throughout the rest of the ventricle. In those patients with systemic hypertension and clinically apparent heart failure, these ratios fell within the normal range throughout the ventricle indicating that hypertrophy was inadequate and that wall stress was abnormally high. In contrast, in the dilated,

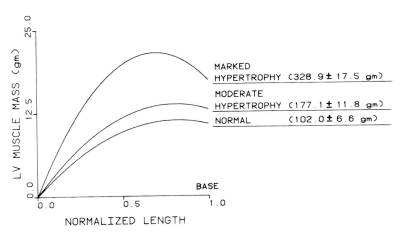

FIG. 4. The distribution in LV muscle mass as a function of normalized apex-to-base length.

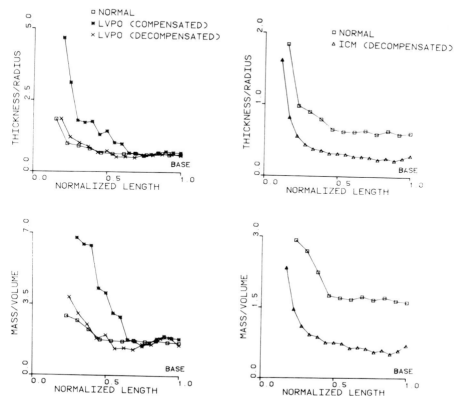

FIG. 5. The thickness-to-radius and mass-to-volume ratios as functions of normalized apex-to-base length for the normal human left ventricle (LV), the chronic pressure overload (LVPO) of systemic hypertension, and idiopathic congestive cardiomyopathy (ICM). The ventricles were subgrouped as compensated and decompensated according to whether or not there was clinically evident heart failure.

myopathic hearts (see right panels of Fig. 5) h/r and M/V were less than normal for the entire ventricle indicating that the increased muscle mass was inadequately apportioned relative to chamber size. Longitudinal systolic stress would be elevated above normal in the failing hearts of both groups, particularly in the failing myopathic hearts where it might reach 2 to 3 times normal. Systolic stress has been reported to be elevated in patients with cardiac failure secondary to a variety of conditions (15–19).

CARDIAC STRUCTURE AND THE STRESS–STRAIN RELATION

The stress–strain relationship of the myocardium is determined by the stress–strain relation of its muscle fibers and connective tissue matrix and their respective volume content. By identifying the various structural elements of the myocardium, the relative volume fraction (F) of each element, and their respective elastic moduli (K), the elastic behavior of the myocardium may be defined (e.g., K_1F muscle + K_2F collagen + K_3F elastin) (2,3). While cardiac muscle occupies 50 to 85% of myocardial volume, collagen is much stiffer than muscle, so that a small increment in the amount of connective tissue will adversely affect myocardial distensibility during both diastole and systole. At the present time, there is only a limited amount of quantitative information concerning the elastic moduli and relative volume fractions of the connective tissue elements in either normal or diseased hearts. We have initiated a series of investigations to determine this information and to correlate alterations in cardiac structure with the development of cardiac failure.

Collagen and the Hypertrophied Heart

The collagen volume fraction of the hypertrophied myocardium accompanying systemic hypertension was calculated using morphometric methods. The relevant clinical information has been reported previously (7). In brief, there were 9 hearts obtained from patients with systemic hypertension and electrocardiographic evidence of left ventricular hypertrophy. Five of these patients had no evidence of failure (compensated hypertrophy) and four had clinically apparent heart failure (decompensated hypertrophy). The hearts were prepared as previously reported (7), with full thickness cubes of myocardium obtained from the LV free wall and interventricular system. The sections were stained using Masson trichrome with the resultant blue-stained connective tissue assumed to predominantly represent collagen. The sections were also divided into thirds to examine relative difference between the subendo- and subepicardial distribution of collagen. The collagen volume fractions for normal hearts and the compensated and decompensated pressure overloaded hearts are given in Table 1. These findings indicate that the collagen content of the hypertrophic heart was greater than normal and that there was a significant increase in collagen in decompensated as compared to compensated

TABLE 1. *Percent collagen volume fraction in normal human hearts and hearts with systemic hypertension*

Heart	LV Free wall	LV Free wall and septum
Normal	2.4	2.5
Compensated hypertrophy	3.2[a]	3.3[a]
Decompensated hypertrophy	4.2[a,b]	3.8[a,b]

[a] Significantly different ($p < 0.05$) from normal.
[b] Significantly different ($p < 0.05$) from compensated hypertrophy.

hearts. This was true for both the LV free wall alone and free wall plus septum. Interestingly, there was no statistically significant difference in collagen distribution between the subendo- or subepicardium.

The functional importance of this structural remodeling of the myocardium is unknown. It is tempting to speculate that, because of the increased collagen volume fraction, the elastic properties of the myocardium were altered, accounting for the defect in cardiac function and the appearance of heart failure. The increase in myocardial collagen accompanying the left ventricular pressure overload of systemic hypertension may occur as a sequel to muscle fiber hypoxia and necrosis or in response to elevated wall stress, analogous to bone formation. Further studies will be required to clarify these issues.

SUMMARY

The heart is a muscular pump composed of cardiac muscle fibers embedded in a network of connective tissue. The viscoelastic properties of its muscular and connective tissue elements, together with its functional architecture, determine the mechanical behavior of the heart. Systolic stress, which determines the strain or deformation of the myocardium, is elevated in chronic cardiac disease. This is true whether the disease is hypertensive, myopathic, or valvular in origin, or associated with a segment of infarcted myocardium, which elevates the stress in the remaining viable segments. Myocardial hypertrophy, and the attendant increase in muscle mass, is a mechanism for normalizing stress. The adequacy of the hypertrophy in fact will be determined by whether or not systolic stress returns to normal. The remodeling process of hypertrophy may create regional differences in cardiac shape and the composition of the myocardium as we have seen in the hypertensive heart. Myocardial failure is accompanied by an elevated wall stress and inadequate distribution of the hypertrophied myocardium relative to the configuration and size of the left ventricle. An increased collagen content in the hypertrophied heart may stiffen the myocardium and also contribute to the failure state. Further investigation into the stimulus to hypertrophy, the transition from compensated to decompensated hypertrophy, and the role of connective tissue in the genesis of heart failure will be required to answer these questions.

ACKNOWLEDGMENTS

This work was supported in part by Program Project Grant HL-08805 from the National Heart, Lung, and Blood Institute, National Institutes of Health, Bethesda, Maryland. Drs. Weber and Janicki are the recipients of Research Career Development Awards HL-00187 and HL-00411, respectively, from the National Heart, Lung, and Blood Institute.

We wish to thank J. Dowell, D. Ward, and N. Dehghani for their dedicated and skillful technical assistance. In addition, we want to express our graditude to Dr. G. Pietra, Director of the Autopsy Service of the Hospital of the University of Pennsylvania, for his cooperation during the study. The secretarial assistance of S. Wahl in preparing this manuscript is appreciated.

REFERENCES

1. Borg, T. K., and Caulfield, J. B. (1981): *Fed. Proc.*, 40:2037–2041.
2. Weber, K. T., and Hawthorne, E. W. (1981): *Fed. Proc.*, 40:2005–2010.
3. Weber, K .T., Janicki, J. S., Shroff, S., and Pearlman, E. S. (1983): In: *Myocardial Hypertrophy and Failure*, edited by N. R. Alpert, pp. 85–102. Raven Press, New York.
4. Linzbach, A. J. (1960): *Am. J. Cardiol.*, 5:370–382.
5. Schwarz, F., Flameng, W., Schaper, J., and Hehrlein, F. (1978): *Am. J. Cardiol.*, 42:895–903.
6. Pfeffer, J. M., Pfeffer, M. A., Fishbein, M. C., and Frohlich, E. D. (1979): *Am. J. Physiol.*, 237:H461–H468.
7. Pearlman, E. S., Weber, K. T., Janicki, J. S., Pietra, G., and Fishman, A. P. (1982): *Lab. Invest.*, 46:158–164.
8. Woods, R. H. (1892): *J. Anat. Physiol.*, 26:362–370.
9. Burton, A. C. (1957): *Am. Heart J.*, 54:801–809.
10. Weber, K. T., Janicki, J. S., Reeves, R. C., and Hefner, L. L. (1976): *Am. J. Physiol.*, 230:419–426.
11. Weber, K. T., and Janicki, J. S. (1977): *Am. J. Physiol.*, 232:H241–H249.
12. Weber, K. T., Janicki, J. S., Hunter, W. C., Shroff, S., Pearlman, E. S., and Fishman, A. P. (1981): *Prog. Cardiovasc. Dis.*, 24:210–243.
13. Weber, K. T., and Janicki, J. S. (1979): *Am. Heart. J.*, 98:371–384.
14. Janicki, J. S., Weber, K. T., Gochman, R. F., Shroff, S., and Geheb, F. J. (1981): *Am. J. Physiol.*, 241:H1–H11.
15. Sandler, H., and Dodge, H. T. (1963): *Circ. Res.*, 13:91–104.
16. Hood, W. P. Jr., Rackley, C. E., and Rolett, E. L. (1968): *Am. J. Cardiol.*, 22:550–558.
17. Gould, K. L., Lipscomb, K., Hamilton, G. W., and Kennedy, J. W. (1974): *Am. J. Cardiol.*, 34:627–634.
18. Grossman, W., Jones, D., and McLaurin, L. P. (1975): *J. Clin. Invest.*, 56:56–64.
19. Gunther, S., and Grossman, W. (1979): *Circulation*, 59:679–688.

Perspectives in Cardiovascular Research, Vol. 8,
edited by R. C. Tarazi and J. B. Dunbar.
Raven Press, New York © 1983.

Influence of Cardiac Hypertrophy on Myocardial Compliance

William Grossman and Beverly H. Lorell

Department of Medicine, Harvard Medical School, Beth Israel Hospital, and Brigham and Women's Hospital, Boston, Massachusetts 02115

Cardiac hypertrophy is an almost invariant response to chronic pressure or volume loading of the heart. It generally develops in a pattern specific to the inciting stress (1–4) with sustained pressure overload leading to concentric hypertrophy (predominant increase in mass relative to volume), while volume overload leads to the development of eccentric hypertrophy (balanced increase in mass and volume). Eccentric hypertrophy is so named because the heart becomes "eccentric" in the chest cavity, enlarging to the left. Eccentric hypertrophy is a uniform process affecting all walls of the involved cardiac chamber, and should not be confused with "asymmetric" hypertrophy, where one wall of a particular cardiac chamber becomes hypertrophied relative to the other walls of that chamber.

That the hypertrophied heart can perform increased work has been clearly demonstrated (2,5,6); however, the burden of a sustained increase in systolic or diastolic load is commonly associated with congestive heart failure and depressed ventricular pump function. The explanation for this impaired systolic function has been the subject of intense study in recent years, and is discussed by others in this book. In this chapter, we shall concentrate on reviewing the diastolic abnormalities that may accompany cardiac hypertrophy.

DIASTOLIC FUNCTION

The importance of diastolic relaxation and compliance to adequate systolic function is not always appreciated. As should be obvious, the extent of cardiac muscle activation with each systole is dependent on the completeness of relaxation during the preceding diastole; also, ventricular systolic ejection is dependent on adequate ventricular diastolic filling. Although simple, these fundamental facts of cardiac physiology are not always considered in attempts to understand the causes of depressed systolic function.

DIASTOLIC RELAXATION OF HYPERTROPHIED MYOCARDIUM

There is now considerable evidence that ventricular relaxation is impaired in advanced cardiac hypertrophy, at least in the concentric and idiopathic asymmetric varieties (7–10). An example of marked impairment of diastolic relaxation in a patient with hypertrophic cardiomyopathy (HCM) is shown in Fig. 1. This patient exhibited a very high early left ventricular (LV) diastolic pressure which showed a continuous fall into mid-diastole, despite the fact that LV volume (as assessed by a simultaneous LV cineangiogram) was increasing steadily throughout this interval. This prolonged fall in LV diastolic pressure indicates marked slowing of the normal process of myocardial relaxation, which was largely corrected by administration of the Ca^{2+} channel-blocking agent nifedipine (9). Systolic function (as assessed by ejection fraction) was depressed in this patient and improved simultaneously with the improved relaxation following nifedipine. Thus, impaired relaxation in advanced myocardial hypertrophy may be a cause of increased ventricular filling pressures and reduced ventricular forward output. The basic mechanism for such impaired relaxation is unknown, but its response to Ca^{2+} channel-blocking agents suggests intracellular Ca^{2+} overload as an underlying factor. A similar mechanism has been proposed for impaired myocardial relaxation in association with myocardial hypoxia/ischemia (7,11,12), and it is possible that subendocardial ischemia of the markedly hypertrophic ventricle may cause (or contribute to) the impaired relaxation.

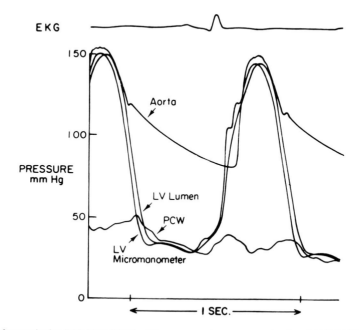

FIG. 1. Left ventricular (**LV**) high fidelity micromanometer pressure tracing, LV fluid-filled lumen catheter pressure tracing, and simultaneous pulmonary capillary wedge (**PCW**) pressure tracing in a patient with non-obstructive HCM with congestive heart failure. The continuous fall of pressure into mid-diastole when LV volume was increased suggests marked impairment of LV relaxation. (From Lorell et al., ref. 9, with permission.)

Hanrath and co-workers (8) have studied LV relaxation and filling pattern in different forms of LV hypertrophy. They examined a relaxation time index, defined as the time from minimal LV dimension to mitral valve opening (MVO). This index was 13 ± 15 msec in normal subjects, but was prolonged in patients with hypertrophic obstructive cardiomyopathy (HOCM) (93 ± 37 msec) and in patients with chronic left ventricular pressure overload (CPO) (66 ± 31 msec). The duration of the rapid filling phase and the increase in dimension during this period were significantly reduced in HOCM and CPO (Fig. 2). These data were felt by Hanrath and co-workers to support the concept of an abnormality in myocardial relaxation and early ventricular filling in conditions associated with cardiac hypertrophy.

St. John Sutton and colleagues (10) studied 29 patients with HCM and found evidence of abnormal relaxation in more than half. In this study, wide variation in diastolic function allowed separation of patients into 3 groups on

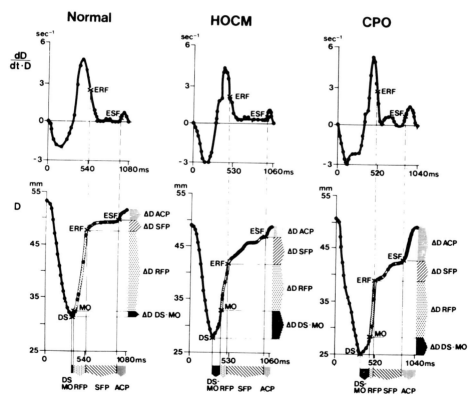

FIG. 2. Computer output of the echograms of the LV cavity of a normal subject, a patient with HOCM, and a patient with chronic LV pressure overload (CPO). **D**, dimension; **dD/dt · D**, normalized derivative of dimension; **DS**, end-systolic dimension; **MO**, mitral valve opening; **ERF**, end of rapid filling; **ESF**, end of slow filling; **ACP**, atrial contractive period. See text for details. (From Hanrath et al., ref. 8, with permisison.)

the basis of LV peak filling rate. The results showed that in HCM, peak LV filling rate is determined primarily by the rate of free wall thinning, because of the severe septal hypertrophy and hypokinesia. With reduction in LV peak filling rate and impaired free wall thinning, there was an increased incidence of angina and of atrial fibrillation, suggesting that these diastolic abnormalities may have clinical importance. Of interest is the fact that in their study, the diastolic abnormalities were not always accompanied by systolic dysfunction in the same myocardial region (Fig. 3).

Abnormalities in diastolic relaxation have been reported in patients with congestive cardiomyopathy who showed reductions in the rate of circumferential fiber lengthening as well as in maximum negative dP/dt (13). If these relaxation abnormalities are characteristic of the heart failure state (perhaps due to catecholamine depletion), then it is possible that the intrinsic abnormalities in relaxation that appear to be associated with cardiac hypertrophy (in the absence of heart failure) could be exacerbated in advanced stages, when heart failure supervenes.

DIASTOLIC COMPLIANCE OF HYPERTROPHIED MYOCARDIUM

In addition to altered relaxation, cardiac hypertrophy may cause substantial abnormalities of ventricular compliance. As pointed out by Mirsky (14,15)

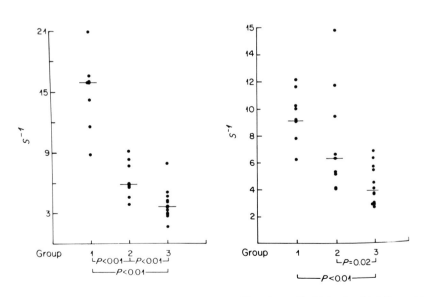

FIG. 3. Normalized rates of posterior wall thinning (**left**) and systolic thickening (**right**) expressed in sec −1 (**S^{-1}**) in three groups of patients with idiopathic hypertrophic subaortic stenosis (IHSS). Group 1 was defined as those with increased peak LV filling rates; group 2, patients with normal filling rates; group 3, patients with decreased filling rates. Systolic function is normal or greater-than-normal throughout groups 1 through 3, but diastolic function deteriorates disproportionately, so that it is normal in group 2 but severely abnormal in group 3. (From St. John Sutton et al., ref. 10, with permission.)

and others (16,17), decreased chamber compliance leads to an increase in end-diastolic pressure if adequate sarcomere stretch is to be maintained. In the case of chronic volume-overload hypertrophy, cardiac muscle stiffness (the opposite of compliance) is usually normal (14,15,18), although chamber stiffness may be increased. However, in some patients with volume-overload hypertrophy, both muscle and chamber stiffness are increased (14,19), and in such instances very high ventricular filling pressures may be required to maintain adequate diastolic sarcomere stretch. If the abnormal diastolic compliance does not improve following surgical correction, LV systolic function may not improve or deteriorate, since the high preload associated with the volume-overload state is no longer present, and end-diastolic sarcomere stretch may be inadequate for effective systolic contraction.

In pressure-overload hypertrophy, substantial increases in chamber stiffness are common (18,20–23). While this increased chamber stiffness is in large part due to the increased ventricular wall thickness in concentric hypertrophy (22,23), an increase in intrinsic muscle stiffness (as assessed by stress-strain analysis) may occur in some patients with this condition (23). In experimental studies, Alpert et al. (24) have shown that pressure-overload hypertrophy of the right ventricle (induced by banding of the pulmonary artery) is associated with a change in the modulus of elasticity of isolated cardiac muscle, consistent with increased muscle stiffness (Fig. 4). Similar findings have been reported by Natarajan et al. (25). This increased muscle stiffness may be due to increased collagen and fibrous tissue in this particular model of pressure-overload hy-

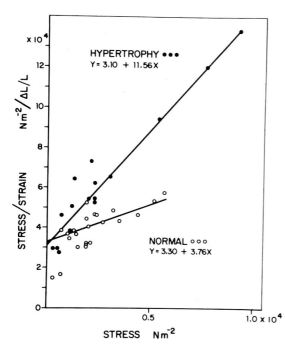

FIG. 4. Ratio of stress to strain (modulus of elasticity) versus stress of resting right ventricular papillary muscles taken from rabbits with chronic pulmonary artery banding (**hypertrophy**) and normal controls (**normal**). The hypertrophied muscle exhibits a substantial increase in passive stiffness. (From Alpert et al., ref. 24, with permission.)

pertrophy. Bishop and Melsen (26) have described myocardial necrosis and fibrosis in cats with experimental cardiac hypertrophy induced by pulmonary artery banding.

Also, Lund et al. (27) compared collagen content and muscle fiber diameter in heart of the spontaneously hypertensive rat (SHR), aortic-constricted normotensive rat (NTR), and a control group of normal rats. They found that the development of cardiomegaly with spontaneous hypertension is caused primarily by an increase in muscle mass with relatively less proliferation of the connective tissue elements. Unlike the findings in SHR, the collagen response in the aortic-constricted rat paralleled the muscle response, as cardiomegaly and increased muscle fiber diameter were associated with maintenance of hydroxyproline concentration similar to that in normotensive controls (27). They concluded that the connective tissue response to cardiomegaly produced by spontaneous hypertension is significantly different from the response produced by aortic constriction. Thus, it is possible that pressure-overload hypertrophy in humans, if it developed slowly, could be associated with little increase in connective tissue and with normal muscle stiffness. However, rapidly progressive or advanced pressure overload could cause myocardial injury and connective tissue proliferation with an increase in muscle stiffness, particularly if myocardial ischemia is superimposed on the hypertrophic stimulus (27).

It should be pointed out that, although fibrosis in association with advanced cardiac hypertrophy could explain the increased muscle stiffness seen in some patients, a study by Schwarz and co-workers (28) relating myocardial structure and histology (from LV transmural biopsies taken at the time of cardiac surgery) with diastolic compliance found that "myocardial cell diameter, but not myocardial fibrosis, is a major determinant of end-diastolic properties of the left ventricle in chronic aortic valve disease" (28). Thus, much work needs to be done in order to understand fully the factors in cardiac hypertrophy that cause abnormalities of diastolic relaxation and compliance, as these abnormalities clearly influence systolic performance.

REFERENCES

1. Linzbach, A. J. (1960): *Am. J. Cardiol.*, 5:370–382.
2. Sandler, H., and Dodge, H. T. (1963): *Circ. Res.*, 13:91–104.
3. Grossman, W., Jones, D., and McLaurin, L. P. (1975): *J. Clin. Invest.*, 56:56–65.
4. Grossman, W. (1980): *Am. J. Med.*, 69:576–584.
5. Kennedy, J. W., Twiss, R. D., Blackmon, J. R., and Dodge, H. T. (1968): *Circulation*, 38:838–845.
6. Pfeffer, M. A., Pfeffer, J. M., and Frolich, E. D. (1976): *Circ. Res.*, 38:423–429.
7. Grossman, W., and Barry, W. H. (1980): *Fed. Proc.*, 39:148–155.
8. Hanrath, P., Mathey, D. G., Siegert, R., and Bleifeld, W. (1980): *Am. J. Cardiol.*, 45:15–23.
9. Lorell, B. H., Paulus, W., Grossman, W., Wynne, J., Cohn, P. F., and Braunwald, E. (1980): *N. Engl. J. Med.*, 303:801–803.
10. St. John Sutton, M. G., Tajik, A. J., Gibson, D. G., Brown, D. J., Seward, J. B., and Guiliani, E. R. (1978): *Circulation*, 57:512–520.

11. Paulus, W. J., Serizawa, T., and Grossman, W. (1982): *Circ. Res.,* 50:218–227.
12. Serizawa, T., Carabello, B. A., and Grossman, W. (1980): *Circ. Res.,* 46:430–439.
13. Grossman, W., McLaurin, L. P., and Rolett, E. L. (1979): *Cardiovasc. Res.,* 13:514–522.
14. Mirsky, I. (1976): *Progress Cardiovasc. Dis.,* 18:277–306.
15. Mirsky, I., and Pasipoularides, A. (1980): *Fed. Proc.,* 39:156–161.
16. Levine, H. J. (1972): *Circulation,* 46:423–426.
17. Braunwald, E., and Ross, J., Jr. (1963): *Am. J. Med.,* 34:147–150.
18. Grossman, W., McLaurin, L. P., and Stefadouros, M. A. (1974): *Circ. Res.,* 35:793–800.
19. Gault, J. H., Covell, J. W., Braunwald, E., et al. (1970): *Circulation,* 42:773–780.
20. Gaasch, W. H., Battle, W. E., Oboler, A. A., Banas, J. S., and Levine, H. J. (1973): *Circulation,* 42:746–762.
21. Gibson, D. G., and Brown, D. J. (1974): *Br. Heart J.,* 36:1066–1077.
22. Grossman, W., McLaurin, L. P., Moos, S. P., et al. (1974): *Circulation,* 48:801–809.
23. Peterson, K. L., Tsuji, J., Johnson, A., et al. (1978): *Circulation,* 58:77.
24. Alpert, N. R., Hamrell, B. B., and Halpern, W. (1974): *Circ. Res. (Supplement II),* 34:71–82.
25. Natarajan, G., Bove., A. A., Coulson, R. L., Carey, R. A., and Spann, J. F. (1979): *Am. J. Physiol.,* 237:H676–H680.
26. Bishop, S. B., and Melsen, L. R. (1976); *Circ. Res.,* 39:238.
27. Lund, D. D., Twietmeyer, T. A., Schmid, P. G., and Tomanek, R. J. (1979): Independent changes in cardiac muscle fibers and connective tissue in rats with spontaneous hypertension, aortic constriction and hypoxia. *Cardiovasc. Res.,* 13:39–44.
28. Schwarz, F., Flameng, W., Schaper, J., and Hehrlein, F. (1978): *Am. J. Cardiol.,* 42:895–903.

Perspectives in Cardiovascular Research, Vol. 8,
edited by R. C. Tarazi and J. B. Dunbar.
Raven Press, New York © 1983.

Electrical Properties of Hypertrophied Ventricular Muscle of Rats with Renal Hypertension

R. S. Aronson and E. C. H. Keung

Department of Medicine, Division of Cardiology, Albert Einstein College of Medicine, Bronx, New York 10461

Cardiac hypertrophy is associated with electrocardiographic, ultrastructural, biochemical, and contractile alterations. However, until recently, the electrical properties of hypertrophied cardiac fibers has received relatively little attention. This is surprising because the surface sarcolemma and transverse tubular system (T-system) are important components in excitation–contraction coupling, and low resistance electrical connections between fibers ensure the orderly spread of excitation. Therefore, alterations in the properties of these membrane systems, or changes in electrical coupling between fibers, may contribute to the altered physiology of hypertrophied myocardium. For these reasons, we have done a series of electrical studies to characterize the membrane properties of hypertrophied myocytes.

The few previous studies on the electrophysiologic alterations associated with cardiac hypertrophy have reported a variety of changes in the action potential, but have not agreed on the nature of the alterations and on when they occurred during the course of hypertrophy. Most of the previous studies of the electrophysiologic effects of cardiac hypertrophy have used a model in which right ventricular hypertrophy is induced in cats by banding the pulmonary artery (1–7). The results have varied according to whether or not congestive heart failure was present and on the duration of pressure overload. In the absence of congestive heart failure, an increase in action potential duration was the only consistent electrical change reported (5–7).

It has also been reported that spontaneously hypertensive rats (8–10) and rats made hypertensive with deoxycorticosterone acetate (10) have longer action potentials than control rats.

The variability in the results of these studies is probably related to the model used, the duration of stress used to produce hypertrophy, and the animal species used. For example, in the right ventricular hypertrophy model, the acute pressure overload imposed probably causes variable degrees of damage to a chamber that normally functions against low pressures. In the spontaneously hypertensive rat model, the nature of the hypertrophy and the relation between elevated blood pressure and hypertrophy are not entirely clear (11).

Therefore, we have chosen to study the electrophysiologic effects of hypertrophy induced by a model that imposes a more gradual pressure overload on the heart. A useful model for producing this kind of pressure overload is renal hypertension in the rat. This is done by placing a silver clip around the left renal artery of experimental rats (12,13).

Additional advantages of this model include the availability of ultrastructural (14–16) and mechanical (17) data for correlation with electrical alterations and the similarity of hypertension in the rat to hypertensive disease in humans.

TRANSMEMBRANE ACTION POTENTIALS

Our first approach to investigating the electrophysiologic effects of cardiac hypertrophy was to compare transmembrane action potentials recorded from papillary muscles of hypertensive (HBP) and normal (SHAM) rats (13). We used standard microelectrode techniques to obtain electrical recordings. Preparations were driven at 1.0 Hz and perfused with Tyrode's solution ($K_o^+ = 4.0$ mM, $Ca_o^{2+} = 2.4$ mM) at 34 to 35°C.

Table 1 gives the characteristics of the animal groups. Both blood pressure and heart weight were significantly greater in HBP rats, but body weight did not differ significantly. The 37% increase in heart weight of HBP rats of body weight similar to SHAM rats indicates the presence of cardiac hypertrophy.

Figure 1 shows representative action potentials recorded simultaneously from three different pairs of HBP and SHAM papillary muscles. In each case, the HBP action potential is clearly longer than the SHAM action potential. Furthermore, the shape of the prolonged course of repolarization in HBP action potentials shows a much wider variation than the course of normal repolarization in SHAM action potentials.

Table 2 gives parameters of HBP and SHAM action potentials. As suggested by the records in Fig. 1, the action potential duration (APD) measured to both 50% (APD_{50}) and 75% (APD_{75}) of complete repolarization was significantly prolonged in HBP preparations. On the other hand, resting membrane potential, amplitude, and overshoot were not significantly different for HBP and SHAM action potentials. In addition, the maximum rate of rise of the upstroke

TABLE 1. *Characteristics of animal group*[a]

Model	BP (mm Hg)	HW (g)	BW (g)
HBP	210 ± 22 (48)[b]	1.36 ± 0.13 (47)[b]	391.9 ± 47.7 (48)
SHAM	127 ± 23 (49)	0.99 ± 0.14 (50)	427.6 ± 49.2 (51)

[a] HBP = hypertensive animals, SHAM = control animals, BP = systolic blood pressure, HW = heart weight, BW = body weight. Data are presented as the mean ± SD (number of animals).
[b] $P < 0.01$, HBP versus SHAM.
From Aronson, ref. 13, by permission of the American Heart Association, Inc.

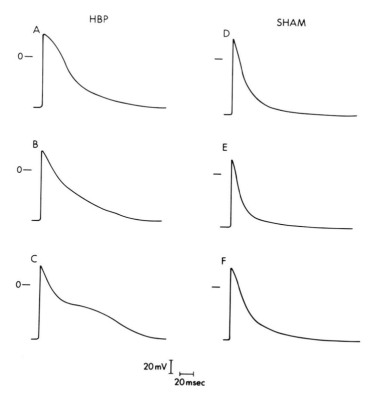

FIG. 1. Configuration of representative action potentials recorded from normal (SHAM) and hypertrophied (HBP) papillary muscles. Traces of HBP action potentials (**A–C**) and SHAM action potentials (**D–F**) recorded simultaneously from three pairs of muscles taken from different animals. Note that HBP action potentials show marked and consistent lengthening as well as considerable variability in the course of repolarization. *Horizontal bars* show zero potential. (From Aronson, ref. 50, by permission of the American Heart Association, Inc.)

of HBP action potentials (160 ± 35 V/sec; $N = 11$) was not significantly different from that of SHAM action potentials (154 ± 34 V/sec; $N = 12$).

These results show that hypertrophy induced by renal hypertension in the

TABLE 2. *Action potential parameters for animal groups[a]*

Model	RMP (−mV)	AMP (mV)	OS (mV)	APD_{50} (msec)	APD_{75} (msec)
HBP	78.8 ± 5.5 (49)	108.5 ± 7.1 (49)	29.7 ± 5.4 (49)	49.8 ± 16.6 (49)[b]	85.2 ± 23.1 (49)[b]
SHAM	81.5 ± 6.1 (53)	111.6 ± 7.4 (53)	30.0 ± 6.0 (53)	21.3 ± 6.1 (53)	37.0 ± 11.6 (53)

[a] HBP = hypertensive preparations, SHAM = control preparations, RMP = resting membrane potential, AMP = amplitude, OS = overshoot, APD_{50} and APD_{75} = action potential duration to 50 and 75% of repolarization to the RMP. Data are presented as the mean ± SD (number of preparations).

[b] $P < 0.01$ HBP versus SHAM.

From Aronson, ref. 13, by permission of the American Heart Association, Inc.

rat is associated with a specific, consistent, and significant increase in action potential duration. Another recent study (18) in which the same model was used reported a similar striking increase in duration of HBP action potentials without significant changes in other parameters.

The prolonged time course of repolarization in hypertrophied fibers could be due to delayed activation of an outward repolarizing current, slower inactivation of an inward depolarizing current, or some combination of these changes. These currents are carried by ions so that alterations in the ionic composition of the external fluid or the use of ionic channel-blocking agents can be used to gain some information about the mechanism underlying the prolonged action potentials seen in hypertrophied myocardium.

Accordingly, we did a series of experiments in which we increased the concentration of possible inward charge carriers (Ca^{2+}, Sr^{2+}), decreased the concentration of an inward charge carrier (Na^+), and blocked the outward current channel with tetraethylammonium (TEA) (13). The results of these experiments are given in Table 3, and show that exposure to Tyrode's solution with increased Ca^{2+} or low Na^+ produced a differentially greater decrease in APD_{50} and APD_{75} in HBP than in SHAM papillary muscles. In contrast, exposure to Sr^{2+}-containing and TEA-containing Tyrode's solution caused an increase in APD_{50} and APD_{75}, but the lengthening effect was not differentially greater in HBP than in SHAM action potentials. The fact that the shortening action of high Ca^{2+} is not mimicked by high Sr^{2+} indicates that this action is unique to Ca^{2+} and not simply a nonspecific effect of charge neutralization. These results all suggest that slowed inactivation of a Ca^{2+}-dependent inward current, as opposed to delayed activation of an outward current, is at least partly responsible for the longer action potentials associated with cardiac hypertrophy.

To obtain more information about the relative contribution of time- and

TABLE 3. *Effects of changing ionic composition and TEA on the duration of HBP and SHAM action potentials*

Composition	APD_{50}		APD_{75}	
	Treatment	Interaction	Treatment	Interaction
12 Ca_o	−	−	−	−
0.5 Na_o	−	−	−	−
12 Sr_o	+	0	+	0
TEA	+	0	+	0

APD_{50} and APD_{75}, action potential duration measured to 50 and 75% of complete repolarization; 12 Ca_o, 12 mm external Ca^{2+}; 0.5 Na_o, 50% of normal external Na^+; 12 Sr_o, 12 mm external Sr^{2+}; TEA, tetraethylammonium chloride. − indicates a significant decrease; + indicates a significant increase; 0 indicates no significant change. Significance was assessed by analysis of variance. A significant treatment difference is one that occurs in APD as the result of treatment, independent of the group to which the rat belongs. A significant interaction refers to a significant differential action of the treatment on APD of HBP as compared to SHAM preparations.

voltage-dependent inward and outward currents to the longer action potentials of hypertrophied ventricular muscle, we determined the changes in relative membrane resistance during the time course of the action potential (19). For these experiments, we used small endocardial strips (4–5 mm long; ≤ 1 mm diameter) and the method described by Weidmann (20). One microelectrode was used to inject an anodal constant current pulse (0.8–1.0 μA) and a second electrode was used to record the resulting voltage deflection. The electrodes were ≤ 0.1 mm apart. The current pulses lasted 20 msec and were synchronized to the external stimulus that induced the upstroke. Anodal pulses were applied throughout the course of the action potential by progressively increasing the delay from the stimulus to the onset of the current pulse. Superimposing successive sweeps on a storage oscilloscope gave a record in which the upper edge of the trace corresponded to an action potential in the absence of applied current and the lower edge showed the action potentials displaced by anodal current.

Figure 2 shows the records obtained from this kind of experiment. The relative membrane resistance is proportional to the amplitude of the voltage deflection produced by the current pulses (20). Therefore, the degree of separation between the upper and lower edges of the trace is a rough measure of the relative membrane resistance at each moment during the action potential.

The relative membrane resistance became progressively larger during the course of repolarization in both HBP and SHAM action potentials, but the time course of this increase was different. In the SHAM action potential, the

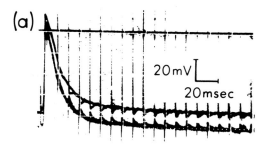

(a)

20 mV

20 msec

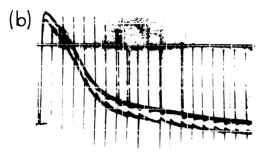

(b)

FIG. 2. Relative membrane resistance during a SHAM (**a**) and HBP (**b**) action potential. The *continuous horizontal line* represents zero membrane potential. The separation between the upper and lower edges of the traces is a measure of the relative membrane resistance. The larger the separation, the larger the relative membrane resistance. The *large spikes* are capacitative artifacts indicating the make and break of each anodal current pulse. Note that the separation between traces becomes larger much later during repolarization of the HBP than during repolarization of the SHAM action potential. See text for further discussion.

separation started to increase approximately 12 msec after the upstroke. In contrast, in the HBP action potential, the separation did not begin to increase until 55 msec after the upstroke.

These measurements of the relative membrane resistance during HBP and SHAM action potentials have some interesting implications. The finding that the membrane resistance increases progressively during repolarization suggests that the action potential duration in ventricular muscle of the rat is more likely to depend on inactivation of an inward current than on activation of an outward current. If the low relative membrane resistance during the early phase of repolarization were due to activation of an outward current, then the progressive increase in relative membrane resistance would indicate that this current inactivates during the course of repolarization. Such a sequence of events is not compatible with the view that repolarization is dominated by activation of an outward current. On the other hand, slow inactivation of an inward current is not only compatible with the recorded sequence of changes in relative membrane resistance, but also would allow a background outward current to repolarize the action potential. The fact that the relative membrane resistance did not start to increase until long after the onset of the action potential in the HBP fiber, as compared to the SHAM fiber, is also in accord with our hypothesis that delayed inactivation of an inward current is an important factor in lengthening HBP action potentials.

In addition to the time- and voltage-dependent ionic currents we have already considered, there is evidence that an electrogenic outward current due to activity of the Na^+-K^+ pump may influence the time course of repolarization in cardiac fibers (21). Therefore, we performed experiments specifically to determine whether altered activity of the Na^+-K^+ pump contributes to the prolonged time course of repolarization in hypertrophied ventricular muscle (19).

These experiments involved reducing pump activity with ouabain (10^{-6}, 10^{-5}, and 10^{-4} M) and stimulation of pump activity by sodium loading produced by exposure to K^+-free solution (21,22).

Exposure to ouabain caused dose-dependent shortening of both HBP and SHAM action potentials. This result does not support the view that the lengthening of HBP action potentials is due to reduced outward electrogenic current generated by the pump for the following reason. Inhibition of pump activity should lengthen SHAM action potentials and have little or no effect on HBP action potentials if a lack of outward pump current were primarily responsible for the longer duration of HBP action potentials.

Stimulation of pump activity by sodium loading did not significantly affect the action potential duration of either SHAM or HBP fibers. One would expect enhanced pump activity to shorten SHAM action potentials and to have little if any influence on HBP action potentials if lack of electrogenic pump activity was an important factor contributing to the lengthening of HBP action potentials.

NONUNIFORM ELECTROPHYSIOLOGICAL PROPERTIES IN HYPERTROPHIED RAT MYOCARDIUM

To investigate further the nature and distribution of the electrical alterations associated with cardiac hypertrophy, we studied the duration and the effects of stimulation on the action potentials recorded from three different regions of the left ventricle: (a) papillary muscles, (b) endocardial preparations, and (c) epicardial preparations (23). To determine the effects of increasing stimulation frequency, preparations were stimulated at five cycle lengths (23).

Typical action potentials recorded at three stimulation cycle lengths are shown in Fig. 3. As illustrated in Fig. 4, the degree of shortening and the

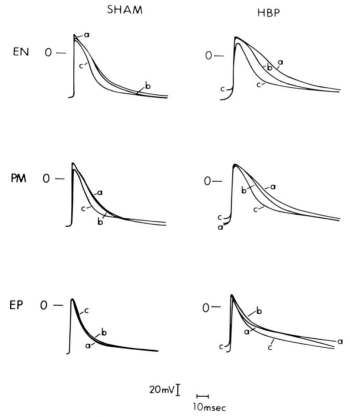

FIG. 3. Tracings of representative action potentials showing the effect of stimulation cycle length on configuration. Stimulation cycle length = 1000 (**a**), 300 (**b**) and 150 (**c**) msec. Tracings are from endocardial (**EN**), papillary muscle (**PM**), and epicardial (**EP**) fibers of SHAM and HBP rats. Note that HBP action potentials of endocardial and papillary muscle fibers are clearly longer than those of SHAM fibers at longer stimulation cycle lengths. Prolongation of epicardial HBP action potentials is seen only during the latter half of repolarization. (From Keung and Aronson, ref. 23, by permission of the American Heart Association, Inc.)

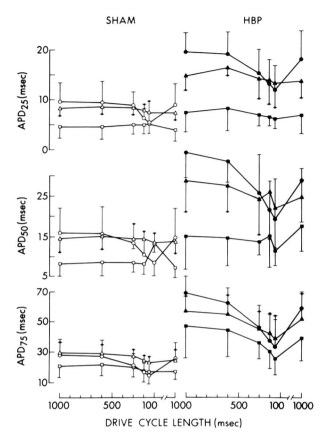

FIG. 4. Effects of stimulation cycle length on the action potential duration of endocardial (*circles*), epicardial (*squares*), and papillary muscle (*triangles*) action potentials of HBP (*solid symbols*) and SHAM (*open symbols*) rats. Values are presented as mean ± SD, $N = 7$. A *small dot* is used to mark the bars representing SD for papillary muscles. (From Keung and Aronson, ref. 23, by permission of the American Heart Association, Inc.)

relative change in the contour of the action potential vary according to the recording site and group. The data in Fig. 4 show that endocardial and papillary muscle HBP action potentials were consistently longer than SHAM action potentials at all stimulation cycle lengths, but that the epicardial HBP action potentials were similar to epicardial SHAM action potentials, except for APD_{75}.

Statistical analysis of the data in Fig. 4 by two-way analysis of variance and single-degree of freedom contrast showed that APD_{25}, APD_{50}, and APD_{75} of endocardial and papillary muscle preparations were significantly longer ($p < 0.05$) for HBP and SHAM action potentials at all stimulation cycle lengths. On the other hand, APD_{25} and APD_{50} of epicardial action potentials were not significantly longer for HBP than SHAM preparations at any stimulation cycle length. However, APD_{75} of epicardial action potentials was significantly longer for HBP than SHAM preparations at all cycle lengths except 150 msec. Thus, our data show that whereas the entire course of repolarization is significantly longer in endocardial and papillary muscle action potentials of HBP than SHAM fibers, epicardial action potentials are similar in duration in HBP and SHAM fibers during the first half of repolarization. However, during the latter half of repolarization, epicardial action potentials are again longer in HBP than SHAM fibers.

In addition to the absolute differences in duration between HBP and SHAM action potentials discussed above, the response of action potential duration to decreasing stimulation cycle length is different in HBP and SHAM muscles. Statistical analysis of our data showed a strong interaction between animal group (SHAM and HBP) and stimulation cycle length independent of recording site. That is, APD_{50} and APD_{75} of all HBP preparations shorten to a greater extent than SHAM preparations. Similar statistical analysis showed a strong interaction between recording site and stimulation cycle length, independent of animal group. When stimulation cycle length is decreased, endocardial action potentials shortened to a larger extent than papillary muscle and epicardial action potentials. The action potentials of HBP fibers resemble those of endocardial fibers in that both demonstrate a quantitatively greater degree of shortening in response to increasing stimulation frequency.

Possible mechanisms for the greater sensitivity of endocardial action potentials, especially HBP, to increasing stimulation frequency include slower deactivation kinetics of an outward current, slow reactivation kinetics of an inward current, greater accumulation of K^+ in extracellular space, and augmented electrogenic repolarization current generated by enhanced activity of the Na^+-K^+ pump (21,24). Available evidence (24,25) and recent results from our laboratory indicate that the duration of ventricular action potentials depends much more strongly on inactivation of a slow inward current than on activation of an outward K-current or an electrogenic outward current. This suggests that the greater degree of rate-dependent shortening of endocardial action potentials in general, and action potentials of hypertrophied muscle in particular, may be due to a greater rate-dependent alteration in a slow inward current.

PASSIVE ELECTRICAL PROPERTIES

To investigate the alterations in passive electrical properties in hypertrophied rat myocardium, we determined the electrical constants of epicardial and endocardial preparations from both normal and hypertrophied rat hearts (26). This was done by comparative analysis of the spatial decay of steady state electrotonic voltage deflection produced by injection of a hyperpolarizing constant current pulse. We used short preparations (0.8 mm) to minimize the difficulties that arise from the steep falloff in electrotonic voltage with distance in long preparations in which current spread is multidimensional. We derived an equation to describe the spatial voltage decrement in our short preparations by assuming that current spreads in two dimensions and that the preparations were finite. We used this equation to obtain the curve that best fit the data for each type of preparation. The variables obtained from the equation for each curve enabled us to calculate the apparent membrane resistance $(R_m)_{app}$ and internal longitudinal resistivity (R_i).

$(R_m)_{app}$ was significantly larger in epicardial $(565 \pm 222 \text{ ohm} \cdot \text{cm}^2)$ than endocardial $(375 \pm 137 \text{ ohm} \cdot \text{cm}^2)$ preparations from normal hearts. This regional difference disappeared in hypertrophied hearts (epicardium, 421 ± 138; endocardium, $383 \pm 121 \text{ ohm} \cdot \text{cm}^2$). R_i was similar for normal endocardial $(272 \pm 169 \text{ ohm} \cdot \text{cm})$ and epicardial $(326 \pm 152 \text{ ohm} \cdot \text{cm})$ preparations, as well as for hypertrophied endocardial $(251 \pm 108 \text{ ohm} \cdot \text{cm})$ and epicardial $(312 \pm 59 \text{ ohm} \cdot \text{cm})$ preparations. We determined the effective membrane capacity (C_{eff}) by measuring the ratio of applied charge to the displacement of membrane potential. C_{eff} was larger for normal hearts (epicardium, 9.7 ± 2.5; endocardium, $7.5 \pm 3.0 \ \mu F/cm^2$) than for hypertrophied hearts (epicardium, 4.1 ± 1.4; endocardium, $4.7 \pm 1.2 \ \mu f/cm^2$). From the values for C_{eff}, we calculated the effective membrane resistance, $(R_m)_{eff}$. $(R_m)_{eff}$ was larger for normal (epicardium, $5,392 \pm 2,613$; endocardium, $3,013 \pm 2,096$ $\text{ohm} \cdot \text{cm}^2$) than for hypertrophied (epicardium, $1,552 \pm 633$; endocardium, $1,838 \pm 826 \text{ ohm} \cdot \text{cm}^2$) preparations. Our results show that the amount of electrically effective membrane area is decreased in hypertrophied myocardium despite the increased total area per hypertrophied cell. One functional implication of this finding is that activation of contraction by spread of surface electrical depolarization into the T-tubules may be impaired in hypertrophied cardiac muscle.

THE ELECTROCARDIOGRAM IN EXPERIMENTAL CARDIAC HYPERTROPHY

The diagnosis of left ventricular hypertrophy by alterations in the electrocardiogram (ECG) is of importance since such ECG changes may represent the only clinical sign of left ventricular hypertrophy. Criteria for the diagnosis of left ventricular hypertrophy usually include an increase in QRS magnitude, lengthening of the QRS duration, and alterations in the ST and T waves (32–34). The ECG criteria for left ventricular hypertrophy are based largely on empirical observation and often lack specificity or selectivity when assessed in conjunction with correlative autopsy data (32–33,35).

Therefore, we thought it would be interesting to determine whether or not left ventricular hypertrophy induced by renal hypertension in rats is associated with characteristic ECG changes and whether such changes, if present, might correlate with the alterations we have observed in action potentials of hypertrophied ventricular muscle (36). This was done by recording ECGs from age-matched HBP and SHAM rats with subdermal electrodes. The rats were anesthetized lightly and six standard limb leads were recorded at a paper speed of 60 mm/sec. After obtaining the ECGs, the hearts were removed and action potentials were recorded from epicardial and endocardial preparations.

Figure 5 shows lead II records from an HBP and SHAM ECG. Under control conditions, prior to induction of hypertension, the QRS complex in both HBP and SHAM records is followed immediately by a T wave without an identifiable intervening ST segment. This kind of pattern is well known in the rat ECG and has been attributed to the lack of a plateau or slow phase of repolarization in the normal rat ventricular action potential (37). In contrast, by 6 weeks after induction of hypertension, the HBP ECG shows a marked change. The peaked T wave that usually follows the QRS in the normal rat ECG has been replaced by an almost isoelectric segment lasting until the next P wave. In contrast, the SHAM ECG obtained at 6 weeks after operation shows a similar T wave pattern to that of the control ECG. At 10 weeks after operation, the HBP ECG continues to show an almost isoelectric segment between the end of the QRS and the following P wave. On the other hand, the SHAM ECG at 10 weeks is generally similar in overall appearance to earlier records, except for a decrease in T wave size.

Previous studies (38–39) suggested that the T wave corresponded to the repolarization of the ventricle and resulted from the shorter duration of the action potentials in the epicardial than the endocardial region. However, in SHAM and HBP rat ECGs the magnitude of the T wave did not consistently correlate with the difference in action potential duration between endocardial and epicardial action potentials. For example, in one SHAM rat, at the physiological stimulation rate of 400 beats/min, there was no difference in duration between epicardial and endocardial action potentials, although a prominent T wave was observed in the ECGs. In one HBP rat, flattened T waves were associated with a significant difference in duration between epicardial and endocardial action potentials. In seven HBP and seven SHAM rats studied, we observed a highly variable relationship between the T wave configuration and the regional differences in action potential duration (36).

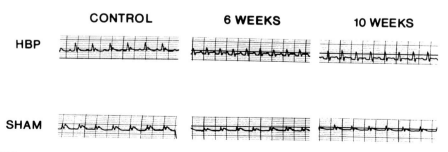

FIG. 5. Limb lead II ECG records obtained from HBP and SHAM rats. Control records were obtained prior to operation to produce hypertension. Records obtained at 6 and 10 weeks after operation are labeled accordingly. Calibrations: Each large *vertical division*, 0.5 mV; *horizontal division*, 100 msec.

It is likely that the T wave configuration may be influenced not only by difference in action potential duration, but also by other factors. These include altered time sequence of propagation of the repolarization wave front in hypertrophied myocardium (40) and the magnitude and polarity of the solid angles subtended by the limits of a boundary of an activation front (41,42). Finally, the lack of correlation between differences in action potential duration and T wave configuration could be due to the fact that we did not sample enough action potentials or that we did not record from those parts of the heart that are responsible, *in situ*, for the shape of the T wave.

AFTERPOTENTIALS AND TRIGGERED ACTIVITY

In normal ventricular muscle, repolarization of the action potential returns the membrane potential to the diastolic level that prevailed prior to excitation. The fiber then remains electrically quiescent until it is excited again. The usual course of events during repolarization and "electrical diastole" can be altered by two kinds of afterdepolarizations (43–45): (a) delayed afterdepolarizations that occur after completion of repolarization and carry the membrane potential to a level more positive than that recorded later in diastole; and (b) early afterdepolarizations that interrupt the normal course of repolarization, thereby preventing the membrane potential from returning to the level prevailing before the action potential upstroke. Such afterpotentials are important because they can give rise to nonstimulated action potentials that might in turn account for some kinds of abnormal rhythmic activity in the heart (43–45).

We have found that afterdepolarizations can be induced selectively in hypertrophied myocardium from rats with renal hypertension (45). Figure 6

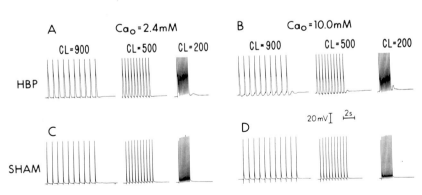

FIG. 6. Effects of stimulation cycle length (**CL**) and Ca_o on afterpotential characteristics. **A** and **B** show that the magnitude and configuration of delayed afterdepolarization in HBP fibers vary according to the CL and Ca_o. **C** and **D** show that SHAM fibers did not develop afterpotentials at any cycle length at either Ca_o. (From Aronson, ref. 45, by permission of the American Heart Association, Inc.)

shows that, under the same experimental conditions, HBP fibers develop delayed afterdepolarizations but SHAM fibers do not.

Our studies showed that the delayed afterdepolarizations became larger when the stimulation frequency, number of preceding driven beats, or $(Ca^{2+})_o$ was increased. The coupling interval from the upstroke of the last driven action potential to the peak of the delayed afterdepolarization decreased when the stimulation frequency or number of preceding driven beats increased. Hypertrophied fibers treated with high $(Ca^{2+})_o$ that gave rise to triggered activity had a characteristic relation between delayed afterpotential magnitude and drive cycle length. In hypertrophied muscles treated with TEA, triggered activity developed from an early afterdepolarization, but terminated with a delayed afterdepolarization. The occurrence of afterpotentials in hypertrophied, but not in normal, myocardium appears to reflect the development of an important electrophysiologic alteration that may predispose hypertrophied fibers to develop arrhythmias.

The delayed afterdepolarizations recorded from HBP muscles have certain features in common with apparently similar electrical activity reported to occur in other cardiac tissues under a variety of experimental conditions (43–45). Although the mechanism underlying delayed afterdepolarization is not clear, our results and those of previous studies suggest that they depend in some way on Ca^{2+}. This view is supported by the findings that their magnitude is increased when external Ca^{2+} is increased and decreased by "slow channel blockers" like verapamil and Mn^{2+} (43–46). In addition, these delayed afterdepolarizations are accompanied by aftercontractions (47–48) suggesting an important role for Ca^{2+}.

The mechanism underlying early afterdepolarizations also is unknown. It would seem that relative lack of a repolarizing outward current is possibly involved, but further studies are required to determine the precise mechanism.

FUNCTIONAL IMPLICATIONS OF THE ELECTRICAL PROPERTIES ASSOCIATED WITH VENTRICULAR HYPERTROPHY

It seems reasonable to briefly consider the possible functional implications of the electrical properties of hypertrophied ventricular muscle. One possible connection between altered electrical activity and mechanical function is that the longer action potentials of hypertrophied muscle may represent a compensatory mechanism for preserving the contractile strength of hypertrophied ventricular muscle. In rats with hypertrophy induced by renal hypertension, developed tension is maintained at normal levels despite a decrease in velocity of shortening (17,49). The ability to maintain normal levels of tension development appears to be related to the prolonged time to peak tension invariably seen in hypertrophied muscles (17,49). It is possible that the longer duration of contraction in hypertrophied ventricular muscles is due to the longer action potentials associated with hypertrophy.

The afterpotentials and triggered activity associated with cardiac hypertrophy could predispose hypertrophied hearts to a wide variety of rhythm disorders. The fact that afterdepolarizations can initiate sustained rhythmic activity in our experimental model of cardiac hypertrophy as well as in human atrial fibers from diseased hearts (50) suggests that triggered activity may be an important mechanism underlying arrhythmias.

The occurrence of afterdepolarizations in hypertrophied muscle may also have effects on the mechanical performance of the heart. Since delayed afterdepolarizations are associated with aftercontractions, it is possible that such aftercontractions might influence the diastolic pressure–volume relations in the intact heart. Furthermore, if early afterdepolarizations are also associated with tension development, then it is possible that such a mechanism might actively increase diastolic pressure in hypertrophied hearts.

The graded transmural changes in action potential duration suggest that the response of the membrane to pressure overload is not uniform. Alternatively, the graded changes from endocardium to epicardium also might imply that the stress responsible for inducing hypertrophy is not uniformly distributed across the wall of the heart.

Our analysis of the passive membrane properties of hypertrophied muscle indicates that the electrical coupling between hypertrophied fibers is as effective as that between normal fibers. This is indicated by the similar values for R_i in normal and hypertrophied muscles. Therefore, it is unlikely that uncoupling of cells occurs up to the stage of hypertrophy we studied. This implies that spread of excitation should not be seriously impaired in hypertrophied hearts.

Our finding that C_{eff} is only about half the normal value in hypertrophied myocardium has an important functional implication with regard to excitation-contraction coupling. It seems most likely that the low values for C_{eff} in hypertrophied muscle are due to a lack of effective charging of the T-tubular system. This means that despite morphological evidence of more abundant T-tubular membrane in hypertrophied myocardium (15), a large portion of this membrane is not functional electrically. Therefore, it is possible that activation of contraction by spread of surface electrical depolarization into the T-tubular may be impaired in hypertrophied cardiac muscle.

ACKNOWLEDGMENTS

This work was supported in part by National Institutes of Health Young Investigator Grant HL 21167 and Molly Berns Senior Investigator of the New York Heart Association Award, supported through the Kreindler-Berns Foundation, awarded to Dr. Aronson. Dr. Aronson is a recipient of an Established Investigator Award from the American Heart Association.

REFERENCES

1. Spann, J. F., Jr., Buccinno, R. A., Sonnenblick, E. H., and Braunwald, E. (1967): *Circ. Res.*, 21:341–354.
2. Kaufmann, R. L., Homburger, H., and Wirth, H. (1971): *Circ. Res.*, 28:346–357.
3. Bassett, A., and Gelband, H. (1973): *Circ. Res.*, 32:15–26.
4. Gelband, H., and Bassett, A. (1973): *Circ. Res.*, 32:625–634.
5. Tritthart, H., Leudcke, H., Bayler, R., Stierle, H., and Kaufmann, R. (1975): *J. Mol. Cell. Cardiol.*, 7:163–174.
6. Ten Eick, R., Gelband, H., Kahn, J., and Bassett, A. (1977): *Circulation (Abstract)*, 56:III–47.
7. Ten Eick, R., Gelband, H., Goode, M., and Bassett, A. (1978): *Circulation (Abstract)*, 58:II–47.
8. Hayashi, H., and Shibata, S. (1974): *Eur. J. Pharmacol.*, 27:355–359.
9. Heller, L. J., Stauffer, E. K., and Fox, W. D. (1978): *Fed. Proc. (Abstract)*, 37:349.
10. Heller, L. J., and Stauffer, E. K. (1979): *Fed. Proc. (Abstract)*, 38:975.
11. Cutilletta, A., Benjamin, M., Culpepper, W. S., and Oparil, S. (1978): *J. Molec. Cell. Cardiol.*, 10:689–703.
12. Wolinsky, H. (1971): *Circ. Res.*, 28:622–637.
13. Aronson, R. S. (1980): *Circ. Res.*, 47:443–454.
14. Loud, A. V., Anversa, P., Giacomelli, F., and Wiener, J. (1978): *Lab. Invest.*, 38:586–596.
15. Anversa, P., Loud, A. V., Giacomelli, F., and Wiener, J. (1978): *Lab. Invest.*, 38:597–609.
16. Wendt-Gallitelli, M. F., Ebrecht, G., and Jacob, R. (1979): *J. Molec. Cell. Cardiol.*, 11:275–287.
17. Capasso, J. M., Strobeck, J. E., and Sonnenblick, E. H. (1981): *Amer. J. Physiol.*, 241:H435–H441.
18. Gulch, R. W., Baumann, R., and Jacob, R. (1979): *Basic Res. Cardiol.*, 74:69–82.
19. Aronson, R. S., and Keung, E. C. H. (1983): *Perspectives of Cardiovascular Research, Vol. 6*, edited by N. Alpert, pp. 233–243. Raven Press, New York.
20. Weidmann, S. (1951): *J. Physiol. (Lond.)*, 115:227–236.
21. Gadsby, D. C., and Cranefield, P. F. (1979): *J. Gen. Physiol.*, 73:819–837.
22. Kerkut, G. A., and York, B. (1971): *The Electrogenic Sodium Pump.* Scientechnica Ltd., Bristol.
23. Keung, E. C. H., and Aronson, R. S. (1981): *Circ. Res.*, 49:150–158.
24. Carmeliet, E. (1977): *J. Physiol. (Paris)*, 73:903–923.
25. Beeler, G. W., and Reuter, H. (1977): *J. Physiol.*, 268:117–210.
26. Keung, E. C. H., Keung, C., and Aronson, R. S. (1983): *Am. J. Physiol.*, 243:H917–H926.
27. Berkinblit, M. B., Kovalev, S. A., Smolyaninor, V. V., and Chaylakhyan, L. M. (1971): In: *Models of the Structural–Functional Organization of Certain Biological Systems*, edited by I. M. Gelfant, V. S. Gurfinkel, S. V. Formin, and M. L. Tsetlin, Ch. 3. M.I.T. Press, Cambridge.
28. Jack, J. J. B., Noble, D., and Tsien, R. W. (1975): *Electrical Current Flow in Excitable Cells.* Clarendon Press, Oxford.
29. Woodbury, J. W., and Crill, W. E. (1961): In: *Nervous Inhibitors, Proceedings of an International Symposium*, edited by Lord Florey, pp. 124–135. Pergamon Press, Oxford.
30. Tanaka, I., and Sasaki, Y. (1966): *J. Gen. Physiol.*, 49:1089–1110.
31. Shiba, H. (1971): *J. Theor. Biol.*, 30:59–68.
32. Selzer, A., Ebnother, C. L., Packard, P., Stone, A. O., and Quinn, J. E. (1958): *Circulation*, 17:255–265.
33. Romhilt, D. W., and Estes, E. H. (1968): *Am. Heart J.*, 75:752–758.
34. Cooksey, J. D., Dunn, M., and Massie, E. (1977): *Clinical Vectorcardiography and Electrocardiography.* Year Book Medical Publishers, Chicago.
35. Holt, J. H., Barnard, C. L., and Kramer, J. O. (1971): In: *Cardiac Hypertrophy*, edited by N. R. Alpert, pp. 611–621. Academic Press, New York.
36. Keung, E. C. H., and Aronson, R. S. (1981): *Cardiovasc. Res.*, 15:611–614.
37. Hoffman, B. F., and Cranefield, P. F. (1960): *Electrophysiology of the Heart.* McGraw-Hill, New York.
38. Fukushima, I. (1970): *Jap. Circ. J.*, 34:465–467.

39. Noble, D., and Cohen, I. (1978): *Cardiovasc. Res.*, 12:13–27.
40. Durrer, D., Van Dam, R. T., Freud, G. E., Meijler, F. L., and Roos, J. P. (1969): In: *Electrical Activity of the Heart*, edited by G. W. Manning and S. P. Ahuja, pp. 53–68. Charles C Thomas, Springfield, Illinois.
41. Holland, R. P., and Arnsdorf, M. F. (1977): *Prog. Cardiovasc. Dis.*, 19:431–457.
42. Scher, A. M., and Spach, M. S. (1979): In: *Handbook of Physiology: The Cardiovascular System, Volume I, The Heart*, edited by R. M. Berne, pp. 357–392. Williams and Wilkens, Baltimore.
43. Cranefield, P. F. (1975): *The Conduction of the Cardiac Impulse: The Slow Response and Cardiac Arrhythmias.* Futura, Mount Kisco, New York.
44. Cranefield, P. F. (1977): *Circ. Res.*, 41:415–423.
45. Aronson, R. S. (1981): *Circ. Res.*, 48:720–727.
46. Rosen, M. R., and Danilo, P., Jr. (1980): *Circ. Res.*, 46:117–124.
47. Ferrier, G. R. (1976): *Circ. Res.*, 38:156–162.
48. Heller, L. J. (1979): *Am. J. Physiol.*, 6:H649–H654.
49. Capasso, J. M., Strobeck, J. E., Malhotra, A., Scheuer, J., and Sonnenblick, E. H. (1982): *Am. J. Physiol.*, 242:H882–H889.
50. Mary-Rabine, L., Hordoff, A. J., Danilo, P., Jr., Malm, J. R., and Rosen, M. R. (1980): *Circ. Res.*, 47:267–277.

*Perspectives in Cardiovascular
Research, Vol. 8,*
edited by R. C. Tarazi and J. B. Dunbar.
Raven Press, New York © 1983.

Cardiac Reflexes

Vernon S. Bishop and Eileen M. Hasser

*Department of Pharmacology, The University of Texas Health Science Center
at San Antonio, San Antonio, Texas 78284*

Reflexes originating from receptors in the cardiopulmonary region have two major afferent pathways. One input is to the medulla by way of the vagus and the other is to the upper thoracic region by way of the cardiac sympathetic afferents. There are approximately 2,000 to 2,500 vagal afferents from the right side of the cat's heart. Approximately 25% of these are myelinated (1) and serve receptors located primarily in the atria and vein-atrial junctions (2–4). The remaining vagal fibers are unmyelinated and are distributed throughout the heart in atria and ventricles (5,6). The sympathetic fibers are located in the atria and ventricles and along the coronary arteries. There are also approximately 300 myelinated sympathetic afferent fibers in the inferior cardiac nerve (7). Because of the large number of unmyelinated sympathetic efferents the number of unmyelinated afferents have not been determined. However, it seems reasonable to assume that vagal and sympathetic input to the central nervous system is similar (8).

Activation of cardiac afferent sympathetic nerves appears to produce a reflex response that is primarily excitatory (9–12), although inhibitory responses have been observed (13,14). Sympathetic afferents in the heart are excited by a variety of chemical substances such as bradykinin (15) and veratridine (11). Both unmyelinated and myelinated endings in the atria and ventricles are responsive to increases in pressure (17–19); the unmyelinated fibers also appear to be excited by increases in ventricular contractility (19). Reduction in coronary perfusion pressure is known to increase the discharge of sympathetic afferents as well (16). The excitatory response to activation of sympathetic afferents results in increased cardiac efferent activity, heart rate, increased left ventricular dP/dt_{max} and arterial pressure (Fig. 1) (20). The cardiac effects are eliminated by beta-adrenergic receptor blockade and the systemic effects by alpha-adrenergic blockade. Low frequency electrical stimulation of cardiac sympathetic afferents inhibits renal nerve activity and causes renal vasodilation (21). Thus, in addition to a cardiocardiac component, the cardiac sympathetic afferents can also increase or decrease sympathetic outflow to other cardiovascular regions. In addition, there is a medullary component that inhibits vagal efferent activity (22).

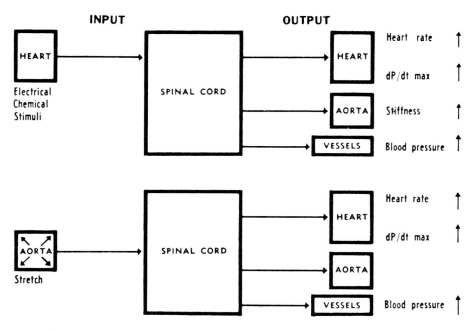

FIG. 1. Cardiovascular responses to stimulation of afferent sympathetic fibers. (From Malliani et al., ref. 20, with permission.)

CARDIAC REFLEX STUDIES IN ANIMAL MODELS

The cardiocardiac sympathetic reflex has been demonstrated in several studies. In spontaneously breathing cats with chronic spinal section at C-8 (vagal efferent blocked with atropine), a reflex tachycardia was observed during acute volume loading (23). The response was blocked by the sectioning of the upper thoracic dorsal roots. Thus, in the spinal cat, a Bainbridge-type response can be mediated by sympathetic afferents. Another study in conscious dogs demonstrated that stretch of the thoracic aorta induced a reflex increase in arterial pressure and heart rate (24). The rise in arterial pressure was mediated through alpha receptors while the tachycardia was mediated by activation of beta receptors and vagal withdrawal. This observation, together with previous studies, suggests that spinal excitatory reflexes exhibit positive feedback characteristics (25). The importance of the cardiac sympathetic reflexes has been discounted by many investigators because many of the excitatory responses are small and supraspinal structures may override these reflexes (26). However, as noted by Malliani et al. (25), the positive feedback nature of the sympathetic reflexes may be important in the modulation of negative feedback systems. For example, when veratridine is administered into the coronary artery of conscious dogs with intact vagal and sympathetic afferents, the classical Bezold-Jarisch reflex is observed (27). There is a pronounced bradycardia, hypotension, and a decrease in left ventricular (LV) dP/dt. However, interruption of the vagal afferents by bilateral vagal cold block prevents the bradycardia and hypotension to intracoronary veratridine. Also LV dP/dt is increased, suggesting that the decrease in LV dP/dt observed when the vagi were intact may have been modulated by the sympathetic afferents.

The contribution of cardiac sympathetic fibers to the regulation of the circulation in normal physiological states is not yet known. However, it is conceivable that an excitatory reflex may contribute to the pathophysiology observed in many clinical states (25). These include hypertensive episodes and cardiac arrhythmias during myocardial ischemia (28,29) and hypertension after coronary bypass surgery (30).

Activation of vagal afferents may elicit excitatory (3) or inhibitory responses, depending upon the receptors activated (31). Unencapsulated endings, which are located in the atria and vein atria junctions, are connected to myelinated vagal afferents, and are activated during atrial contraction and filling (2,3). Linden and co-workers (32) have demonstrated that activation of atrial receptors with myelinated afferents leads to tachycardia and an increase in cardiac sympathetic efferent discharge to the sino-atrial node. Stretch of the atria also results in a decrease in renal sympathetic outflow to the kidney, but sympathetic outflow to other regions appears to be unaltered. The increase in urine flow is independent of changes in plasma antidiuretic hormone (ADH) (3). A vagally mediated excitatory response, which is characterized by hypertension and tachycardia, is also observed when serotonin is injected in the proximal portion of the left coronary artery (33).

The activity of receptors with unmyelinated vagal afferents is sparse and irregular (34,35); collectively, however, they constitute a major input to the CNS. In general, the cardiovascular response to activation of unmyelinated vagal afferents is inhibitory; electrical activation of unmyelinated vagal afferents causes prompt bradycardia, hypotension, and a reduction in sympathetic outflow to the periphery (36). The atrial receptors, which are often silent, may discharge during the V wave of atrial pressure, particularly during end-inspiration and early expiration when the transmural pressure is high (34). The discharge of these receptors also increases with atrial pressure during volume expansion. The threshold for those in the right atrium is approximately 2 mm Hg, and 5 to 12 mm Hg for those in the left atrium. Thus, atrial receptors subserved by both myelinated and unmyelinated vagal afferents respond to atrial volume changes within the physiological range.

LV receptors with unmyelinated vagal afferents discharge during early systole. However, receptor activity appears to correlate better with changes in LV end-diastolic pressure (LVEDP) than with changes in left ventricular systolic pressure (LVSP) (35). The discharge rate of these receptors is increased by interventions that improve systolic performance of the left ventricle (increases in total force and rate of force developed), such as preload and inotropic agents. Interventions that reduce the inotropic state, such as beta-blocking agents, also decrease the discharge rate. The curvilinear relationship between receptor activity and LVEDP is similar to the relationship between developed force and preload. Thus, the correlation of receptor activity to increases in LVEDP may be explained in part by the Frank-Starling mechanism.

Vagal afferents from the cardiopulmonary region (lungs, atria, and heart) exert a tonic inhibitory influence on sympathetic outflow from the vasomotor center (36). Interruption of the vagal afferent activity in anesthetized rabbits, cats, and dogs results in an increase in heart rate, arterial pressure, and renal, mesenteric and hindlimb vascular resistance (36,37). The magnitude of the vasoconstriction observed during interruption of the vagal afferents varies inversely with the carotid sinus pressure and is related directly to the existing sympathetic outflow (36–38). These responses occur whether the animals are atropinized or the vagi are cut below the diaphragm, indicating that the tonic influence is due to the interruption of vagal afferents from the cardiopulmonary region. Results from experiments utilizing selective blockade of vagal afferents indicate that the tonic inhibitory influence is due to activity in the unmyelinated vagal afferents (6).

The tonic inhibitory influence of vagal afferents has also been observed in conscious dogs (39,40). Interruption of vagal afferents by vagal cold block in these dogs with aortic baroreceptors denervated results in significant increases in arterial pressure and peripheral resistance. The increases in arterial pressure and peripheral vascular resistance during vagal block are significantly greater in sinoartic denervated dogs than when the arterial baroreflex is intact (Fig. 2). Thus it appears that there is an important central interaction between arterial baroreceptors and cardiopulmonary receptors with vagal afferents. The interaction is such that the inhibitory influence of cardiopulmonary afferents is increased when the arterial baroreflex is reduced, whether acutely or chronically (37–42).

The effects of cardiopulmonary vagal afferents on sympathetic outflow to

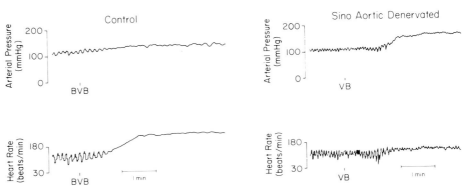

FIG. 2. Analogue recording of heart rate and mean arterial pressure in the control state and during bilateral vagal block (BVB) before (**left**) and after (**right**) sinoaortic denervation.

different vascular beds are not uniform. A number of studies have shown that these afferents exert a preferential effect on sympathetic outflow to the kidney (41,42). These afferents also inhibit the secretion of renin (43,44), ADH (45,46), and catecholamines from the adrenal medulla (47).

There are a number of studies indicating that ventricular receptors with unmyelinated afferents are sensitive to alterations in ventricular contractility (35,48). It is also known that increases in intraventricular pressure (49) and myocardial contractility (48,50) can produce a reflex peripheral vasodilation that has its afferents in the vagi (50). A recent study in our laboratory demonstrated that the increase in arterial pressure during vagal cold block in anesthetized cats was related to the existing cardiac sympathetic activity (48) (Fig. 3). Furthermore, vagal cold block also produced an increased left ventricular contractility in these animals. It has been postulated that cardiac sympathetic activity may modulate vagal afferent activity from cardiopulmonary receptors through changes in ventricular contractility. This could serve as a negative feedback system to regulate myocardial contractility such that increases in cardiac sympathetic activity would increase cardiac vagal afferent activity. This, in turn, could act to restrain sympathetic outflow to the heart and thus buffer myocardial contractility. A similar feedback system has been suggested by Fox et al. (50).

Our laboratory tested this hypothesis in conscious dogs in which the aortic baroreceptors were denervated (51). Dogs were instrumented for the measurement of left ventricular pressure, LV dP/dt_{max}, and arterial pressure. Thermodes were implanted around the cervical vagi; bilateral cold block of the vagi

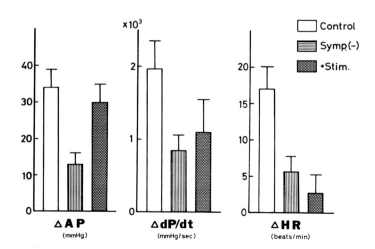

FIG. 3. Effect of cardiac sympathectomy and sympathetic stimulation on circulatory responses to vagal blockade. Responses are illustrated as changes in arterial pressure (ΔAP), LV dP/dt_{max} (ΔdP/dt), and heart rate (ΔHR). (From Shimizu et al., ref. 48, with permission of the American Heart Association.)

resulted in significant increases in arterial pressure and heart rate, but did not alter LV dP/dt_{max}. At doses that had no systemic effects, intracoronary administration of catecholamines caused a dose dependent increase in dP/dt_{max} when the vagi were intact and during vagal cold block (Fig. 4); however, the inotropic effects were always greater when the vagi were blocked. Ganglionic blockade produced a similar degree of inotropic potentiation to epinephrine. These observations are consistent with a negative feedback reflex, and provide evidence for the existence of a cardiocardiac vago-sympathetic negative feedback reflex that can be initiated by an increase in myocardial contractility. This reflex would offer a mechanism by which the autonomic nervous system can sense and modulate the contractile state of the ventricular myocardium.

MYOCARDIAL ISCHEMIA AND INFARCTION

Anesthetized Studies

The cardiovascular changes due to acute myocardial ischemia and infarction in either anesthetized or conscious animals are often rapid and dramatic. During acute ischemia or infarction of the heart, potential sources of cardiac reflexes are implicated by the numerous dynamic changes that take place. These changes include increases in end-diastolic and atrial pressures and decreases in myocardial contractility with akinetic and dyskinetic regions of contractions. In the isolated perfused hindlimb and kidney, vasodilatation is usually observed during coronary occlusions. Neural recordings from cardiac vagal and sympathetic afferents indicate that myocardial ischemia activates myelinated and unmyelinated vagal afferents as well as sympathetic afferents (52–57). Activation of cardiac receptors subserved by unmyelinated vagal afferents may inhibit sympathetic outflow to the cardiovascular system (31,51,58–60), while

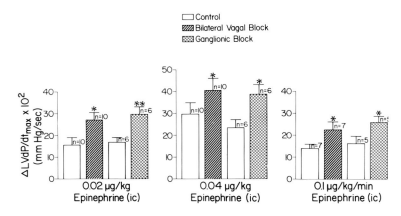

FIG. 4. Comparison of the increases in LV dP/dt_{max} during BVB and ganglionic blockade due to intracoronary (ic) epinephrine. Mean ± SE; n = number of dogs. (From Barron and Bishop, ref. 27, with permission of the American Heart Association.)

increasing cardiac parasympathetic efferent activity. Activation of myelinated vagal afferents from receptors within the atrium may increase sympathetic activity to the sinus node and decrease sympathetic activity to the kidney (30,32); activation of cardiac sympathetic nerves may exert an excitatory effect on the heart and systemic circulation (19,53,61,62). Finally, one must consider that hypotension associated with myocardial ischemia may elicit arterial baroreflex adjustments. Thus, reflexes from vagal and sympathetic afferents, as well as arterial baroreflexes, may contribute to the integrated reflex responses in myocardial ischemia or infarction.

Myocardial embolization by mercury or air decreases renal sympathetic nerve activity in dog (63,64). This decrease in renal sympathetic nerve activity is abolished by vagotomy. A more recent study (59) in anesthetized dogs shows that in the absence of arterial baroreflexes, renal sympathetic nerve activity is reduced by circumflex occlusion and, to a lesser degree, by left anterior descending occlusion.

There are conflicting reports concerning the effects of coronary occlusion on cardiac sympathetic efferent nerve activity. In cats with intact arterial baroreceptors, studies report both decreases (65) and increases (66,67) in cardiac sympathetic nerve activity. Constantin (65) observed decreases in blood pressure and cardiac sympathetic efferent nerve activity during coronary occlusion, both of which were abolished by vagotomy. Malliani et al. (67) observed increases in nerve activity recorded from the gray ramus at T-3. Vagotomy and spinal section at C-1 did not alter the response, suggesting that cardiocardiac sympathetic reflexes operate at the spinal level. In anesthetized sinoaortic denervated dogs, however, cardiac sympathetic efferent activity decreased during coronary occlusion. An increase was observed only in animals with high spinal sections, suggesting that supraspinal inhibitory pathways prevented the excitatory reflex from cardiac sympathetic afferents (26).

The difference between the two studies may lie in the species or the techniques utilized by these investigators to determine sympathetic nerve activity. Malliani et al. (67) recorded from fibers at T-3, while Felder and Thames (26,58) recorded the integrated nerve activity from a bundle of nerves in the preganglionic fibers in the ansa subclavia.

Conscious Studies

The characteristic responses to brief occlusion of the left circumflex coronary artery are a rise in heart rate and left atrial pressure, a modest but significant fall in arterial pressure, and a slight increase in peripheral resistance (68,69). The tachycardia is initiated from receptors in or near the heart, and the magnitude of the response is a combination of the responses from these receptors and the arterial baroreceptors. The efferent pathway involves both the vagi and the right cardiac sympathetic nerves; the site of origin of the reflex has not been determined. In view of the study by Linden (3), it is possible that the tachycardia is initiated by stretch of left atrial receptors with myelinated vagal afferents. If this is the case, then the efferent limb would be in the right cardiac sympathetic nerves.

In the conscious dog, the arterial baroreceptors have been shown to play an important role in the maintenance of perfusion pressure during coronary occlusion (68). The elimination of these baroreceptors unmasked a vasodilatory response which reduced peripheral resistance and, consequently, arterial pressure. The contribution of vagal afferent activity in the cardiovascular responses to coronary occlusions was determined in the conscious dog using vagal cold block techniques (40). With intact arterial baroreceptors, coronary occlusion during vagal block results in similar decreases in arterial pressure but peripheral resistance increases significantly. After sinoaortic denervation, however, the dramatic hypotension observed during coronary occlusion is reversed partially by vagal block and the decline in peripheral resistance is prevented (Fig. 5). These studies clearly demonstrate that vagal afferents collectively exert a tonic inhibitory influence on the cardiovascular system in the conscious dog and that they interact with the arterial baroreflexes in regulating the vascular responses during coronary occlusions.

There is evidence of autonomic disturbances in man at the onset of acute myocardial infarction. Pantridge (29) observed evidence of sympathetic over-reactivity (tachycardia and/or hypertension) or parasympathetic over-reactivity (bradycardia and/or hypotenson) in 8% of the patients studied within 30 min of onset of myocardial infarction. Signs of excessive sympathetic activity were more frequent in cases of anterior infarction, whereas signs of vagal over-

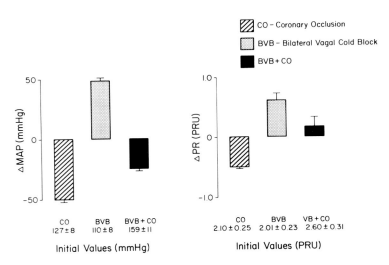

FIG. 5. Effects of bilateral vagal cold block on the changes in mean arterial pressure (ΔMAP) and peripheral resistance (ΔPR) in coronary occlusion, bilateral vagal cold block, and coronary occlusion during bilateral vagal cold block. (From Bishop and Peterson, ref. 40, with permission.)

reactivity were more frequent in cases in inferior infarction. In the dog, the inhibitory responses (neural and depressor) to circumflex occlusion exceeded those observed during occlusion of the left anterior descending coronary artery (70). Thus, in both man and dog, the inhibitory responses observed during reductions in coronary flow are caused by cardiac receptors which appear to be localized in the inferoposterior of the left ventricular wall.

HEART FAILURE

A major concern in cardiovascular physiology is the contribution of neural reflexes in the neurohumoral adjustments that occur in heart failure. This problem has obvious clinical relevance to the management of patients with heart failure. In patients and experimental animals with congestive heart failure, there is evidence of an increase in sympathoadrenal activity (71); in addition, the regulation of renin and ADH may be altered (74,75). In dogs with right heart failure, there is a marked redistribution of peripheral blood flow away from the splanchnic and renal vascular beds during exercise (72,73). It has been postulated that increased sympathetic drive is due to reduced inhibitory input from the arterial baroreceptors (76). However, because of the potential of the cardiopulmonary receptors to influence sympathetic activity and renin and ADH release, the inputs from these receptors also may contribute to the neurohumoral response observed in heart failure (79).

In experimental chronic congestive heart failure, atrial receptors with myelinated vagal afferents show a reduced response to increases in atrial pressure (78). The threshold atrial pressure for receptor activation is increased, and the sensitivity to changes in pressure is reduced. This resetting and reduction of sensitivity is due to decreases in atrial compliance and to morphological changes of the receptor endings (79). These changes appear to be reversible when the symptoms of heart failure are removed (80). There are no data to indicate whether the sensitivity of cardiac receptors with unmyelinated fibers also is altered in heart failure.

A decreased sensitivity and/or increased threshold of cardiopulmonary receptors would reduce the braking influence of these receptors on sympathetic outflow. Both the tonic and reflex inhibitory influences would be decreased. This could explain the increased sympathoadrenal drive observed during exercise in patients with heart failure, since the normal opposition exerted by the cardiopulmonary reflexes to activation of somatic afferents would be significantly less (81).

Clinical observations have provided evidence in man that also suggests that resetting of the cardiopulmonary receptors may occur in heart failure (77, 78,82,83). Head-up tilting normally decreases forearm bloodflow, but increases it in patients with heart failure (77,83). A speculative explanation is that the tonic activity of ventricular receptors is low in heart failure patients with low ventricular ejection fractions. During head-up tilt, however, the reduction in filling pressure improves ventricular function, leading to an activation of ventricular receptors. This would inhibit sympathetic outflow to the forearm, thereby causing vasodilatation (83).

HYPERTENSION

There are very little data concerning the role of cardiac receptors in hypertension. Malliani and co-workers (25) have postulated that cardiovascular sympathetic afferents may initiate positive feedback reflexes that could lead to and sustain an elevated arterial pressure. Under normal circumstances, the reflex may serve to modulate the range of operation, the gain and stability of negative feedback mechanisms. Under pathological states, however, sympathosympathetic loops may escape central suppression, resulting in increased efferent sympathetic activity.

The role of cardiac vagal afferents in the regulation of circulation in hypertension has been investigated only recently. Resetting of the cardiopulmonary receptors has been reported in renal-hypertensive dogs (84) and in spontaneously hypertensive rats (85,86). The vasodilatory responses to sudden increases in ventricular pressure have been studied in dogs. When compared to normotensive dogs, renal hypertensive dogs required a greater increase in left ventricular pressure to elicit a similar degree of vasodilatation of the perfused gracilis muscle (84).

Thoren and co-workers (55,86) investigated the characteristics of unmyelinated cardiac fibers in normotensive rats (NCR) and spontaneously hypertensive rats (SHR). In rat, there are no myelinated vagal afferents, and all unmyelinated fibers originate from the atria. The pressure threshold for activation of the left atrial fibers was twice as high in the SHR as in the NCR. The resting left atrial pressure of the SHR was also twice as high as the NCR. The reflex inhibition of renal sympathetic nerve activity was reset to higher atrial pressures in the SHR. The sensitivity of the atrial receptors to changes in pressure and the resulting reflex response were similar in the SHR and NCR. Thus, the low pressure receptors in the SHR responded normally to changes in pressure but higher pressures were required. The mechanism responsible for the resetting of cardiopulmonary receptors in the hypertensive dog and SHR is not known. In the rat, the resetting appears to be due in part to a reduced atrial distensibility and altered receptor function. However, in both the hypertensive dog and SHR, cardiac hypertrophy may have contributed to the resetting by altering the coupling of the receptor endings with the myocardium (85,86).

In borderline hypertensive humans with no evidence of cardiac hypertrophy, the forearm vasoconstriction due to unloading of the cardiopulmonary receptors by lower body negative pressure is significantly greater than in normotensive subjects (87). The augmented inhibitory influence may be related to a decreased sensitivity of the arterial baroreceptors and an increased left ventricular systolic pressure which may increase vagal afferent activity.

SUMMARY

Numerous studies have shown that reflexes initiated from cardiac receptors with vagal and sympathetic afferents can contribute to the neurohumoral regulation of the circulation. However, there are many questions still to be answered concerning the importance of these reflexes in the overall regulation of the circulation. These include: (a) Are cardiac reflexes important in the long term control of the circulation? (b) Is resetting of cardiac receptors in pathological states beneficial to the overall circulation? (c) In certain pathological states, are cardiac reflexes beneficial to the circulation or do they interact with other regulatory mechanisms in an antagonistic manner resulting in a deterioration of the circulation?

ACKNOWLEDGMENTS

This study was supported by National Institutes of Health grant HL 12415 and Air Force Contract AFOSR 73-2525.

REFERENCES

1. Agostoni, E., Chinnock, J. E., Daly, M. de B., and Murray, J. G. (1957): *J. Physiol. (Lond.)*, 135:182–205.
2. Nonidez, J. F. (1937): *Am. J. Anat.*, 61:203–231.
3. Linden, R. J. (1975): *Prog. Cardiovasc. Dis.*, 18:201–221.
4. Brown, A. M. (1965): *J. Physiol. (Lond.)*, 177:203–214.
5. Coleridge, H. M., Coleridge, J. C. G., Dangel, A., Kidd, C., Luck, J. C., and Sleight, P. (1973): *Circ. Res.*, 33:87–97.
6. Thoren, P., Donald, D. E., and Shepherd, J. T. (1976): *Circ. Res. (Suppl.)*, 39:2–9.
7. Emery, D. G., Foreman, R. D., and Coggeshall, R. E. (1976): *J. Comp. Neurol.*, 166:457–468.
8. Brown, A. M. (1979): *Am. J. Cardiol.*, 44:849–851.
9. Brown, A. M., and Malliani, A. (1971): *J. Physiol. (Lond.)*, 212:685–705.
10. Peterson, D. F., and Brown, A. M. (1971): *Circ. Res.*, 28:605–610.
11. Malliani, A., Parks, M., Tuckett, R. P., and Brown, A. M. (1973): *Circ. Res.*, 32:9–14.
12. Malliani, A., Peterson, D. F., Bishop, V. S., and Brown, A. M. (1972): *Circ. Res.*, 30:158–166.
13. Brown, A. M., and Malliani, A. (1971): *J. Physiol. (Lond.)*, 212:685–705.
14. Brown, A. M. (1964): Ph.D. Thesis. University of London, London.
15. Uchida, Y., and Murao, S. (1974): *Jap. Heart J.*, 15:84–91.
16. Ueda, H., Uchida, Y., and Kamisaka, K. (1969): *Jap. Heart J.*, 10:70–81.
17. Kostreva, D. R., Zuperku, E. J., Purtock, R. V., Coon, R. L., and Kampine, J. P. (1975): *Am. J. Physiol.*, 229:911–915.
18. Malliani, A., Recordati, G., and Schwartz, P. J. (1973): *J. Physiol. (Lond.)*, 29:457–469.
19. Casti, R., Lombarda, F., and Malliani, A. (1979): *J. Physiol. (Lond.)*, 292:135–148.
20. Malliani, A., Lombardi, F., Pagani, M., Recordati, G., and Schwartz, P. J. (1975): *Brain Res.*, 87:239–246.
21. Purtock, R. V., Von Colditz, J. H., Seagard, J. L., Igler, F. O., Zupecker, E. J., and Kampine, J. P. (1977): *Am. J. Physiol.*, 233:H580–H586.
22. Schwartz, P. J., Pagani, M., Lombardi, F., Malliani, A., and Brown, A. M. (1973): *Circ. Res.*, 32:215–220.
23. Bishop, V. S., Lombardi, F., Malliani, A., Pagani, M., and Recordati, G. (1976): *Am. J. Physiol.*, 230:25–29.
24. Pagani, M., Pizzinelli, P., Furlan, R., Guzzetti, S., and Malliani, A. (1980): *Circ. Res. (Suppl.)*, 62:569.

25. Malliani, A., Pagani, M., and Brgamaschi, M. (1979): *Am. J. Cardiol*, 44:860–865.
26. Felder, R. B., and Thames, M. D. (1979): *Circ. Res.*, 48:728–736.
27. Barron, K. W., and Bishop, V. S. (1982): *Am. J. Physiol.*, 242:H810–H817.
28. Malliani, A., and Lombardi, F. (1978): In: *Neural Mechanisms in Cardiac Arrhythmias*, edited by P. J. Schwartz, A. M. Brown, A. Malliani, and A. Zanchetti, pp. 209–219. Raven Press, New York.
29. Pantridge, J. F. (1978): In: *Neural Mechanisms in Cardiac Arrhythmias*, edited by P. J. Schwartz, A. M. Brown, A. Malliani, and A. Zanchetti, pp. 7–17. Raven Press, New York.
30. Tarazi, R. C., Estafanous, F. G., and Fouad, F. M. (1978): *Am. J. Cardiol.*, 42:1013–1018.
31. Oberg, B., and Thoren, P. (1973): *Acta Physiol. Scand.*, 87:121–132.
32. Linden, R. J., Mary, D. A. S. G., and Weatherwill, D. (1980): *J. Physiol. (Lond.)*, 300:31–40.
33. James, T. N., Hageman, G. R., and Urthaler, F. (1979): *Am. J. Cardiol.*, 44:852–859.
34. Thoren, P. (1976): *Circ. Res.*, 38:357–362.
35. Thoren, P. (1977): *Circ. Res.*, 40:415–421.
36. Donald, D. E., and Shepherd, J. T. (1978): *Cardiovasc. Res.*, 12:449–469.
37. Oberg, B., and White, S. (1970): *Acta Physiol. (Scand.)*, 80:395–403.
38. Mancis, G., Shepherd, J. T., and Donald, D. E. (1975): *Circ. Res.*, 37:200–208.
39. Bishop, V. S., and Barron, K. W. (1980): In: *Arterial Baroreceptors in Hypertension*, edited by P. Sleight, pp. 91–97. Oxford University Press, London.
40. Bishop, V. S., and Peterson, D. F. (1978): *Circ. Res.*, 43:840–847.
41. Mancia, G., Shepherd, J. T., and Donald, D. E. (1976): *Am. J. Physiol.*, 230:19–24.
42. Mancia, G., Shepherd, J. T., and Donald, D. E. (1975): *Circ. Res.*, 37:200–208.
43. Thames, M. D., Jarecki, J., and Donald, D. E. (1978): *Circ. Res.*, 42:237–245.
44. Mursch, D. A., and Bishop, V. S. (1980): *Fed. Proc.*, 39:3025A.
45. Thames, M. D., and Schmid, P. G. (1979): *Am. J. Physiol.*, 237:H299–H304.
46. Thames, M. D., and Schmid, P. G. (1980): *Am. J. Physiol.*, 239:H784–H788.
47. Heesch, C. M., and Bishop, V. S. (1982): *Circ. Res.*, 51:391–399.
48. Shimizi, W. T., Peterson, D. F., and Bishop, V. S. (1979): *Am. J. Physiol.*, 237:H528–H534.
49. Salisbury, P. F., Cross, C. E., and Rieben, P. A. (1960): *Circ. Res.*, 8:530–534.
50. Fox, I. J., Gerasch, D. A., and Leonard, J. J. (1977): *J. Physiol. (Lond.)*, 273:405–425.
51. Barron, K. W., and Bishop, V. S. (1981): *Circ. Res.*, 49:159–169.
52. Brown, A. M. (1967): *J. Physiol. (Lond.)*, 190:35–53.
53. Malliani, A., and Brown, A. M. (1970): *Brain Res.*, 24:352–355.
54. Recordati, G., Schwartz, P. J., Pagani, M., Malliani, A., and Brown, A. B. (1971): *Experientia*, 27:1423–1424.
55. Thoren, P. (1976): *Am. J. Cardiol.*, 37:1046–1051.
56. Uchida, Y., and Murao, S. (1974): *Am. J. Physiol.*, 226:1094–1099.
57. Zucker, I. H., and Gilmore, J. P. (1974): *Am. J. Physiol.*, 227:360–363.
58. Felder, R. B., and Thames, M. D. (1979): *Circ. Res.*, 45:728–738.
59. Thames, M. D., and Abboud, F. M. (1979): *J. Clin. Invest.*, 63:395–402.
60. Thames, M. D., Kloppenstein, H. S., Abboud, F. M., Mark, A. L., and Walker, J. L. (1978): *Circ. Res.*, 43:512–519.
61. Malliani, A., Schwartz, P. J., and Zanchetti, A. (1969): *Am. J. Physiol.*, 217:703–709.
62. Malliani, A., Pagani, M., Recordath, G., and Schwartz, P. J. (1971): *Am. J. Physiol.*, 220:128–134.
63. Kezdi, P., Kordenat, R. K., and Misra, S. N. (1974): *Am. J. Cardiol.*, 33:853–860.
64. Uchida, Y., and Sakamoto, A. (1974): *Japan Circ. J.*, 38:491–495.
65. Constantin, L. (1963): *Am. J. Cardiol.*, 11:205–217.
66. Gillis, R. A. (1979): *Am. Heart J.*, 81:677–684.
67. Malliani, A., Schwartz, P. J., and Zanchetti, A. (1969): *Am. J. Physiol.*, 217:703–709.
68. Peterson, D. F., and Bishop, V. S. (1974): *Circ. Res.*, 34:226–232.
69. Peterson, D. F., Kaspar, R. L., and Bishop, V. S. (1973): *Circ. Res.*, 32:652–659.
70. Thames, M. D., Kloppenstein, H. S., Abboud, F. M., Mark, A. L., and Walker, J. L. (1978): *Circ. Res.*, 43:512–519.
71. Chidsey, C. A., Harrison, D. C., and Braunwald, E. (1962): *N. Engl. J. Med.*, 267:650–654.
72. Higgins, C. B., Vatner, S. F., Franklin, D., and Braunwald, E. (1972): *Circ. Res.*, 31:186–194.
73. Millard, R. W., Higgins, C. B., Franklin, D., and Vatner, S. F. (1972): *Circ. Res.*, 31:881–888.

74. Belleau, L., Mion, H., Simard, S., Granger, P., Bertranou, E., Nowaczynski, W., Boucher, R., and Genest, J. (1970): *Can. J. Physiol. Pharmacol.*, 48:450–456.
75. Genest, J., Granger, P., DeChamplain, J., and Boucher, R. (1968): *Am. J. Cardiol.*, 22:35–42.
76. Barger, A. C., Muedowney, F. P., and Libowitz, M. R. (1959): *Circulation*, 20:273–285.
77. Abboud, F. M., and Schmid, P. G. (1978): In: *Heart Failure*, edited by A. P. Fishman, pp. 249–260. Hemisphere Publishing Corporation, Washington, D.C.
78. Greenberg, T. T., Richmond, W. H., Stocking, R. A., Gupta, P. D., Meehan, J. P., and Henry, J. P. (1973): *Circ. Res.*, 32:424–433.
79. Zucker, I. H., Earle, A. M., and Gilmore, J. P. (1977): *J. Clin. Invest.*, 60:323–331.
80. Zucker, I. H., Earle, A. M., and Gilmore, J. P. (1979): *Am. J. Physiol.*, 237:H555–H559.
81. Thames, M. D., and Abboud, F. M. (1979): *Am. J. Physiol.*, 237:H560–H565.
82. Brigiden, W., and Sharpey-Schafter, E. P. (1950): *Clin. Sci.*, 9:93–100.
83. Abboud, F. M., Thames, M. D., and Mark. A. L. (1981): In: *Disturbances in Neurogenic Control of the Circulation*, edited by F. M. Abboud, H. A. Fozzard, J. P. Gilmore, and D. J. Reis, pp. 65–86. Williams and Wilkins, Baltimore, Maryland.
84. Kezdi, P. (1976): *Clin. Sci.*, 51:353–355.
85. Thoren, P., Noresson, E., and Ricksten, S. E. (1979): *Acta Physiol. Scand.*, 107:13–18.
86. Ricksten, S. E., Noresson, E., and Thoren, P. (1979): *Acta Physiol. Scand.*, 106:17–22.
87. Mark, A. L., and Kerber, R. E. (1982): *Hypertension,* 4:39–46.

Perspectives in Cardiovascular Research, Vol. 8,
edited by R. C. Tarazi and J. B. Dunbar.
Raven Press, New York © 1983.

Capillary Reserve and Tissue O_2 Transport in Normal and Hypertrophied Hearts

Carl R. Honig and Thomas E. J. Gayeski

Department of Physiology, University of Rochester Medical Center, Rochester, New York 14642

The pathophysiology of cardiac hypertrophy depends largely on the volume of blood provided per volume of tissue. Accordingly, this chapter's focus is the coronary capillary reserve in normal and hypertrophied hearts. The function of this reserve is reconsidered in light of recent measurements of intracellular O_2 gradients (1).

DEFINITIONS AND METHODS

Total Capillary Density

The conventional unit for capillary density (C.D.) is capillaries/mm². This approximation to capillaries/mm³ is convenient, and can be converted to capillaries/mm³ by dividing by capillary length. It is essential to bear in mind, however, that capillary length, diameter, and local capillary density have probability distributions with physiologically important variances (19). Indeed, the variability of these parameters is often of greater interest than the means. Classical histologic methods can only approximate the total number of capillaries per volume of myocardium because of difficulties introduced by fiber orientation (2). Stereologic techniques are required to overcome this problem (2,3).

Attainable Capillary Density

Vetterlein et al. (16) have shown that in the steady state the number of capillaries accessible to a dye covalently bound to plasma protein is identical to the total C.D. measured with histologic methods. Thus, there is no reserve of unperfused capillaries whatsoever if a plasma label is employed. In contrast, a large number of capillaries is not perfused with erythrocytes in heart and adult skeletal muscle (Table 1) (4–11). This is true even if all vessels are maximally dilated by adenosine, hypoxemia, or asphyxia (8). Cell-free capillaries result in part from the behavior of particles at bifurcations. Both in model systems (12) and *in vivo* (13), particles such as erythrocytes are preferentially collected by the branch with higher linear velocity. Indeed, above a critical ratio of velocities in the two branches all the cells enter the fast branch. The resulting high capillary hematocrit increases resistance, slows flow, and thereby redistributes cells into the opposite branch. In this way, time-variant stochastic hemodynamic and rheologic factors (12,13) make it impossible to perfuse all capillaries with erythrocytes simultaneously, even in the complete absence of vasomotor tone.

Functional Capillary Density and Capillary Reserve

In the presence of normal vasomotor tone, the number of capillaries actively perfused with erythrocytes is substantially less than the maximum attainable C.D. The former is termed the functional C.D., and the difference between the two is the capillary reserve (see Table 1).

The foregoing implies that capillaries not perfused with erythrocytes are of no consequence for transport. This is obviously true for O_2; at normal Pa_{O_2} and hemoglobin concentration, dissolved O_2 accounts for only 1.5% of the total. Transport of other substances depends on the rate of plasma flow. Judging from the rate of movement of platelets *in vivo* (13), the flow rate is low in capillaries devoid of erythrocytes. This is, of course, expected. If the terminal arteriole is constricted sufficiently to prevent passage of erythrocytes, resistance to flow of plasma around obstructed cells will be high. If, on the other hand, the arteriole is dilated, only the low-velocity channel at bifurcations will be free of cells (12,13). The large volume flow in the fast branch more than compensates for the low fractional content of plasma.

Clearance measurements offer a test of the contribution of cell-free capillaries to transport of small diffusion-limited molecules. Rb^{86} clearance (14) and multiple indicator dilution (15) yield an expansion factor of approximately 2 for C.D. in dog gracilis. Precisely the same expansion factor for dog gracilis was obtained independently, by direct enumeration of red cell-containing capillaries (7,8), indicating that cell-free capillaries have little effect on transport. It follows that a "perfused" capillary should be defined as one in which there is a flow of erythrocytes. As a corollary, plasma labels as used to date provide no information about the capillary reserve.

Recently, Vetterlein et al. (16) and Renkin and co-workers (17) reported the time course of accumulation of plasma label in capillaries after an abrupt injection. Values for functional C.D. in rat heart after 5 sec were almost identical to those obtained in our laboratory from measurements of red cell-containing capillaries *in situ* (4–6,11,18). Presumably, the capillaries first stained were those in which there was fast flow and, therefore, a stream of erythrocytes. Unfortunately, the apparent functional C.D. in myocardium becomes identical to the anatomical value at 10 sec, so in this tissue timing would appear to be too critical to permit use of the initial accumulation for quantitation.

Species, Preparative Artifact, and Cardiac Motion

All microscopy of the intact microcirculation *in vivo* is based on small animals—rat, hamster, rabbit, etc. Only in such creatures is the surface fascia (or pericardium) thin enough to permit visualization of microvessels. Unfortunately, hearts of small species are poor models of the human coronary circulation. Resting oxygen consumption ($\dot{V}_{O_2}$) and heart rate in small animals are very high, so the expansion factors for flow, $\dot{V}_{O_2}$, and C.D. are correspondingly limited. This means that measurements must be sufficiently precise to detect small changes. What is more important is that the extent of change may not be extrapolated to hearts of dog or man. We particularly emphasize that the rat heart continues to grow through adult life (19,20), whereas growth of the human heart virtually stops at maturity (21); consequently, the effects of abnormal growth (hypertrophy) could be quite different in small and large species. Finally, anesthetics strongly depress active vasomotion, and those used in small animals, notably chloralose and/or urethane, can abolish completely vasomotion and active capillary control (22). It is therefore likely that coronary functional C.D. is overestimated and the reserve underestimated in all experiments reported to date. Use of decerebrate anesthetic-free preparations (*unpublished data*) should provide more realistic data in the future.

Until quite recently, the problem of cardiac motion made measurements of coronary microvascular pressures, red cell velocities, and vessel diameters virtually impossible. To overcome this problem Steinhausen et al. (23) used closely spaced steel pins to prevent movement of the beating ventricle. In our experience, even lightly touching the epicardial surface abolishes the capillary reserve because of dilation of precapillary vessels. Pressures or diameters from such vasodilated preparations are of limited value. The effect of manipulation has been well recognized since the time of Krogh (9) and has recently been quantified for coronary vessels by Nellis et al. (24). Their data demonstrate that it is essential to allow the heart to move without restraint through the cardiac and respiratory cycles. The elegant techniques developed in Nellis' laboratory employ a strobed light source synchronized with the heart. This allows the observer to see a vessel only at the same point in the cycle, thus "stopping" the motion. The entire cycle can be explored by slowly advancing the strobe. Pressures in microvessels are measured with a micromanipulator programmed to synchronize motion of a micropipette with vessel motion. Vessels as small as 50 μ have been so cannulated. The principal result to date is that the transcoronary pressure drop occurs mainly in large arterioles (>50 μ). This suggests that the properties of precapillary networks deduced from models of the somatic circulation may be applicable qualitatively to the normal heart (25).

THE NORMAL CORONARY CAPILLARY RESERVE

Rat Hearts *in Situ*

Vessels up to 20 μ from the epicardial surface can be visualized by use of reflected light. Measurements exploit the color contrast between 15 mM hemoglobin and 0.5 mM myoglobin to identify capillaries on Ektachrome film. Steinhausen et al. (23) recently suggested—without supporting data—that recruitment in such experiments is an artifact of differential sensitivity of film to light absorbed by oxygenated versus deoxyhemoglobin. In fact, no such difference exists, and recruitment can be readily observed at high as well as low arterial saturation (Fig. 1).

Functional intercapillary distance (ICD) is measured on stop-motion ciné photomicrographs of unrestrained hearts. The anatomical C.D. can be obtained from photos in which the optical properties of endothelium render all capillaries visible ("white" appearance) (25). The maximum attainable value is that observed after reversible asphyxia or hypoxemia (Pa$_{O_2}$ 30–40 torr). Means in each animal are based on 100 to 800 individual measurements. Distance measurements are transformed to capillary densities assuming a square array. Since no regular geometry exists, and local spacings vary markedly (Fig. 3), the calculated densities are satisfactory descriptors. (Technique and statistics are available in refs. 4 and 11.)

Right Versus Left Ventricle

Data in Table 1 are representative of 250 g normoxic rats. Virtually identical values for left ventricular C.D. and reserve were obtained independently by Korecky and co-workers (27) using a similar stop-motion technique. Notice that the number of available capillaries is greater, but the number actively perfused is smaller, in right versus left ventricle. Consequently, the reserve is more than twice as great in right ventricle (4). These differences appear to reflect the fact that the left ventricle grows approximately twice as rapidly as

TABLE 1. *Components of capillary reserve*

Animal model	Anatomic maximum (cap/mm^2)	Attainable maximum (cap/mm^2)	Attainable surface area (cm^2/g)	Functional in normoxia (cap/mm^2)	Reserve (cap/mm^2)	Approximate utilization (%)
Rat						
RV	4,400	3,800	560	2,500	1,300	65
LV	4,000	3,400	500	2,900	500	85
40% LV						
hypertrophy	3,200	2,600	380	2,400	150	90–100
Dog						
LV	3,400	2,800	410	1,700	1,100	60
Gracilis	1,800	1,200	180	550	650	50

Values pertain to 200–300-g rats. Estimates for dog heart are based on assumptions given in text.

the right (5). Moreover, the slopes of regressions of functional and minimum intercapillary distances on right ventricular weight are not significantly different from 0. A high C.D. and large reserve capacity for O_2 and substrate transport may help to explain the relatively benign course of right ventricular hypertrophy in animal models and in human disease.

In sharp contrast, normal growth is a major determinant of capillary spacing in left ventricle (Fig. 2) (5). Regressions are based on 3,483 individual values in 30 rats. Note that the right ordinate is nonlinear. During the period of rapid growth from 40 to 100 days of age, minimum ICD increases 2.5 μ, whereas total C.D. drops 1,250/mm². Between the equivalent of 3 and 30 years of human life total C.D. is roughly halved, and the capillary reserve changes from approximately 1,300 to 300/mm² (72–87% utilization, respectively). Thus, the older rat not only possesses many fewer capillaries, but also uses a larger fraction of those that it has. This doubtless contributes to the progressive decline of aerobic capacity in aging rats. We emphasize, however, that although the reserve is small, it remains essential for adaptation to stress throughout life, as explained below.

Role of O_2

The only important determinant of coronary C.D. other than age and growth is the partial pressure of O_2 (P_{O_2}) (4,5,11). P_{CO_2} and pH are without effect (17), as is arterial pressure over the normal range. The effect of O_2 can be studied conveniently by varying Pa_{O_2}. Change in tissue P_{O_2} per se produces qualitatively similar changes (11). The relation between Pa_{O_2} and ICD is well fitted by the parabolic least-squares regressions shown in Fig. 1. ICD is low in both hypoxemia and extreme hyperoxemia. The longest distances (lowest densities) are typical of arterial tensions between 150 and 350 mm Hg. Moreover, such tensions produce marked heterogeneity of capillary spacing and "holes" in the array. These maladaptive changes reflect O_2-induced constriction of terminal arterioles (10), and should be borne in mind when O_2 is used in patients or in animal models of disease. Note in Fig. 1 that regressions for rapidly growing 100 to 200 g rats and for mature rats weighing 300 to 600 g are not different except for their intercepts which, of course, denote minimum ICD, and anatomical C.D. These values are virtually identical to those obtained from the linear regressions of ICD on ventricular weight shown in Fig. 2. The combined effect of Pa_{O_2} and growth on mean ICD is given by the following multiple regression:

$$ICD = 8.78 + 0.015 \text{ body wt} + 0.0243\, Pa_{O_2} - 0.0000644\, (Pa_{O_2})^2$$

Capillary Reserve in Canine Hearts

In an exemplary study, Bassingthwaighte et al. (2) applied modern morphometry to silicone casts of the canine coronary microvasculature. Mea-

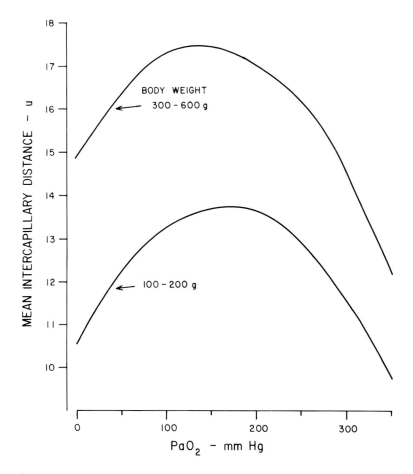

FIG. 1. Parabolic least squares regressions showing recruitment in hypoxemia and hyperoxemia, and the effect of growth. (From ref. 5, by permission of the American Heart Association, Inc.).

surements were carefully controlled for anisotropic shrinkage. Maximum capillary densities within muscle bundles ranged from 3,100 to 3,800 mm^2. Because of the opaque pericardium, it is impossible to visualize canine coronary capillaries *in situ*, so functional C.D. must be inferred from indirect measurements. Values given in Table 1 are estimates based on the following logic.

If the maximum attainable C.D. is about the same fraction of the total in dog and rat hearts, we obtain roughly 2800 mm^2. Though functional C.D. per se cannot be measured in dog hearts, its expansion factor has been determined by two methods based on different physical principles. Durán (28,29) calculated a factor of 2 (functional C.D. half the maximum attainable value) by use of the first-circulation multiple indicator dilution method. Rb[86] clearances (30) yield values of 1.4 to 1.7. Very similar expansion factors were obtained from

measurements of small vessel blood volume (31). Regardless of which published expansion factor one selects, the coronary capillary reserve is substantially larger in dog, and presumably in man, than in rat. The high degree of
capillary utilization in small species doubtless reflects high basal metabolic rate
and the O_2 cost of 350 to 400 beats/min at rest. In contrast, the large capillary
reserve of dog left ventricle permits 90% O_2 extraction in maximum exercise
despite a 4.5-fold increase in flow (32). This extraordinary extraction is essential
to achieve the observed sixfold increase in myocardial $\dot{V}_{O_2}$. We shall see that
such extraction need not be accompanied by anoxia, because myoglobin can
stabilize cell P_{O_2} near 1 torr. This tension should suffice for maximal $\dot{V}_{O_2}$.

Capillary Reserve in Hypertrophy

There is general agreement that capillary growth is not proportional to
growth of muscle fibers in pathologic cardiac hypertrophy (6,21,33). The extensive literature on this topic is summarized by Rakusan (19), and will not
be considered further. It is remarkable that in physiological, i.e., exercise-induced hypertrophy, vigorous growth of capillaries maintains or even expands
the cardiac capillary reserve (20). The stimulus is unknown, though a humoral
factor has recently been suggested (34).

The only direct measurements of functional C.D. in hypertrophy were made
in our laboratory on female Sprague-Dawley rats subjected to salt loading and
unilateral nephrectomy (6). We sought to determine whether or not functional
C.D. is maintained by recruitment as anatomical C.D. decreases. We observed
8 pairs of rats, each consisting of an experimental rat and a pair-fed littermate
control. Control and experimental rats were not different with respect to
Pa_{O_2}, Pa_{CO_2}, pHa, heart rate, or mean arterial pressure. Pulse pressure, however,
was much greater in experimental rats. Treatment was initiated at 45 days of
age when animals weighed approximately 160 g. Measurements were made
8 to 9 weeks later, and 1 to 3 weeks before cardiac failure developed in a pilot
study. All left ventricles in the treated group were significantly larger than
normal. The average extra growth was 252 mg, or 43% of left ventricular
weight predicted from body weight.

Results are summarized in Fig. 2. Means for control animals fall within
95% confidence intervals for the corresponding regressions, indicating the small
sample we studied is representative. The fact that the mean for minimum ICD
(anatomical maximum C.D.) in experimental animals is very close to its regression line means that the effect of hypertrophy on the anatomic C.D. is the
same as if the ventricle had enlarged to the same weight more slowly by normal
growth. The anatomical ICD was 2.4 μ longer than predicted, due to loss of
800 capillaries/mm^2. The regression of functional ICD fell below a 99% confidence interval, indicating that the hypertrophied hearts were indeed using
most or all of their capillary reserve. A weighted, paired 2-way analysis of
variance also indicated that minimum and functional ICD were not significantly different in treated animals.

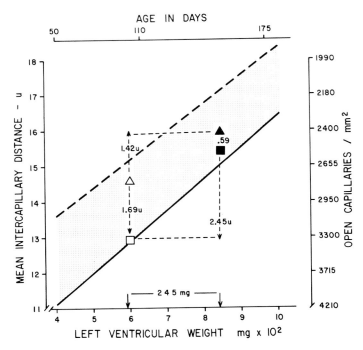

FIG. 2. Regressions of minimum ICD (*solid line*) and functional ICD (*dashed line*) are used to analyze effects of hypertrophy. *Open* and *closed* symbols: means for control and experimental animals, respectively. *Squares*: minimum ICD and anatomical maximum C.D. *Triangles*: functional ICD and C.D. (From ref. 6, by permission of the American Heart Association, Inc.)

Even though hypertrophied hearts were using virtually all capillaries at the time of measurement, comparison of functional ICD and C.D. in control and experimental rats indicates that C.D. was approximately $200/mm^2$ lower than predicted for age and weight. If the experiment had been allowed to continue, ICD would have increased along the solid regression line, and additional capillaries would have been deleted from the array. All animals not sacrificed for capillary measurements died in cardiac failure 1 to 3 weeks after the capillary reserve should have been exhausted.

Recall that normal rat hearts reach even larger size than observed in hypertrophy; this growth is far slower; the equivalent of 6 years of human life would be required to reach the ventricular weight of our experimental rats. Normal growth is accompanied by a progressive decrease in heart rate, and in whole body and cardiac $\dot{V}_{O_2}$. Consequently, a smaller total and functional C.D. can be tolerated. In this respect, the hypertrophy model we studied is simply inappropriately accelerated growth.

The reader is cautioned that the analyses in Figs. 1 and 2 predict means in a population of animals, not individual values of ICD or local C.D. in a particular rat. The within-animal variability is shown in Fig. 3. Heterogeneity of capillary distribution in this animal model is clearly not greater than expected, had the ventricle achieved equal size through normal growth. This may not be the case, however, in humans (21).

Hypertrophy and O_2 Transport

An abnormally long diffusion path (i.e., ICD) is thought to underlie the pathophysiology of cardiac hypertrophy. The basic unstated assumption is that diffusion is solely responsible for O_2 transport from capillary to mitochondria. This assumption may not be valid for heart and exercising skeletal muscle (1).

Muscles contract at constant volume (35). Consequently, shortening increases lateral spacing of myofilaments and causes flow of myoplasm normal to the fiber axis. This convection could dissipate radial diffusion gradients, and convection in the fiber axis due to sliding of filaments could minimize longitudinal O_2 gradients. If convection is large relative to ordinary and/or facilitated diffusion, myoglobin will fix P_{O_2} throughout the cell at a value determined by the instantaneous balance between O_2 delivery and $\dot{V}_{O_2}$. Since the P_{50} of myoglobin is one-fifth that of hemoglobin, convection could produce a steep gradient in P_{O_2} from the capillary to bulk myoplasm. We have developed a cryomicrospectrophotometric method capable of trapping and measuring the O_2 saturation of myoglobin in single cells (12). Spatial resolution is 3 μ, adequate to resolve O_2 gradients in a 50-μ skeletal muscle cell. Freezing rate (initially 10 μ/msec) and other technical details indicate that gradients are not dissipated during preparative procedures. Figure 4 illustrates an experiment

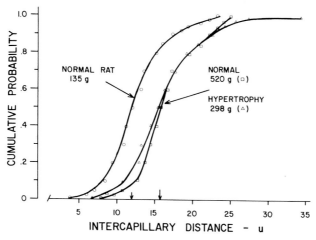

FIG. 3. Representative frequency distributions of individual values of ICD in a large and a small normal rat and in a rat with hypertrophy.

to determine directly whether O_2 gradients during contraction resemble those predicted by diffusion equations.

A dog gracilis muscle was freeze-clamped during twitch contraction at 8/sec. Flow and $\dot{V}_{O_2}$ were 134 and 15.1 ml/100 g min, respectively; Pv_{O_2} was 27 torr. Though saturation in the cell population varied widely, the value in a particular cell was always spatially uniform. Mb saturation was not detectably different near or remote from capillaries. Measurement error was <5%, so the saturation and corresponding P_{O_2} (parentheses, Fig. 4) were unmistakably different from 0. Because of the shape of the myoglobin dissociation curve, our method is most precise for P_{O_2} below the P50, which is 5.3 torr at 37°C. Calculations for free diffusion result in nonlinear oxymyoglobin gradients ranging from approximately 80% saturation 3 to 5 μ from a capillary, to zero at 10 to 15 μ away. The flat gradient in Fig. 4 is totally inconsistent with those calculations, and suggests that contracting muscle is a well-stirred system.

Note particularly in Fig. 4 that P_{O_2} is the same at the left pole of the cell where capillaries are closely spaced and at the opposite pole where they are farther apart. This means that all five capillaries interact, and together determine cell P_{O_2}. This means that local C.D., rather than ICD, is the critical variable.

To grasp the significance of Fig. 4, one must recognize that the transcapillary O_2 gradient is the main determinant of transcapillary O_2 flux. The beautiful match between the affinity constants of hemoglobin, myoglobin, and cytochrome a,a3 permits maximum O_2 flux without compromise of aerobic metabolism. We calculate that the observed transcapillary gradient increases O_2 flux approximately 10-fold over that predicted for diffusion alone. The aggregate surface area of external mitochondrial membranes is approximately 50 times the capillary surface area in dog heart, even at maximum C.D. Since

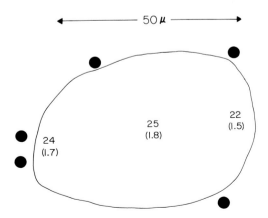

FIG. 4. Myoglobin saturation and P_{O_2} (*parentheses*) at 3 locations in a 50-μ cell. Values were determined in duplicate. Differences are within error of measurement.

the O_2 flux across the capillaries must equal that into mitochondria, the flux density is highest at the capillary. Given adequate flow, capillary surface area sets a limit for O_2 delivery.

O_2 release from red cells and capillaries is influenced by time as well as surface area and the concentration gradient. A probability model (36) indicates that the minimum time for O_2 release from capillaries is only slightly shorter than capillary transit time in myocardium. Consequently, during hyperemia an increase in the cross-sectional area of the capillary bed (recruitment) is required to slow the red cells and maintain transit times longer than the release time for O_2. $\dot{V}_{O_2}$ is the product of flow and extraction. Consequently, the extraordinary ability of myocardium to increase its $\dot{V}_{O_2}$ is due to maintenance of high O_2 extraction despite large increases in blood flow. Thus, capillary recruitment and myoglobin serve as multipliers of the effects of hyperemia, and are essential for adaptation to stress.

If the foregoing conceptions are correct, hypertrophy is not a disease of diffusion distance as assumed in the past. Instead, C.D., surface area, and transcapillary O_2 flux are the critical variables. Compromise of these by hypertrophy is compensated by recruitment during the initial stages of the disease at the cost of adaptation to stress. It follows that a capillary growth factor (34) applicable to myocardium would have the potential for eliminating a root cause of cardiac failure in pathological hypertrophy.

ACKNOWLEDGMENT

This research was supported by grant HLB03290 from the U.S. Public Health Service.

REFERENCES

1. Gayeski, T. E. J., and Honig, C. R. *Adv. Exper. Med. Biol. (in press)*.
2. Buss, D. D., Hyde, D. M., and Stovall, M. Y. *Basic Res. Cardiol. (in press)*.
3. Bassingthwaighte, J. B., Yipintsoi, T., and Harvey, R. B. (1974): *Microvasc. Res.*, 7:229–249.
4. Henquell, L., and Honig, C. R. (1976): *Microvasc. Res.*, 12:35–41.
5. Henquell, L., Odoroff, C. L., and Honig, C. R. (1976): *Am. J. Physiol.*, 231:1852–1859.
6. Henquell, L., Odoroff, C. L., and Honig, C. R. (1977): *Circ. Res.*, 41:400–408.
7. Honig, C. R., Odoroff, C. L., and Frierson, J. L. (1980): *Am. J. Physiol.*, 238:H31–H42.
8. Honig, C. R., Odoroff, C. L., and Frierson, J. L. (1983): *Am. J. Physiol.*, 243:H196–H203.
9. Krogh, A. (1919): *J. Physiol. (Lond)*, 52:457–474.
10. Lindbom, L., Tuma, R. F., and Arfors, K-E. (1980): *Microvasc. Res.*, 19:197–208.
11. Martini, J., and Honig, C. R. (1969): *Microvasc. Res.*, 1:244–256.
12. Fung, Y-C. (1973): *Microvasc. Res.*, 5:34–48.
13. Schmid-Schoenbein, G. W., Skalak, R., Usami, S., and Chien, S. (1980): *Microvasc. Res.*, 19:18–44.
14. Renkin, E. M., Hudlická, O., and Sheehan, R. M. (1966): *Am. J. Physiol.*, 211:86–98.
15. Durán, W. N. (1977): *Circ. Res.*, 41:642–647.
16. Vetterlein, F., and Schmidt, G. (1980): *Basic Res. Cardiol.*, 75:526–536.
17. Renkin, E. M., Gray, S. D., and Dodd, L. R. (1981): *Am. J. Physiol.*, 241:H174–H186.
18. Bourdeau-Martini, J., and Honig, C. R. (1973): *Microvasc. Res.*, 6:286–296.
19. Rakusan, K., and Poupa, O. (1966): *Cardiologia*, 49:293–298.
20. Tomanek, R. J. (1970): *Anat. Rec.*, 167:55–62.

21. Roberts, J. T., and Wearn, J. T. (1941): *Am. Heart J.*, 21:617–633.
22. Faber, J. E., Harris, P. D., Wiegman, D. L., Miller, F. N., and Joshua, I. G. (1980): *Microvasc. Res.*, 20:108.
23. Steinhausen, M., Tillmanns, H., and Thederan, H. (1978): *Pflügers Arch.*, 378:9–14.
24. Nellis, S. H., Liedtke, A. J., and Whitesell, L. (1981): *Circ. Res.*, 49:342–353.
25. Mayrovitz, H. N., Wiedeman, M. P., and Noordergraaf, A. (1975): *Microvasc. Res.*, 10:322–339.
26. Henquell, L., and Honig, C. R. (1976): *Microvasc. Res.*, 12:259–274.
27. Korecky, B., Hai, C. M., and Rakusan, K. (1983): *Cand. J. Physiol. Pharmacol.*, 60:23–32.
28. Durán, W. N., Alvaraz, O. A., and Yudilevich, D. L. (1973): *Microvasc. Res.*, 6:347–359.
29. Durán, W. N., Marsicano, T. H., and Anderson, R. W. (1977): *Am. J. Physiol.*, 232:H276–H281.
30. Renkin, E. M. (1967): In: *Coronary Circulation and Energetics of the Myocardium*, edited by G. Marchetti and B. Taccardi. Karger, New York.
31. Weiss, H. R., and Winbury, M. M. (1974): *Am. J. Physiol.*, 226:838–843.
32. von Restorff, W., Holtz, J., and Bassenge, E. (1977): *Pflügers Arch.*, 372:181–185.
33. Arai, S., Machida, A., and Nakamura, T. (1968): *J. Exp. Med.*, 95:35–54.
34. Cutteno, J. T., Jr., Bartrum, R. J., Hollenberg, N. K., and Abrams, H. L. (1975): *Basic Res. Cardiol.*, 70:568–573.
35. Elliott, G. F., Lowy, J., and Millman, B. M. (1967): *J. Mol. Biol.*, 25:31–45.
36. Honig, C. R., and Odoroff, C. L. (1981): *Am. J. Physiol.*, 240:H199–H208.

*Perspectives in Cardiovascular
Research, Vol. 8,*
edited by R. C. Tarazi and J. B. Dunbar.
Raven Press, New York © 1983.

Myocardial Blood Flow in Experimental Left Ventricular Hypertrophy

Robert J. Bache and Thomas R. Vrobel

*The Department of Medicine, Cardiovascular Section, University of Minnesota
Medical School, Minneapolis, Minnesota 55455*

Myocardial hypertrophy appears to be an appropriate compensatory mechanism by which the heart adapts to a chronically increased work load. Nevertheless, considerable data suggest that significant functional impairment may occur in the chronically pressure-overloaded hypertrophied ventricle, which may ultimately lead to cardiac failure (1,2). It has been suggested that the basis for this functional abnormality may reside in failure of the coronary vasculature to increase in proportion to the degree of myocardial hypertrophy (3). Thus, patients with left ventricular hypertrophy may develop angina pectoris and electrocardiographic repolarization abnormalities that are suggestive of subendocardial ischemia in the absence of occlusive coronary artery disease (4). Not infrequently, during exercise stress testing, patients with myocardial hypertrophy develop ST-segment abnormalities suggestive of inadequate subendocardial perfusion (5). In addition, Zoll and co-workers (6) demonstrated that hypertrophied hearts without coronary artery disease frequently develop an abundant intercoronary collateral circulation, the stimulus for which is thought to be myocardial ischemia. In support of these clinical data, pathologic studies have demonstrated that fibrosis of subendocardial myocardium or papillary muscle may occur in the severely hypertrophied left ventricle despite anatomically normal coronary arteries (7). These data suggest that myocardial ischemia may occur in the pathologically hypertrophied left ventricle in the absence of occlusive coronary artery disease, and that the perfusion abnormality is likely to be most severe in the subendocardium.

Early studies of myocardial blood flow in patients with stable left ventricular hypertrophy due to aortic stenosis or arterial hypertension, as well as in animals with experimental cardiac hypertrophy, generally yielded normal values for both mean coronary blood flow and oxygen consumption per unit myocardial mass (i.e., total coronary flow and total myocardial oxygen consumption are increased in proportion to the increase in myocardial mass) (8–12). These findings support the concept that, in stable left ventricular hypertrophy, the increased wall thickness distributes the systolic load over a larger cross-sectional area of myocardium, thereby returning systolic stress and oxygen consumption per unit mass to near normal levels. However, the techniques used in these early studies yielded only measurements of mean blood flow, and therefore did not eliminate the possibility that areas of underperfused myocardium may exist despite normal overall values for coronary blood flow and myocardial oxygen consumption. In addition, the finding of apparently normal myocardial blood flow during basal conditions does not exclude the possibility that blood flow may be unable to increase adequately during periods of cardiac stress when myocardial oxygen requirements are increased.

MYOCARDIAL BLOOD FLOW AND DEGREE OF HYPERTROPHY

Recent studies in animals with experimental left ventricular hypertrophy have examined the transmural distribution of myocardial blood flow for evidence of perfusion abnormalities confined to the subendocardium and have also assessed the ability of myocardial blood flow to increase during coronary vasodilation. Studies of regional myocardial blood flow with radioactive microspheres in dogs with left ventricular hypertrophy due to renovascular hypertension and in adult dogs subjected to ascending aortic banding have demonstrated normal blood flow per unit myocardial mass and a normal transmural distribution of blood flow across the left ventricular wall (13–15). However, the degree of hypertrophy in these experimental models is relatively modest, with only an approximately 25 to 50% increase in relative left ventricular mass.

In contrast to these studies, results reported by Rembert et al. (16) and our laboratory (17) demonstrated that the transmural distribution of myocardial blood flow differed from the norm in dogs with a more severe degree of left ventricular hypertrophy produced by surgically creating supravalvular aortic stenosis in puppies. In this experimental model, a mild degree of supravalvular aortic stenosis was produced in dogs approximately 6 weeks of age. As the aortic constriction remained fixed in the face of normal body growth, the degree of systolic overload gradually increased, to result in an 80 to 100% increase in relative left ventricular mass. In these animals with marked left ventricular hypertrophy, relative subendocardial flow during resting conditions was significantly less than normal, with the ratio of subendocardial/subepicardial flow (endo/epi) being 1.10 ± 0.08 as compared with 1.25 ± 0.07 in normal control dogs ($p < 0.05$) (17). Unlike normal hearts, myocardial blood flow rates were highest in the midwall of the hypertrophied left ventricle (16,17).

This abnormality of the transmural distribution of myocardial blood flow during resting conditions in dogs with hypertrophy was not caused by lack of ability for further vasodilation in the subendocardium, since blood flow in this area was able to increase substantially during reactive hyperemia, exercise, or pharmacologic vasodilation (16–18). It is possible that this alteration of the transmural distribution of perfusion relates, rather, to a change in the pattern of systolic stress that occurs when the left ventricle becomes markedly hypertrophied. Since coronary autoregulation appears to regulate myocardial blood flow in response to local metabolic needs, blood flow may be expected to reflect local myocardial oxygen consumption (19). In the normal heart, the higher blood flow rate in the subendocardium appears to reflect greater systolic stress in this area, which in turn results in higher myocardial oxygen consumption (20). This pattern does not appear to be altered in hearts with moderate degrees of left ventricular hypertrophy (13–15). In contrast, the markedly hypertrophied left ventricle models tended to have higher flow rates in the midwall of the left ventricle, while blood flow to the subendocardium was not significantly different from subepicardial flow, suggesting that the pattern of systolic stress (and therefore myocardial oxygen consumption) may be different from normal (16,17).

Several investigators have examined the ability of myocardial blood flow in the hypertrophied heart to increase in response to coronary vasodilator stimuli. Holtz and co-workers (18) and Rembert et al. (16) studied myocardial blood flow during reactive hyperemia in dogs with marked left ventricular hypertrophy due to supravalvular aortic stenosis produced in puppies. These investigators found that although the maximum mean blood flow rates per unit myocardial mass were normal during reactive hyperemia in the hypertrophied hearts, the transmural distribution of blood flow during reactive hyperemia was abnormal, with a substantial reduction of the endo/epi blood flow ratio in hypertrophied (but not in normal) hearts. Similarly, during pharmacologic vasodilation with carbocromin, dipyridamole, or adenosine, a similar ability to increase mean blood flow has generally been found in normal and hypertrophied ventricles, but the increase in subendocardial flow tended to be less than normal during maximum coronary vasodilation, suggesting impairment of subendocardial vasodilator reserve capacity in hypertrophied hearts (18).

MYOCARDIAL BLOOD FLOW DURING EXERCISE

Holtz et al. (18), studying dogs with marked left ventricular hypertrophy produced by banding the ascending aorta of puppies, found that mild treadmill exercise, which increased heart rates to approximately 160 beats/min, resulted in a normal increase in mean blood flow per unit myocardial mass. However, the increase in blood flow to the subendocardial myocardium was subnormal in the dogs with hypertrophy, suggesting that exercise was associated with a subendocardial perfusion deficit. We have examined the effect of graded treadmill exercise on myocardial perfusion in dogs with left ventricular hypertrophy produced by banding the ascending aorta at 6 weeks of age. Animals were studied at rest and during three levels of treadmill exercise to achieve heart rates of approximately 190, 230, and 260 beats/min. The external workload required to achieve these heart rates was not different between normal dogs and animals with left ventricular hypertrophy. In the dogs with supravalvular aortic stenosis, left ventricular systolic pressure was elevated to 202 ± 18 mm Hg at rest, and increased progressively with increasing levels of exercise to achieve a maximum pressure of 343 ± 18 mm Hg during heavy exercise ($p < 0.01$).

It is clear from this finding that the left ventricular systolic pressure observed during resting conditions does not reflect that degree of systolic overload that may occur during strenuous exercise. Although left ventricular end-diastolic pressure tended to be higher in the animals with left ventricular hypertrophy during resting conditions, this difference became much more prominent during exercise. Thus, left ventricular end-diastolic pressure did not increase significantly in the control dogs, but underwent progressive increases with each increasing level of exercise in the animals with hypertrophy, reaching a maximum of 37 ± 6 mm Hg during heavy exercise ($p < 0.001$). Although mean aortic pressure increased significantly during exercise in the normal animals, aortic pressure distal to the constricting band did not increase at any exercise level in the dogs with left ventricular hypertrophy.

Mean blood flow per gram of myocardium increased similarly during exercise in normal and hypertrophied hearts. When the regional pattern of myocardial perfusion was examined, however, it was found that significant differences existed between blood flow to the anterior and posterior left ventricular wall of the dogs with left ventricular hypertrophy, but not in the normal animals (Fig. 1). The normal dogs showed regular progressive increases in myocardial blood flow with increasing levels of stress, to reach maximum flow rates of 4 to 5 times the resting level. These increases in flow were essentially uniform across the left ventricular wall, so that no significant differences existed between the four transmural layers at any level of exercise. In contrast, although the mean increase in blood flow in the hypertrophied heart was at least as great as that in the normal heart, the transmural distribution of perfusion was significantly different (Fig. 1). During resting conditions, blood flow rates tended to be highest in the midwall of the left ventricle. In the anterior left ventricular wall, this preferential flow to the midwall appeared to be magnified with increasing intensity of exercise, while blood flow to the innermost myocardial layer was maintained equal to subepicardial flow. The response of blood flow in the posterior left ventricle of the hypertrophied heart was different from the anterior wall and different from the normal control animals. Although the mean increase in blood flow was normal, the increased flow was directed preferentially to the outer left ventricular wall with a subnormal increase in perfusion of the subendocardium, which was especially prominent during the heaviest level of exercise (Fig. 1). Although the mechanism responsible for this difference in myocardial blood flow during exercise in the anterior and posterior walls of the hypertrophied left ventricle are not entirely clear, it is possible that the posterior left ventricle and its papillary muscle are especially vulnerable

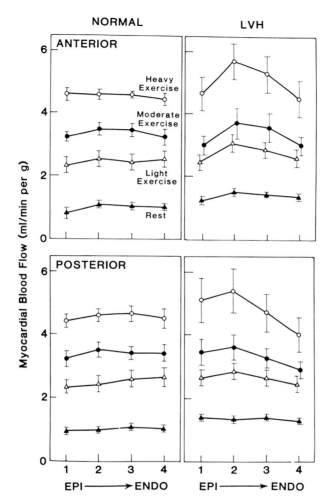

FIG. 1. Mean left ventricular myocardial blood flow (ml/min per g) ± SEM to 4 transmural layers from epicardium to endocardium of the anterior and posterior left ventricular wall from 9 normal control dogs and 8 dogs with left ventricular hypertrophy produced by supravalvular aortic stenosis. Data were obtained at rest and during three levels of treadmill exercise. EPI = subepicardium; ENDO = subendocardium.

to underperfusion merely because this is the region most remote from its blood supply. Thus, the deepest layers of the most terminal portion of the coronary arterial bed may be most sensitive to perfusion deficits produced by exercise stress. It is possible that this perfusion abnormality would become increasingly severe, and perhaps more generalized, during more strenuous exercise or in the presence of a greater degree of hypertrophy.

EFFECT OF HEART RATE ON MYOCARDIAL BLOOD FLOW

Because the subendocardium is principally dependent upon perfusion during diastole, abbreviation of the interval of diastole during tachycardia might be especially likely to reveal subendocardial perfusion abnormalities in the hypertrophied heart (21,22). Mueller et al. (13) studied the effects of cardiac pacing on the transmural distribution of myocardial blood flow in dogs with a moderate degree of left ventricular hypertrophy secondary to experimental renovascular hypertension. They found that cardiac pacing resulted in similar increases in myocardial blood flow both in control animals and in dogs with left ventricular hypertrophy. Pacing resulted in a modest redistribution of blood flow away from the subendocardium in the animals with left ventricular hypertrophy, but the endo/epi blood flow ratio remained greater than 1.0, suggesting that adequate subendocardial perfusion was maintained at a heart rate of 200 beats/min (13).

We have examined the response of myocardial blood flow to a wider range of heart rates produced by cardiac pacing in dogs with an 87% average increase in relative left ventricular mass produced by aortic banding in puppies (23,24). At a heart rate of 100 beats per min, left ventricular systolic pressure was increased to 241 ± 22 mm Hg in the dogs with aortic banding, as compared with 126 ± 4 mm Hg in the control animals. Increasing the pacing rate to 200 and then 250 beats/min, resulted in significant progressive reductions of left ventricular systolic pressure in the hypertrophied but not in the normal hearts. At a heart rate of 100 beats/min, left ventricular end-diastolic pressure was 15 ± 2 mm Hg in the dogs with hypertrophy, as compared with 5 ± 2 mm Hg in the control animals ($p < 0.01$). Increasing pacing rates did not significantly alter left ventricular end-diastolic pressure in the normal dogs, while pacing at 250 beats/min resulted in a further significant increase of left ventricular end-diastolic pressure to 26 ± 25 mm Hg in the animals with hypertrophy ($p < 0.05$) (24). Mean aortic pressure distal to the constricting band in the dogs with hypertrophy was not significantly different from aortic pressure in the control animals, and aortic pressures did not change significantly with increasing heart rates. However, mean pressure in the aortic segment proximal to the stenosis was significantly higher than distal aortic pressure, and higher than mean aortic pressure in the control dogs at all heart rates ($p < 0.05$).

In the normal dogs, increasing pacing rates were accompanied by progressive increases in mean myocardial blood flow, while subendocardial flow was maintained at least as great as subepicardial flow at all heart rates (Fig. 2) (23,24). Both mean myocardial blood flow and the transmural distribution of perfusion in the hypertrophied hearts were similar to control at pacing rates of 100 and 200 beats/min. However, in the hypertrophied hearts, pacing at 250 beats/min was associated with a significant redistribution of perfusion away from the subendocardium, resulting in blood flow rates significantly less than control in the inner half of the left ventricular wall (Fig. 2).

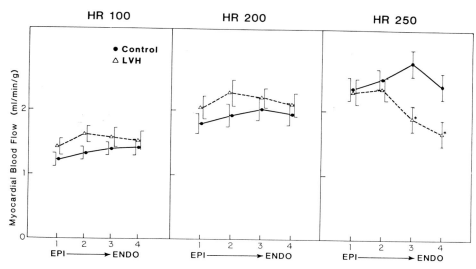

FIG. 2. Mean left ventricular myocardial blood flow (ml/min per g) ± SEM to 4 transmural layers from epicardium (EPI) to endocardium (ENDO) of 7 normal control dogs and 7 dogs with left ventricular hypertrophy (LVH) secondary to supravalvular aortic stenosis. Data were obtained during ventricular pacing at heart rates of 100, 200, and 250 beats/min. *$P < 0.05$, comparing blood flow to corresponding myocardial layers for control dogs and animals with left ventricular hypertrophy.

To assess the residual coronary vasodilator reserve capacity, myocardial blood flow was measured with microspheres during maximum coronary vasodilation produced by infusion of adenosine (1.0 mg/kg per min, i.v.) at the same three heart rates (Fig. 3). During pacing at 100 beats per min, adenosine administration resulted in an approximately fourfold increase in mean myocardial blood flow both in normal and hypertrophied left ventricles. Although blood flow to the subendocardium of the hypertrophied hearts tended to be slightly lower than control, this difference did not achieve statistical significance. However, since mean coronary driving pressure (pressure proximal to the aortic constriction) was significantly higher in the animals with hypertrophy than in the normal dogs, minimum coronary vascular resistance per gram of myocardium was significantly higher in the dogs with hypertrophy than in the normal animals. This impairment of minimum coronary vascular resistance, suggesting that growth of the coronary vasculature did not keep pace with the hypertrophying myocardium, is in agreement with similar findings reported by Mueller et al. (13) in dogs with left ventricular hypertrophy secondary to renovascular hypertension, and by O'Keefe et al. (15) in dogs with constriction of the ascending aorta.

During maximum coronary vasodilation with adenosine in the normal dogs, increasing the pacing rate to 200 and then 250 beats/min was associated with a progressive reduction of blood flow to the deeper myocardial layers, while

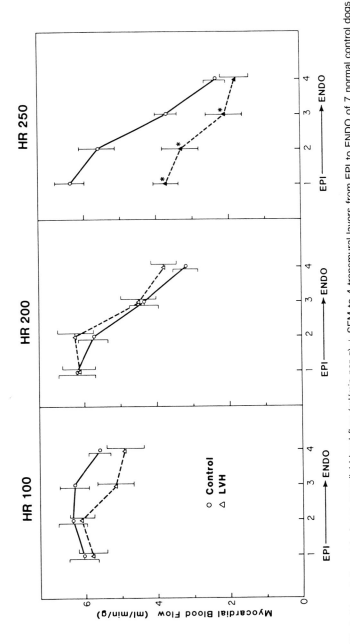

FIG. 3. Mean left ventricular myocardial blood flow (ml/min per g) ± SEM to 4 transmural layers from EPI to ENDO of 7 normal control dogs and 7 dogs with left ventricular hypertrophy secondary to supravalvular aortic stenosis during maximum coronary vasodilation produced by adenosine administration (1.0 mg/kg per min). Data were obtained during ventricular pacing at 100, 200, and 250 beats/min. *$P < 0.05$, comparing flow to corresponding myocardial layers between control dogs and animals with LVH.

subepicardial flow was well maintained at all heart rates (Fig. 3). Since maximum pharmacologic coronary vasodilation abolishes autoregulation, this represents the direct mechanical effects of cardiac contraction during tachycardia on transmural myocardial perfusion. Thus, the reduction of blood flow to the inner myocardial layers appears to result from the decreased interval of diastole available for perfusion of the subendocardium as heart rate is increased (22). In the hypertrophied hearts, pacing at 200 beats/min during adenosine administration resulted in a transmural redistribution of blood flow away from the subendocardium similar to that in normal hearts (Fig. 3). However, pacing at 250 beats/min during maximum coronary vasodilation with adenosine had a much greater effect on myocardial blood flow in the hypertrophied hearts, resulting in reductions of blood flow below control in all transmural layers.

Comparison of blood flow data during normal coronary autoregulation and during maximum vasodilation with adenosine provides insight into the redistribution of perfusion, which occurred during pacing at 250 beats per min in the animals with left ventricular hypertrophy but not in the normal animals. As shown in Fig. 4 during normal autoregulation subendocardial flow was

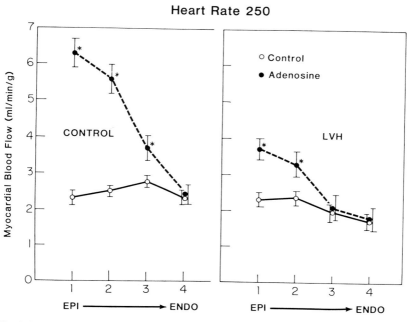

FIG. 4. Mean left ventricular myocardial blood flow (ml/min per g) $\pm$ SEM to 4 transmural layers from EPI to ENDO in 7 normal dogs and 7 animals with LVH secondary to supravalvular aortic stenosis. Data were obtained during ventricular pacing at 250 beats/min during control conditions and during maximum coronary vasodilation produced by adenosine (1.0 mg/kg per min, i.v.). *$P < 0.05$, comparing control conditions (intact coronary vasomotor tone) with maximum coronary vasodilation produced by adenosine administration (24). (By permission of the American Heart Association, Inc.)

maintained equal to subepicardial flow during pacing at 250 beats/min in the control dogs, but preservation of a normal endo/epi flow ratio required all of the available subendocardial vasodilator capacity, as indicated by failure of blood flow to layer 4 (subendocardium) to increase further during adenosine administration. In contrast, during normal autoregulation, blood flow to both layers 3 and 4 was significantly decreased below flow to layer 1 during pacing at 250 beats/min in the animals with hypertrophy. This reduction of blood flow to the inner half of the left ventricular wall was due to impaired coronary vasodilator capacity at a heart rate of 250 beats/min, since blood flow to these layers did not increase significantly in response to adenosine administration (Fig. 4). The finding that myocardial blood flow during maximum coronary vasodilation was not different between normal and hypertrophied ventricles at heart rates of 100 and 200 beats/min indicates that the reduction of coronary vasodilator reserve capacity observed at a heart rate of 250 beats/min was not the result of a structural abnormality, but rather represents a functional difference between normal and hypertrophied hearts which emerged only at a pacing rate of 250 beats/min.

The mechanism for impairment of the coronary vasodilator reserve capacity observed in hypertrophied ventricles at a heart rate of 250 beats per min is of considerable interest. Pacing at 250 beats/min resulted in a significant increase in left ventricular end-diastolic pressure in animals with hypertrophy, but not in control animals. This increase in left ventricular diastolic pressure would be expected to directly impede blood flow to the subendocardium. Reductions of subendocardial perfusion during tachycardia in the hypertrophied heart could potentially become self-perpetuating if the reduced perfusion resulted in subendocardial ischemia. Thus, the occurrence of ischemia could further increase left ventricular diastolic pressure by causing impairment of systolic function as well as by causing increased diastolic tone as a result of impaired myocardial relaxation (25,26). These ischemia-induced decreases in diastolic ventricular compliance might be expected to increase extravascular compression acting on the intramural coronary vessels and thereby impair myocardial perfusion (27). We have recently observed myocardial production of lactate and adenosine metabolites into coronary sinus blood during pacing at 250 beats/min in hypertrophied but not in normal ventricles, indicating that the transmural redistribution of perfusion away from the subendocardium, which occurs during tachycardia in the hypertrophied heart, is in fact associated with myocardial ischemia (28).

SUMMARY

Studies of myocardial blood flow in the experimental animal have generally demonstrated that left ventricular hypertrophy is associated with a perfusion abnormality. Although most laboratories have observed normal myocardial blood rates during basal conditions, most investigators have reported increased minimum coronary vascular resistance per unit myocardial mass during maximum coronary vasodilation. This impairment of coronary vasodilator capacity suggests that the maximum cross-sectional area of the coronary vascular bed may not increase in proportion to the degree of myocardial hypertrophy. In addition to this structural abnormality, evidence has been presented that a functional abnormality may occur during pacing at 250 beats/min, resulting in significant impairment of coronary vasodilator reserve capacity in response to adenosine infusion, which is not present at lower heart rates.

ACKNOWLEDGMENT

This study was supported by U.S. Public Health Service Grants HL21872 and HL20518 from the U.S. Public Health Service.

REFERENCES

1. Cooper, G., Sataba, R. M., Harrison, E., and Coleman, H. M. (1973): *Circ. Res.*, 33:213–223.
2. Pfeffer, M. A., Pfeffer, A. M., and Frohlich, E. D. (1976): *Circ. Res.*, 38:423–429.
3. Linzbach, A. J. (1960): *Am. J. Cardiol.*, 5:370–382.
4. Goodwin, J. F. (1973): *Prog. Cardiovas. Dis.*, 14:199–238.
5. Harris, C. N., Aronow, W. S., Parker, D. P., and Kaplan, M. A. (1973): *Chest*, 63:353–357.
6. Zoll, P. M., Wessler, S., and Schlesinger, M. J. (1951): *Circulation*, 4:797–815.
7. Moller, J. H., Nakeb, A., and Edwards, J. E. (1966): *Circulation*, 34:87–94.
8. West, J. W., Mercken, H., Wendel, H., and Foltz, E. L. (1959): *Circ. Res.*, 7:476–485.
9. Rowe, G. G., Alfonso, S., Lugo, J. E., Castillo, C. A., Boake, W. C., and Crumpton, C. W. (1965): *Circulation*, 32:251–261.
10. Badeer, R. S. (1971): *Am. Heart. J.*, 82:105–119.
11. Malik, A. B., Tomio, A., O'Kane, H., and Geha, A. S. (1973): *Am. J. Physiol.*, 225:186–191.
12. Marchetti, G. V., Merlo, L., Noseda, V., and Visioli, O. (1973): *Cardiovasc. Res.*, 7:519–527.
13. Mueller, T. M., Marcus, M. L., Kerber, R. E., Young, J. A., Barnes, R. W., and Abboud, F. M. (1978): *Circ. Res.*, 42:543–549.
14. Bache, R. J., and Vrobel, T. R. (1979): *Amer. J. Cardiol.*, 44:1029–1033.
15. O'Keefe, D. D., Hoffman, J. I. E., Cheitlin, R., O'Neill, M. J., Allard, J. R., and Shapkin, E. (1978): *Circ. Res.*, 43:43–51.
16. Rembert, J. C., Kleinman, L. H., Fedor, J. M., Wechsler, A. S., and Greenfield, J. C., Jr. (1978): *J. Clin. Invest.*, 62:379–386.
17. Bache, R. J., Vrobel, T. R., Ring, W. S., Emery, R. W., and Anderson, R. W. (1981): *Circ. Res.*, 48:76–87.
18. Holtz, J., Restorff, W., Bard, P., and Bassenge, E. (1977): *Basic. Res. Cardiol.*, 72:286–292.
19. Katz, L. M., and Feinberg, H. (1958): *Circ. Res.*, 6:656–669.
20. Weiss, H. R., Neubauer, J. A., Lipp, J. A., and Sinah, A. K. (1978): *Circ. Res.*, 42:394–401.
21. Hess, D. S., and Bache, R. J. (1976): *Circ. Res.*, 38:5–15.
22. Bache, R. J., and Cobb, F. R. (1977): *Circ. Res.*, 41:648–653.
23. Vrobel, T. R., Ring, W. S., Anderson, R. W., Emery, R. W., and Bache, R. J. (1980): *Am. J. Physiol.*, 239:H621–H627.
24. Bache, R. J., Vrobel, T. R., Arentzen, C. E., and Anderson, R. W. (1981): *Circ. Res.*, 49:742–750.
25. Grossman, W., and Barry, W. H. (1980): *Fed. Proc.*, 39:148–155.
26. Hanrath, P., Mathey, D. G., Siegert, R., and Bleifeld, W. (1980): *Am. J. Cardiol.*, 45:15–23.
27. Apstein, C. S., Mueller, M., and Hood, W. B., Jr. (1977): *Circ. Res.*, 41:206–217.
28. Vrobel, T. R., Arentzen, C. E., Simon, A. B., and Bache, R. J. (1982): *Circulation,* 4:268.

Perspectives in Cardiovascular
Research, Vol. 8,
edited by R. C. Tarazi and J. B. Dunbar.
Raven Press, New York © 1983.

Abnormalities in Coronary Circulation Secondary to Cardiac Hypertrophy

Melvin L. Marcus, Samon Koyanagi, David G. Harrison,
Loren F. Hiratzka, Creighton D. Wright,
Donald B. Doty, and Charles L. Eastham

*Cardiovascular Center, Department of Medicine, Division of Cardiovascular–
Thoracic Surgery, and Department of Surgery, University of Iowa and
Veterans Administration Hospitals, Iowa City, Iowa 52242*

Clinicians have long suspected that hypertrophied hearts have an inadequate coronary circulation. This suspicion was fostered by the observation that some patients with cardiac hypertrophy and anatomically normal epicardial coronary vessels complain of angina pectoris (1,2). In addition, electrocardiographic abnormalities suggestive of myocardial ischemia have been reported frequently in patients with cardiac hypertrophy in the absence of coronary obstructive disease (2,3).

Perfusion abnormalities in hypertrophied hearts may be caused by two mechanisms: (a) hemodynamic alterations related to the cause of the hypertrophy (4), and (b) architectual changes in the coronary vascular bed (5). Hemodynamic alterations can produce abnormalities in both total coronary blood flow and the transmural distribution of myocardial perfusion (4). This chapter will focus on the physiological consequences of structural changes in the coronary vascular bed that occur in hypertrophied ventricles.

STRUCTURAL ALTERATIONS IN THE CORONARY CIRCULATION IN THE HYPERTROPHIED HEART

Cardiac hypertrophy is associated with vascular abnormalities at several levels in the coronary hierarchy. The epicardial coronary vessels do not enlarge appropriately when ventricular hypertrophy occurs in response to a pressure load (6). Since coronary blood flow via the conduit vessels is increased when the heart enlarges, it is likely that large vessel resistance is slightly increased in hypertrophied hearts. If the hypertrophy occurs secondary to systemic hypertension, the wall/lumen ratio of coronary arterioles is increased because of hypertrophy of the vascular wall (7). Hallback-Nordlander et al. (8) have shown that this type of structural change in coronary vessels limits coronary dilation and augments maximal coronary constriction. Capillary density in the myocardium is also altered in hypertrophied hearts. There are reports that, in both left and right ventricular hypertrophy secondary to a pressure load, capillary density decreases by 20 to 30% (9–11). Pathologists have frequently observed that the subendocardium of hypertrophied ventricles is diffusely fibrotic (12). This could result from myocardial ischemia secondary to inadequate coronary perfusion. Thus, there is anatomical evidence that supports the theory that the coronary circulation is inadequate in hypertrophied hearts. However, in general, there is a paucity of precise quantitative information about the anatomical characteristics of the coronary circulation at multiple levels in the coronary heirarchy in hypertrophied hearts.

Several decades ago, investigators measured flow per gram at rest in patients with hypertrophied ventricles, and they reported no abnormalities (13,14). In these studies, the transmural distribution of coronary flow was not assessed, and measurements of flow during stress were not obtained. Fortunately, these early negative results did not deter other investigators from pursuing more sophisticated studies in this area.

EFFECTS OF HYPERTROPHY ON CORONARY CIRCULATION

Conceptual Framework

In 1978, our group published a conceptual diagram concerning the interaction between changes in cardiac mass and coronary vascular growth (Fig. 1) (15). In this diagram, the size of the boxes represents cardiac mass and the circles depict the cross-sectional area of coronary resistance vessels. If cardiac enlargement was accompanied by appropriate vascular growth (top box, Fig. 1), coronary resistance during maximal coronary dilation would decrease, be-

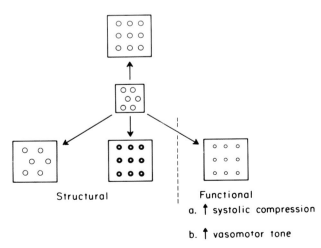

FIG. 1. Interrelationships between growth of cardiac muscle and the coronary vascular bed. See text for details.

cause the resistance across a parallel vascular bed decreases as the number of vascular channels and their cross-sectional area increase. Alternatively, if the change in the size of the cross-sectional area of the coronary vascular bed did not keep pace with an increase in cardiac mass, total vascular resistance would not decrease as the heart enlarged. At least three distinct mechanisms that are not mutually exclusive could limit the cross-sectional area of the coronary vascular bed (see bottom three boxes—Fig. 1). These mechanisms include: (a) decreased vascular growth (bottom left); (b) compromised cross-sectional area secondary to vascular hypertrophy (bottom center); and (c) compression of coronary vascular channels by extravascular forces (bottom right). Under various conditions, all three mechanisms contribute to impaired coronary vascular reserve in hypertrophied ventricles.

PHYSIOLOGICAL STUDIES IN ANIMALS

Since 1975, a large number of experiments in animals have examined the effects of various types of cardiac hypertrophy on coronary reserve. These studies have utilized sophisticated methodology and many different animal models of hypertrophy. Furthermore, many studies examined awake, chronically instrumented animals during a variety of perturbations that produce coronary vasodilation of variable intensity. Most studies focused on the effects of pressure-induced left ventricular hypertrophy on the coronary circulation.

Effects of Pressure-Induced Left Ventricular Hypertrophy on Coronary Circulation

Myocardial Perfusion at Rest

Almost all studies in animal models of left ventricular hypertrophy have shown that when the increase in muscle mass stabilizes following application of a stimulus that produces left ventricular hypertrophy, flow per gram in the enlarged left ventricle is normal (15–27). Sasayama et al. (28) demonstrated that left ventricular wall stress increased substantially immediately following the imposition of the pressure load. In time, increases in ventricular wall thickness return wall stress to control levels. Since the major determinants of myocardial oxygen consumption, wall stress, heart rate, and myocardial contractility are near normal in hypertrophied ventricles, it is not surprising that flow per gram is not altered. Even so, total flow to the enlarged ventricle should be increased. This is the case when hypertrophy is severe or differences in cardiac mass secondary to body mass or animal breed are minimized.

The transmural distribution of resting left ventricular perfusion is usually not altered unless hypertrophy is intense (greater than 75% increase in left ventricular mass). In dogs with severe left ventricular hypertrophy secondary to coarctation of the aorta, endocardial flow is usually equal to or less than epicardial flow, and the greatest flow occurs in the mid-wall layers of the left ventricle (16,17,19,24,25). The unusual transmural distribution of coronary blood flow suggests that severe pressure-induced left ventricular hypertrophy either alters the transmural distribution of wall stress or extravascular compressive forces. This issue is unsettled.

Tachycardia/Exercise

In normal hearts, when heart rate is doubled by pacing, coronary flow increases about twofold, and the ratio of endocardial to epicardial flow usually decreases slightly (15,25). In the pressure-hypertrophied left ventricle, flow invariably increases with pacing, but in some models the increase in endocardial perfusion is limited (15,25).

The effects of exercise on myocardial perfusion in dogs with pressure-induced cardiac hypertrophy have been variable. If hypertrophy is mild and secondary to hypertension, moderate exercise does not elicit any abnormalities in myocardial perfusion (21,29). In dogs (17) and mini-swine (26) with severe hypertrophy secondary to coarctation of the aorta, high-grade exercise was associated with underperfusion of the endocardium. In contrast, Bache et al. (24) noted only minimal perfusion abnormalities to the posterior papillary muscle during intense exercise in dogs with severe hypertrophy secondary to aortic coarctation. In Bache's study, during peak exercise, coronary flow increased fivefold in the hypertrophied ventricle.

In summary, in dogs with pressure-induced left ventricular hypertrophy, pacing or exercise elicits mild abnormalities in the transmural distribution of myocardial perfusion; these abnormalities occur only when the stress imposed is near maximal. It should be noted that coronary vascular resistance during pacing or intense exercise is usually greater than the minimal coronary vascular resistance that can be achieved with pharmacological coronary vasodilation (15,18,25,27).

Minimal Coronary Resistance

All studies that have assessed coronary vascular resistance during maximal coronary dilation have reported that minimal coronary vascular resistance is inappropriately high in animals with pressure-induced left ventricular hypertrophy (15,18,23,25,27). Usually, coronary vascular resistance for the entire ventricle is similar in normal and in enlarged hearts, and minimal coronary vascular resistance per gram is increased. In light of the conceptual framework presented above, this implies that vascular growth has not kept pace with the increase in muscle mass. Although the finding of increased minimal coronary vascular resistance in pressure-induced left ventricular hypertrophy has been consistent, the actual magnitude of the abnormality is quite small.

Coronary Occlusion

Epidemiological studies have shown that when patients with hypertension and left ventricular hypertrophy sustain a myocardial infarction, the incidence of sudden cardiac death is increased threefold and other complications of myocardial infarction, such as heart failure, are more frequent than expected (30). These adverse effects of coronary occlusion could be related to hypertension, left ventricular hypertrophy, or more extensive coronary disease in patients with these concomitant conditions. Koyanagi et al. (31,32) studied the effects of coronary occlusion in awake dogs with left ventricular hypertrophy secondary to renal hypertension. During the first 48 hr following coronary occlusion, death presumed secondary to ventricular fibrillation occurred more frequently in dogs with hypertension and left ventricular hypertrophy than in controls (Fig. 2) (31). Furthermore, infarct size over a wide range of risk areas was increased in the dogs with left ventricular hypertrophy secondary to hypertension (Fig. 3) (32). This study provides the first experimental evidence that hypertrophy and hypertension alone adversely affect the response of myocardium to sudden coronary occlusion. These adverse effects could be related to electrophysiological abnormalities in hypertrophied cardiac muscle (33,34), to abnormalities in coronary reserve, or to native collateral vessels in hypertrophied ventricle.

Volume-Induced Left Ventricular Hypertrophy

Two studies have evaluated coronary reserve in animals with volume-induced left ventricular hypertrophy (35,36). In both, the degree of left ventricular hypertrophy produced was modest, and no major abnormalities in coronary reserve were noted.

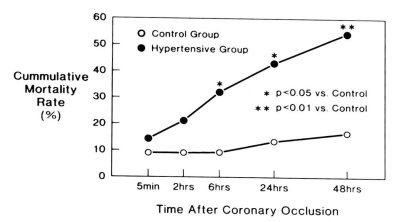

FIG. 2. Effects of sudden coronary occlusion in awake dogs with renal hypertension and left ventricular hypertrophy versus controls. The cumulative mortality rate in the hypertensive dogs with left ventricular hypertrophy was much greater than that observed in controls; the primary cause of death was ventricular fibrillation. This data indicates that renal hypertension and associated left ventricular hypertrophy markedly augment the incidence of sudden cardiac death following coronary occlusion in chronically instrumented dogs. Control group, N = 28; hypertensive group, N = 30. (From Koyanagi et al., ref. 31, with permission.)

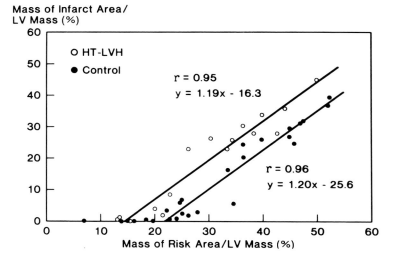

FIG. 3. The relationship between the area at risk determined by quanitative coronary steroan-giography and the area of infarction determined pathologically in chronically instrumented dogs subjected to sudden coronary occlusion. *Open circles*, results in dogs with renal hypertension and left ventricular hypertrophy (HT-LVH) (N = 30); *solid circles*, results in normal control dogs (N = 28). Throughout the entire range of risk areas, infarct size was greater in dogs with HT-LVH than in controls; supporting the theory that hypertension in association with LVH augments the size of myocardial infarcts following sudden coronary occlusion. (From Koyanagi et al., ref. 32, with permission.)

Volume-Induced Right Ventricular Hypertrophy

Murray and Vatner (37,38) produced severe right ventricular hypertrophy (70–110% increase in right ventricular mass) in dogs by creating severe supravalvular pulmonary stenosis. They noted that under resting conditions, right ventricular flow per gram doubled, but the transmural distribution of coronary flow was near normal. Responses to three coronary dilator stimuli—peak exercise, infusion of adenosine, and transient coronary occlusion—indicated that in this model of cardiac hypertrophy, right ventricular coronary reserve was profoundly impaired (38). The magnitude of the coronary abnormalities in dogs with right ventricular hypertrophy reported in this study far exceeds that which has been observed in animal models of left ventricular hypertrophy.

Pressure-Induced Right Ventricular Hypertrophy in Neonatal Animals

Several groups have produced right ventricular hypertrophy in lambs *in utero* or in lambs or calves immediately following birth (39–41). In all studies, supravalvular pulmonary obstruction induced marked right ventricular hypertrophy. The outstanding observation in these studies was that right ventricular coronary reserve was normal or greater than expected. Thus, very early in the animal's development, right ventricular pressure overload produces an increase in muscle mass coupled with an appropriate augmentation in the coronary vasculature.

SUMMARY OF RESULTS OF PHYSIOLOGICAL STUDIES IN ANIMALS

It is now established that, under most conditions, cardiac hypertrophy secondary to a pressure load is associated with normal myocardial perfusion at rest and a mild impairment in coronary vascular reserve. The limitation in coronary vascular capacity is engendered by inadequate growth of new vessels and vascular hypertrophy in coronary resistance vessels if systemic hypertension is present. The interaction between an increase in cardiac muscle mass and structural changes in the coronary vascular bed is mediated by: (a) intensity of hypertrophy; (b) the ventricle involved (right versus left); (c) the type of stress employed (pressure versus volume); and (d) the time in the animal's life cycle when hypertrophy is produced.

The most dramatic abnormalities encountered thus far have been a marked decrease in coronary reserve in adult dogs with pressure-induced right ventricular hypertrophy (37,38) and a striking increase in the adverse effects of sudden coronary occlusion in dogs with left ventricular hypertrophy secondary to renal hypertension (31,32).

PHYSIOLOGICAL STUDIES IN HUMANS

There are three major reasons for studying the effects of cardiac hypertrophy on the coronary circulation in humans. First, the severity of cardiac hypertrophy that presents in humans is much greater than that which can be produced in animals. Most animal models of hypertrophy have less than a twofold increase in ventricular mass. In contrast, patients with severe aortic stenosis occasionally have a two to threefold increase in ventricular mass (42). Second, the duration of cardiac hypertrophy in humans often lasts for a period of many decades. Most animal studies employ preparations that have had cardiac hypertrophy over a small fraction of the animal's lifespan. Third, studies of coronary reserve in patients with cardiac hypertrophy are obviously of greater clinical relevance than animal studies.

Effects of Pressure-Induced Left Ventricular Hypertrophy on Coronary Reserve

Since 1979, we have obtained measurements of coronary reactive hyperemia in patients with cardiac hypertrophy at the time of cardiac surgery (43–50). These studies were facilitated by the development of a Doppler probe, which

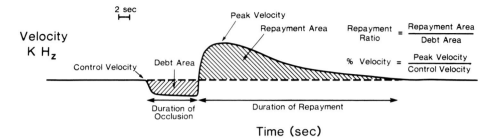

FIG. 4. Diagram of a reactive hyperemic response illustrating the manner in which we determine the repayment ratio, the percent increase in peak velocity, and the duration of the coronary occlusion from recordings of a reactive hyperemic response.

can be coupled to surface coronary vessels with suction (44). With this device, phasic and mean coronary blood flow velocity can be measured and the quantitative characteristics of coronary reactive hyperemia can be assessed. In all of our studies, the characteristics of coronary reactive hyperemia were measured prior to cardiopulmonary bypass. In humans, maximal coronary dilation follows release of a 20-second coronary occlusion (Figs. 4 and 5) (44).

In adult patients with normal coronary vessels and severe left ventricular hypertrophy secondary to valvular aortic stenosis, we have found that the coronary reactive hyperemic response in the left anterior descending coronary artery is strikingly impaired (Fig. 6) (45). In contrast, the coronary reactive hyperemic response in vessels which perfuse the nonhypertrophied right ven-

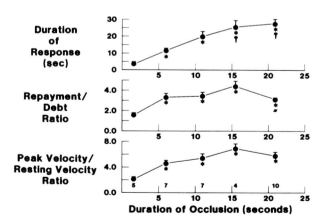

FIG. 5. Quantitative characteristics of coronary reactive hyperemia in humans. Three quantitative characteristics of the coronary reactive hyperemic response are plotted against duration of occlusion. Integers in **bottom panel** indicate the number of responses averaged to obtain each point. On the average, coronary velocity can increase sixfold in response to the ischemia associated with a 20-second coronary occlusion, significantly different from the one-second data (*asterisk*), 6-second data (*dagger*), and 15-second data (*slashed solid circle*) at the .05 level of confidence.

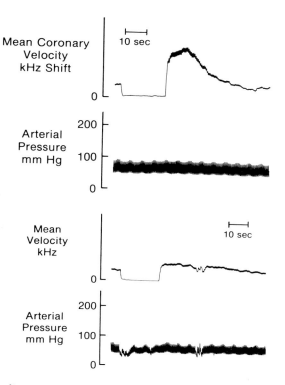

FIG. 6. Recordings of mean coronary velocity and arterial pressure in a right ventricular branch of the right coronary artery of a patient with aortic stenosis (**top** two panels) and the left anterior descending coronary artery of the same patient (**bottom** two panels). Coronary angiography demonstrated that all coronary vessels were angiographically normal. The reactive hyperemic response in the right ventricular branch of the right coronary artery is normal whereas that in the left anterior descending coronary artery is strikingly depressed.

tricle are nearly normal (Fig. 6). In most patients, coronary reserve is reduced to about one-third of normal (45). Immediately following relief of aortic obstruction, the coronary reactive hyperemic response in the left anterior descending coronary artery is not significantly improved (50). This suggests that extravascular compressive forces are not responsible for the observed impairment in coronary reserve.

Strauer (51) and Tauchert et al. (52) have measured flow per gram with argon clearance in the left ventricle of patients with left ventricular hypertrophy secondary in aortic stenosis. Data were obtained at rest and during maximal coronary dilation produced by infusing a potent coronary dilator, dipyridamole. During maximal coronary dilation coronary reserve was substantially decreased. Patients with concomitant cardiac dilation and left ventricular failure demonstrated the greatest abnormalities in coronary reserve.

These studies demonstrated that coronary reserve with severe left ventricular hypertrophy secondary to aortic stenosis is severely impaired. The magnitude of the abnormality in coronary reserve is sufficient to significantly contribute to the pathogenesis of angina in patients with aortic stenosis and normal coronary vessels. Furthermore, it is likely that intermittent episodes of subendocardial ischemia in these patients lead to subendocardial fibrosis, which in turn contributes to the genesis of congestive heart failure.

The results of these human studies are in striking contrast to data reported from investigations in animals. Most animal studies of cardiac hypertrophy have detected a mild decrease in coronary reserves; humans with severe pressure-induced left ventricular hypertrophy have a profound decrease in coronary vasodilator reserve.

Strauer (2) has also examined coronary reserve in patients with various degrees of systemic hypertension and left ventricular hypertrophy. These studies demonstrate that coronary reserve is frequently decreased with cardiac hypertrophy secondary to hypertension even if the magnitude of the hypertrophy is relatively modest (30% increase in left ventricular mass).

Volume-Induced Left Ventricular Hypertrophy

We have examined the characteristics of coronary reactive hyperemia in patients with volume-induced cardiac hypertrophy secondary to severe mitral regurgitation (48). Coronary reserve was significantly diminished in vessels perfusing the hypertrophied left ventricle. Studies with the argon clearance approach also indicate that coronary reserve is decreased in patients with volume-induced left ventricular hypertrophy secondary to mitral or aortic regurgitation (51,52). Thus, left ventricular hypertrophy in humans, secondary to volume-overload, is associated with impaired coronary reserve. Studies in animals have yielded the opposite result.

Volume-Induced Right Ventricular Hypertrophy

Patients with isolated large atrial septal defects and normal pulmonary artery pressure have marked right ventricular dilation and hypertrophy. We have examined the characteristics of coronary reactive hyperemia in vessels perfusing the enlarged right ventricle of patients with atrial–septal defects (46). Two important abnormalities were observed: (a) the maximal dilator response was about one-half of that observed in control patients; and (b) the duration of the coronary reactive hyperemic response was markedly prolonged. The mechanism responsible for the prolongation of the reactive hyperemic response is uncertain.

Pressure-Induced Right Ventricular Hypertrophy

Pressure-induced right ventricular hypertrophy occurs in patients with various types of cyanotic congenital heart disease (tetrology of Fallot, transposition of the great vessels, etc.). We have noted that the coronary reactive hyperemic response in these patient groups, in vessels perfusing the hypertrophied ventricle, is markedly diminished (49). The magnitude of the abnormality observed is similar to the results of animal studies reported by Murray and Vatner (37,38).

SUMMARY OF RESULTS OF PHYSIOLOGICAL STUDIES IN HUMANS

In humans, coronary reserve is markedly decreased in volume or pressure-induced hypertrophy of either the right or left ventricle. Studies in patients with mild-to-moderate hypertension associated with only a 30% increase in left ventricular mass indicate that even under these conditions there is a significant decrease in coronary reserve. It is likely that diminished coronary reserve in hypertrophied ventricles contributes significantly to the pathogenesis of angina and heart failure in patients with hypertrophied ventricles.

FUTURE DIRECTIONS

There are many new areas in this field that warrant additional studies; principally, they are as follows.

(a) To determine if the abnormalities in coronary reserve secondary to cardiac hypertrophy disappear or persist following regression of cardiac hypertrophy.

(b) To characterize precisely the anatomical basis for decreased coronary reserve in hypertrophied hearts. At what level(s) in the coronary hierarchy are anatomical abnormalities present? What are the anatomical abnormalities in the coronary circulation in pressure- versus volume-induced cardiac hypertrophy?

(c) To explore further the adverse interaction between pressure-induced cardiac hypertrophy and coronary occlusion. Are the lethal arrhythmias that occur in this setting related to electrophysiological abnormalities in hypertrophied cardiac muscles? Is the increase in infarct size dependent on the presence of hypertension and hypertrophy versus hypertension alone? Does pressure-induced cardiac hypertrophy alter the characteristics of coronary collateral circulation?

Although studies in this area are difficult and expensive, the problem being addressed is important, and research in this field should be enthusiastically encouraged and supported.

ACKNOWLEDGMENTS

The original studies from the University of Iowa described in this chapter were supported by the following grants: Research Development Award

HL00328; National Institutes of Health grant HL20827, Program Project grant HL 14288 and research funds from the Veterans Administration.

REFERENCES

1. Hurst, J. W., Logue, R. B., Schlant, R. B., and Wenger, N. K., editors (1978): *The Heart, Arteries and Veins (Fourth Ed.).* pp. 1556–1590. McGraw-Hill, New York.
2. Strauer, B. E. (1980): *Hypertensive Heart Disease.* Springer-Verlag, New York.
3. Harris, C. N., Aronow, W. S., Parker, D. P., and Kaplan, M. A. (1973): *Chest*, 63:353–357.
4. Buckberg, G. D., Fixler, D. E., Archie, J. P., and Hoffman, J. I. E. (1972): *Circ. Res.*, 30:67–81.
5. Marcus, M. L., Mueller, T. M., Gascho, J. A., and Kerber, R. E. (1979): *Am. J. Cardiol.*, 44:1023–1028.
6. Stack, R. S., Schirmer, B., and Greenfield, J. C., Jr. (1980): *Circulation (Suppl.)*, 64:(Suppl. III) 64.
7. Yamori, Y., Mori, C., Nishio, T., Ooshima, A., Horie, R., Ohtaka, M., Soeda, T., Saito, M., Abe, K., Nara, Y., Nakao, Y., and Kihara, M. (1979): *Am. J. Cardiol.*, 44:964–969.
8. Hallback-Nordlander, M., Noresson, E., and Thoren, P. (1979): *Am. J. Cardiol.*, 44:986–993.
9. Rakusan, K. (1971): *Achiev. Exp. Pathol.*, 5:272–286.
10. Wearn, J. T. (1928): *J. Exp. Med.*, 47:273–292.
11. Murray, P. A., Baig, H., Fishbein, M. C., and Vatner, S. F. (1979): *J. Clin. Invest.*, 64:421–427.
12. Buchner, F. (1971): *Methods Achiev. Exp. Pathol.*, 5:60–120.
13. Bing, R. J., Hammond, M. M., Handelsman, J. C., Powers, S. R., Spencer, F. C., Eckenhoff, J. E., Goodale, W. T., Hafkenschiel, J. F., and Kety, S. S. (1949): *Am. Heart J.*, 38:1–24.
14. Rowe, G. G., Castillo, C. A., Maxwell, G. M., and Crumpton, C. W. (1961): *Ann. Intern. Med.*, 54:405–412.
15. Mueller, T. M., Marcus, M. L., Kerber, R. E., Young, J. A., Barnes, R. W., and Abboud, F. M. (1978): *Circ. Res.*, 42:543–549.
16. Einzig, S., Leonard, J. J., Tripp, M. R., Burchell, H. B., and Fox, I. J. (1975): *Physiologist (abstract)*, 18:285.
17. Holtz, J., Restorff, W. V., Bard, P., and Bassenge, E. (1977): *Basic Res. Cardiol.*, 72:286–292.
18. O'Keefe, D. D., Hoffman, J. I. E., Cheitlin, R., O'Neill, M. J., Allard, J. R., and Shapkin, E. (1978): *Circ. Res.*, 43:43–51.
19. Rembert, J. C., Kleinman, L. H., Fedor, J. M., Wechsler, A. S., and Greenfield, J. C. (1978): *J. Clin. Invest.*, 62:379–386.
20. White, F. C., Sanders, M., Peterson, T., and Bloor, C. M. (1979): *Am. J. Pathol.*, 97:473–486.
21. Bache, R. J., and Vrobel, T. R. (1979): *Am. J. Cardiol.*, 44:1029–1034.
22. Breisch, E. A., Houser, S. R., Carey, R. A., Spann, J. F., and Bove, A. A. (1980): *Cardiovascular Res.*, 14:469–475.
23. Mittmann, U., Bruckner, U. B., Keller, H. E., Kohler, U., Vetter, H., and Waag, K.-L. (1980): *Basic Res. Cardiol.*, 75:199–206.
24. Bache, R. J., Vrobel, T. R., Ring, W. S., Emery, R. W., and Andersen, R. W. (1981): *Circ. Res.*, 48:76–87.
25. Bache, R. J., Vrobel, T. R., Arentzen, C. E., and Ring, W. S. (1981): *Circ. Res.*, 49:742–750.
26. Attarian, D. E., Jones, R. N., Currie, W. D., Hill, R. C., Sink, J. D., Olsen, C. O., Chitwood, W. R., Jr., and Wechsler, A. S. (1981): *J. Thorac. Cardiovasc. Surg.*, 81:382–388.
27. Marcus, M. L., Mueller, T. M., and Eastham, C. L. (1981): *Am. J. Physiol.*, 241:H358–H362.
28. Sasayama, S., Ross, J., Franklin, D., Bloor, C. M., Bishop, S., and Dilley, R. B. (1976): *Circ. Res.*, 38:172–178.
29. Mueller, T. M., Marcus, M. L., Eastham, C. L., and Tipton, C. M. (1979): *Fed. Proc. (abstract)*, 37:647.
30. Kannel, W. B. (1974): *Prog. Cardiovasc. Dis.*, 17:5.
31. Koyanagi, S., Eastham, C., and Marcus, M. L. (1982): *Circulation*, 65:1192–1197.
32. Koyanagi, S., Eastham, C. L., Harrison, D. G., and Marcus, M. L. (1982): *Circ. Res.*, 50:55–63.
33. Aronson, R. S. (1980): *Circ. Res.*, 47:443.

34. Gelband, H., and Bassett, A. (1973): *Circ. Res.*, 32:625–634.
35. Gascho, J., Mueller, T. M., Eastham, C. L., and Marcus, M. L. (1978): *Clin. Res. (abstract)*, 26:652A.
36. Huntgren, P. B., and Bove, A. A. (1978): *Fed. Proc. (abstract)*, 37:647.
37. Murray, P. A., Baig, H., Fishbein, M. C., and Vatner, S. F. (1979): *J. Clin. Invest.*, 64:421–427.
38. Murray, P. A., and Vatner, S. F. (1981): *Circ. Res.*, 48:27–33.
39. Vlahakes, G. J., Turley, K., Verrier, E. D., and Hoffman, J. I. E. (1980): *Circulation (Suppl.)*, 62:III:415.
40. Archie, J. P., Fixler, D. E., Ullyot, D. J., Buckberg, G. D., and Hoffman, J. I. E. (1974): *Circ. Res.*, 34:143–154.
41. Manohar, M., Thurmon, J. C., Tranquilli, W. J., Devous, M. D., Sr., Theodorakis, M. C., Shawley, R. V., Feller, D. L., and Benson, J. G. (1981): *Circ. Res.*, 48:785–796.
42. Kennedy, J. W., Doces, J., and Stewart, D. K. (1977): Circulation, 56:941–950.
43. Marcus, M. L., Wright, C., Doty, D., Eastham, C., Fastenow, C., Laughlin, D., and Krumm, P. (1976): *Circulation*, 261:59–60.
44. Marcus, M. L., Wright, C., Doty, D., Eastham, C., Laughlin, D., Krumm, P., Fastenow, C., and Brody, M. (1981): *Circ. Res.*, 49:877–891.
45. Marcus, M. L., Doty, D., Wright, C., and Eastham, C. (1980): *Circulation*, 62:III–111.
46. Doty, D., Wright, C., Eastham, C., and Marcus, M. L. (1980): *Circulation*, 62:III–115.
47. Eastham, C., Doty, D., Wright, C., and Marcus, M. L. (1980): *Circulation*, 62:III–64.
48. Eastham, C. L., Doty, D. B., Hiratzka, L. F., Wright, C. B., and Marcus, M. L. (1981): *Circulation (Suppl.)*, 64:IV–127.
49. Marcus, M. L., Doty, D., Hiratzka, L., Wright, C., and Eastham, C. (1981): *Circulation (in press)*.
50. Doty, D., Eastham, C., Hiratzka, L., Wright, C., and Marcus, M. (1982): *Circulation*, 66:I–186–192.
51. Strauer, B-E. (1979): *Am. J. Cardiol.*, 44:999–1006.
52. Tauchert, M., and Hilger, H. H. (1979): In: *The Patho-Physiology of Myocardial Perfusion*, edited by W. Schaper, pp. 141–167. Elsevier/North-Holland, Amsterdam.

Perspectives in Cardiovascular
Research, Vol. 8,
edited by R. C. Tarazi and J. B. Dunbar.
Raven Press, New York © 1983.

Cardiac Hypertrophy in Chronic Ischemic Heart Disease

L. Maximilian Buja, Kathryn H. Muntz, Kirk Lipscomb,
and James T. Willerson

*Departments of Pathology and Internal Medicine (Cardiac Division), The University
of Texas Health Science Center at Dallas, and the Veterans Administration Hospital,
Dallas, Texas 75235*

Using increased heart weight as the diagnostic criterion, autopsy studies have shown that cardiac hypertrophy is an extremely common finding in patients with coronary atherosclerosis and fatal ischemic heart disease (1–4). In our recent experience, of 83 patients with fatal ischemic heart disease, postmortem measurement of heart weight showed 85% at over 400 g (normal heart weight is 300 to 350 g) (3). Clinicopathological studies have identified a number of factors associated with cardiac hypertrophy in patients with coronary heart disease, including hypertension, previous myocardial infarction with subsequent abnormal regional wall motion (with or without ventricular aneurysm formation), congestive heart failure, and mitral regurgitation secondary to papillary muscle dysfunction (1–4). These pathophysiological phenomena may lead to cardiac hypertrophy as a compensatory response to increased afterload or preload. A vicious cycle of chronic ischemic injury, increased afterload or preload, and compensatory hypertrophy can result in "ischemic cardiomyopathy." This condition is characterized clinically by congestive heart failure and cardiomegaly, and pathologically by cardiac hypertrophy and dilation, usually multiple myocardial infarcts and fibrosis and severe multivessel coronary artery disease (5–7).

Thus, previous studies have identified a multifactorial etiology for cardiac hypertrophy in patients with coronary heart disease. Previous work, however, also suggests that there is a significant, but poorly defined, incidence of cardiac hypertrophy in patients with coronary heart disease that cannot be accounted for by the previously described pathophysiological alterations, acting alone or in combination (1,4). This observation has raised the possibility that chronic ischemic injury per se is also a stimulus to cardiac hypertrophy.

AUTOPSY STUDIES

Several older clinicopathological studies emphasized the role of congestive heart failure in the development of cardiac hypertrophy in patients with coronary artery disease (1,4). Recently, Dean and Gallagher (4) examined the relationship between cardiac ischemia and cardiac hypertrophy in 50 autopsied patients who had undergone cardiovascular examination including three separate recordings of blood pressure prior to their final illnesses. Coronary artery disease was assessed from postmortem arteriograms and an "ischemic score" was derived based on the presence of a 50 to 75% reduction, or a greater than 75% reduction, in luminal diameter in each of the major coronary arteries. Following removal of adipose tissue, total heart muscle weight and weights of the individual cardiac chambers were determined. No attempt was made to estimate the proportion of fibrous tissue in the hearts or to perform morphometric analyses of muscle cell size. When all 50 cases were considered, only low levels of statistical significance were obtained between coronary artery (ischemic) score and total heart muscle weight ($r = 0.39$, $p < 0.01$). When only the 34 patients with definite coronary arterial stenoses were considered, a better association occurred between extent and severity of coronary disease (ischemic score) and total heart muscle weight ($r = 0.54$, $p < 0.01$). When the 10 patients with well-documented hypertensive or valvular disease were excluded, a stronger correlation ($r = 0.80$, $p < 0.001$) was noted in the remaining 24 patients. An equally strong correlation ($r = 0.86$, $p < 0.001$) was noted in a group of 17 patients when an additional 7 cases with autopsy evidence of healed myocardial infarction were eliminated. Positive correlations were also noted with left ventricular weight ($r = 0.86$, $p < 0.001$), right ventricular weight ($r = 0.62$, $p < 0.01$), and combined atrial weight ($r = 0.62$, $p < 0.01$). Left ventricular weight also correlated with postmortem estimates of left ventricular volume ($r = 0.68$, $p < 0.001$). None of the patients had murmurs of mitral regurgitation. The only correlation between any measurement of blood pressure and hypertrophy was a weak relationship between maximum systolic blood pressure and left ventricular weight ($r = 0.31$, $p < 0.05$). The results suggested that: (a) an association exists between the degree of coronary arterial stenosis and cardiac mass, and (b) the relationship is not confined to left ventricular hypertrophy, but the association is with whole heart hypertrophy.

CLINICAL STUDIES

Further insight into the relationship between cardiac hypertrophy and ischemic heart disease has come from clinical hemodynamic studies of patients with coronary heart disease. In these studies, intracardiac pressure recordings, coronary arteriography, and biplane angiocardiography are performed at cardiac catheterization. Left ventricular dimensions, volume, and mass are calculated from the ventriculograms (7–9). This mass measurement does not distinguish viable muscle and scar tissue. Moraski and co-workers (8) evaluated the relationship between left ventricular function and severity of coronary disease in 96 patients with and without evidence (history, enzyme, and EKG changes) of transmural myocardial infarction. Left ventricular mass was not significantly increased in patients with one- or two-vessel disease, with or without myocardial infarction, whereas left ventricular mass was significantly increased (by approximately 24%) in all patients with three-vessel disease. There was no difference in left ventricular mass in patients with three-vessel disease, with and without myocardial infarction. Patients with three-vessel disease and no infarcts had a moderately depressed left ventricular ejection fraction (18% decrease) and normal left ventricular compliance. Even though left ventricular mass was similarly increased in patients with three-vessel disease, with and without infarcts, those patients with three-vessel disease and infarcts had a significantly lower left ventricular ejection fraction (36% decrease) and compliance (70% decrease) than did those without myocardial infarcts (18% decrease in left ventricular ejection fraction and 15% decrease in compliance).

Gould et al. (7) evaluated the left ventricle in 85 patients with coronary artery disease or nonobstructive cardiomyopathy without coronary artery disease. There were five groups of patients: group I ($N = 12$), controls without heart disease (ejection fraction 58 ± 6); group II ($N = 19$), coronary artery disease, no discrete areas of segmental myocardial dysfunction on ventriculogram, and minimally reduced left ventricular ejection fraction (52 ± 8); group III ($N = 20$), coronary artery disease, localized areas of akinesia or dyskinesia, and moderately reduced left ventricular ejection fraction (40 ± 8); group IV ($N = 15$), severe, usually three-vessel coronary artery disease, generalized hypokinesis, and severely reduced left ventricular ejection fraction (19 ± 4); and group V ($N = 19$), cardiomyopathy, normal coronary arteries, and abnormal left ventricular function with severely reduced ejection fraction (20 ± 6).

Patients with mild or intermediate degrees of left ventricular dysfunction due to coronary disease had modest increases in left ventricular mass. Values for patients in group I were 93 ± 19; group II: 108 ± 20; and group III: 117 ± 30 g/m^2 body area. Left ventricular mass in patients with severe coronary artery disease (group IV) was markedly increased (159 ± 49 g/m^2) and was not significantly different from the mass in patients with cardiomyopathy (185 ± 36 g/m^2).

Measurements were also made of the ratio of left ventricular mass to end-diastolic volume. A major deviation of this mass-to-volume ratio from control values did not occur. This finding indicates that the ventricular hypertrophy occurred in proportion to the increase in end-diastolic volume (7). Rackley et al. (9) reported a similar relationship in 23 normotensive patients with severe coronary artery disease. This pattern is in contrast to the expected response with a pure afterload stimulus to hypertrophy, such as that provided by hypertension. In the latter situation, concentric hypertrophy with an increased mass-to-volume ratio would occur. However, the patients with coronary artery disease did not show this pattern of hypertrophy.

Patients in groups IV and V showed severely depressed left ventricular function by a variety of parameters of left ventricular performance, including indices of fiber shortening, cardiac work, and rate of doing work (7). Patients with mild to moderate impairment due to coronary artery disease (groups II and III) had intermediate degrees of left ventricular dysfunction. However, peak systolic equatorial wall stress (g/cm^2) was not significantly different in any of the patient groups regardless of the severity of ventricular impairment. This finding suggests that left ventricular wall thickening and hypertrophy occurred appropriately in proportion to ventricular size and pressure in both coronary artery disease and cardiomyopathy.

EXPERIMENTAL STUDIES

There is a paucity of experimental work dealing with the association between myocardial ischemia and myocardial infarction (1). This is in large measure related to the difficulties involved in establishing models of chronic coronary artery disease and myocardial ischemia. However, increased cardiac weight has been observed at 4 to 12 weeks after left coronary artery ligation in rats (10–12). The increased cardiac weight has been shown to result from hypertrophy of myocytes in the non-infarcted left ventricle, ventricular septum, and right ventricle (11). Altered left ventricular systolic function and diastolic pressure-volume relations also occur (12).

PATHOPHYSIOLOGICAL MECHANISMS

Thus, the available evidence from human postmortem, clinical, and experimental studies indicates that: (a) a number of factors—including hypertension, previous myocardial infarction, congestive heart failure, and mitral regurgitation—act as important determinants of the magnitude of cardiac hypertrophy in patients with coronary artery disease; and (b) increased myocardial mass occurs in patients with coronary artery disease in the absence of clinically overt manifestations of these complicating factors, suggesting that chronic recurrent episodes of myocardial ischemia with associated ventricular dysfunction can act as the initiating stimulus for cardiac hypertrophy in patients with coronary artery disease.

Considerable evidence indicates that altered left ventricular function is an important common hypertrophic stimulus which can be activated by the several pathophysiological factors discussed above (Fig. 1). Previous work has indicated that increased wall stress (force per unit area) is an important triggering mechanism that leads to compensatory hypertrophy and subsequent normalization of wall stress (13–16). Several studies have indicated that angina pectoris, induced by rapid atrial pacing or other means in patients with coronary artery disease, is associated with significantly elevated left ventricular end-diastolic pressure and volume (17–19). Previous studies have also demonstrated that this is the result of both impaired left ventricular systolic performance and altered diastolic compliance (17–19).

The data of Gould et al. (7) in patients with chronic coronary heart disease are consistent with the hypothesis that the trigger for hypertrophy involves increased wall stress. These findings suggest that the heart responds by nor-

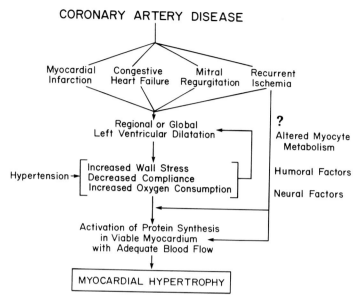

FIG. 1. Pathophysiological mechanisms leading to cardiac hypertrophy in subjects with chronic ischemic heart disease.

malizing the increased stress through the development of hypertrophy and wall thickening in proportion to the degree of ventricular dilatation (7). However, in advanced decompensation, ventricular dilatation may exceed the hypertrophic response, and wall thickening may become relatively less than expected (6).

Although there is considerable evidence that hypertrophy is the result of increased wall stress, the mechanism for translating the increased mechanical work into increased protein synthesis is unknown, and several hypotheses have been proposed (20–26). Increased wall stress may produce changes in membrane proteins that stimulate protein synthesis, perhaps through the adenyl cyclase system (22,23). Increased wall stress may make the myocardial cell mildly hypoxic and the hypoxia, or a metabolite resulting from hypoxia, may lead to increased protein synthesis (20–23). In this respect, there is an excellent correlation between wall tension, oxygen consumption, and hypertrophy (22,23). Other mechanisms that have been proposed include increased membrane permeability to amino acids and a direct effect of increased oxygen consumption on genetic control of respiration (21–23). Humoral or neural factors, such as catecholamines and thyroid hormone, may also play a role in hypertrophy resulting from increased wall stress (20–24).

The question remains, however, as to whether factors other than increased wall stress are also operative in the initiation of cardiac hypertrophy in patients with coronary artery disease. One of the classical theories of myocardial hypertrophy is that transient myocellular hypoxia may act directly to trigger increased protein synthesis by means of an effect on ATP metabolism, break-down of proteins with release of derepressors of genetic control of protein synthesis, or other mechanisms (1,20,22). It also may be hypothesized that local myocardial hypoxia could induce global effects on myocardial protein synthesis via humoral or neural pathways (1,20,21,24). It is of interest in this regard that Dean and Gallagher (4) found a substantial correlation between coronary stenosis and all individual chamber weights, and that the relationship was not confined to the left ventricle, as might be anticipated if the hypertrophic stimulus were purely mechanical. Prominent right ventricular hypertrophy is also a feature of the hypertrophic response following left coronary ligation in rats (10–12). On the other hand, hypertrophy of other cardiac chambers could occur as a secondary response to left ventricular dysfunction and increased left ventricular diastolic pressure. The argument can be made that, if ischemia per se were the primary mediator of hypertrophy, an increased left ventricular mass-to-volume ratio should occur at some point in the course of coronary heart disease. In the clinical studies, however, the left ventricular mass-to-volume ratio in patients with coronary artery disease remained constant, suggesting that the hypertrophy is mechanically appropriate (7–9).

If ischemia serves as a stimulus to cardiac hypertrophy, it can do so only if the myocellular hypoxia is of a certain critical level and of a transient, though recurrent, nature. Experimental studies have indicated that sustained severe hypoxia results in a net decrease in protein synthesis (26). Myocardium subjected to such a stimulus would develop ischemic atrophy rather than hypertrophy. Cardiac hypertrophy in subjects with coronary artery disease must occur in areas of viable myocardium with adequate blood flow for periods of time sufficient for the hypertrophic process to occur (1). However, recurrent ischemic injury may commonly be associated with degeneration and loss of myocytes and fibrosis in the subendocardial region, as well as hypertrophy of myocytes in other areas of the heart. This phenomenon may complicate estimation of ventricular mass from measurements of segmental wall thickness.

CONSEQUENCES OF CARDIAC HYPERTROPHY

Another aspect to consider is the impact of cardiac hypertrophy on the natural history of the disease. In one sense, an increased myocardial mass could have a beneficial effect if factors associated with the hypertrophy (such as a possible increase in the coronary collateral system) could result in a reduction in the relative percentage of myocardial necrosis after the onset of myocardial infarction. Prognosis after myocardial infarction is related to the total mass of myocardium infarcted versus the mass that remains viable (27,28).

On the other hand, several studies have indicated that significantly hypertrophied myocardium may have a reduced capacity to respond to stress in terms of augmentation of perfusion (29–34) and may develop metabolic and functional deterioration when stressed (35). In a unique morphometric study,

Turek et al. (11) found that, in rats with myocardial infarcts, the remaining hypertrophied myocardium had the following characteristics: (a) increased mean muscle fiber diameter, (b) increased mean intercapillary distance, and (c) unchanged fiber/capillary ratio. These results contrasted with those observed in response to hypoxemia produced by exposure to high altitude, where the hypertrophied right ventricle showed shorter intercapillary distances (11). Turek and co-workers concluded that the increased intercapillary distance observed in hypertrophied myocardium following myocardial infarction might result in impaired tissue oxygen transport, particularly during stress (11).

Mueller et al. (36) found that left ventricular hypertrophy produced by renovascular hypertension in dogs was associated with an increase in size of the ischemic region, following acute coronary occlusion. However, the amount of necrosis associated with a given degree of ischemia was similar in the dogs with hypertension and left ventricular hypertrophy and in normotensive controls without left ventricular hypertrophy. There is also evidence that the presence of hypertrophic stimuli can have adverse effects during episodes of acute ischemic heart disease. Roan et al. (37) found that acute hypertension following coronary occlusion in conscious dogs with nonhypertrophied ventricles resulted in transient worsening of the impaired segmental systolic wall thickening in the ischemic left ventricle as well as accentuation of the end diastolic wall thinning in the severely ischemic area. Finally, clinical and epidemiological studies have shown that the electrocardiographic finding of left ventricular hypertrophy is associated with an increased incidence of left ventricular dysfunction (38), left main coronary artery disease (38), and sudden death (39–41).

FUTURE DIRECTIONS

Further understanding of the pathogenesis and significance of cardiac hypertrophy in ischemic heart disease requires several developments. There is a need for more clinical studies with serial monitoring of left ventricular function and stratification of patients with attention to specific pathophysiological factors that may serve as stimuli to hypertrophy. There is also a need for the development of animal models of chronic ischemic heart disease in which the mechanisms of hypertrophy can be studied. Finally, detailed morphometric studies are needed to characterize the anatomic basis of the cardiac enlargement in patients and experimental animals with ischemic heart disease.

ACKNOWLEDGMENTS

Supported in part by NIH Ischemic SCOR grant HL 17669 and Cardiovascular Research Training grant HL 07360.

REFERENCES

1. Badeer, H. (1972): *Am. Heart J.*, 84:256–264.
2. Roberts, C. S., and Roberts, W. C. (1980): *Circulation*, 62:953–959.

3. Buja, L. M., and Willerson, J. T. (1981): *Am. J. Cardiol.*, 47:343–356.
4. Dean, J. H., and Gallagher, P. J. (1980): *Arch. Pathol. Lab. Med.*, 104:175–178.
5. Burch, G. E., Tsui, C. Y., and Harb, J. M. (1972): *Am. Heart J.*, 83:340–350.
6. Schuster, E. H., and Bulkley, B. H. (1980): *Am. Heart J.*, 100:506–512.
7. Gould, K. L., Lipscomb, K., Hamilton, G. W., and Kennedy, J. W. (1973): *Am. J. Med.*, 55: 595–601.
8. Moraski, R. E., Russell, R. O., Jr., Smith, M., and Rackley, C. E. (1975): *Am. J. Cardiol.*, 35:1–10.
9. Rackley, C. E., Dear, H. D., Baxley, W. A., Jones, W. B., and Dodge, H. T. (1970): *Circulation*, 41:605–613.
10. Norman, T. D., and Coers, C. R. (1960): *Arch. Pathol.*, 69:181–184.
11. Turek, Z., Grandtner, M., Kubát, K., Ringnalda, B. E. M., and Kreuzer, F. (1978): *Pflügers Arch.*, 376:209–215.
12. Fletcher, P. J., Pfeffer, J. M., Pfeffer, M. A., and Braunwald, E. (1981): *Circ. Res.*, 49:618–626.
13. Sandler, H., and Dodge, H. T. (1963): *Circ. Res.*, 13:91–104.
14. Hood, W. P., Jr., Rackley, C. E., and Rolett, E. L. (1968): *Am. J. Cardiol.*, 22:550–558.
15. Hood, W. P., Jr., Thomson, W. J., Rackley, C. E., and Rolett, E. L. (1969): *Circ. Res.*, 24:575–582.
16. Grossman, W., Jones, D., and McLaurin, L. P. (1975): *J. Clin. Invest.*, 56:56–64.
17. Mann, T., Brodie, B. R., Grossman, W., and McLaurin, L. P. (1977): *Circulation*, 55:761–766.
18. Mann, T., Goldberg, S., Mudge, G. H., Jr., and Grossman, W. (1979): *Circulation*, 59:14–20.
19. Grossman, W., and Barry, W. H. (1980): *Fed. Proc.*, 39:148–155.
20. Meerson, F. Z. (1969): *Circ. Res. (Suppl.)*, 24 and 25: II1–II163.
21. Fanburg, B. L. (1970): *New Engl. J. Med.*, 282:723–732.
22. Rabinowitz, M., and Zak, R. (1972): *Ann. Rev. Med.*, 23:245–262.
23. Morkin, E. (1974): *Circ. Res. (Suppl.)*, 34 and 35: II37–II48.
24. Cohen, J. (1974): *Circ. Res. (Suppl.)*, 34 and 35: II49–II57.
25. Wikman-Coffelt, J., Parmley, W. W., and Mason, D. T. (1979): *Circ. Res.*, 45:697–707.
26. Schreiber, S. S., Evans, C. D., Oratz, M., and Rothschild, M. A. (1981): *Circ. Res.*, 48:601–611.
27. Page, D. L., Caulfield, J. B., Kastor, J. A., DeSanctis, R. W., and Sanders, C. A. (1971): *N. Engl. J. Med.*, 285:133–137.
28. Alonso, D. R., Scheidt, S., Post, M., and Killip, T. (1973): *Circulation*, 48:588–596.
29. Mueller, T. M., Marcus, M. L., Kerber, R. E., Young, J. A., Barnes, R. W., and Abboud, F. M. (1978): *Circ. Res.*, 42:543–549.
30. O'Keefe, D. D., Hoffman, J. I. E., Cheitlin, R., O'Neill, M. J., Allard, J. R., and Shapkin, E. (1978): *Circ. Res.*, 43:43–51.
31. Rembert, J. C., Kleinman, L. H., Fedor, J. M., Wechsler, A. S., and Greenfield, J. C. (1978): *J. Clin. Invest.*, 62:379–386.
32. Murray, P. A., and Vatner, S. F. (1981): *Circ. Res.*, 48:25–33.
33. Pichard, A. D., Gorlin, R., Smith, H., Ambrose, J., Meller, J. (1981): *Am. J. Cardiol.*, 47:547–554.
34. Bache, R. J., Vrobel, T. R., Ring, W. S., Emery, R. W., and Anderson, R. W. (1981): *Circ. Res.*, 48:76–87.
35. Meerson, F. Z. (1976): *Basic Res. Cardiol.*, 71:630–635.
36. Mueller, T. M., Tomanek, R. J., Kerber, R. E., and Marcus, M. L. (1980): *Am. J. Physiol.*, 239(H6):731–735.
37. Roan, P. G., Buja, L. M., Saffer, S., Hagler, H., Duke, B., Hillis, L. D., and Willerson, J. T. (1982): *Circulation*, 65:115–125.
38. Hamby, R. I., Prakash, M. N., Wyne, U. A., and Hoffman, I. (1980): *Am. Heart J.*, 100:794–801.
39. Kannel, W. B., Gordan, T., Castelli, W. P., and Margolis, J. R. (1970): *Ann. Intern. Med.*, 72:813–822.
40. Kannel, W. B., Doyle, J. T., McNamara, P. M., Quickenton, P., and Gordon, T. (1975): *Circulation*, 51:606–613.
41. Chiang, B. N., Perlman, L. V., Fulton, M., Ostrander, L. D., Jr., and Epstein, F. H. (1970): *Circulation*, 41:31–37.

*Perspectives in Cardiovascular
Research, Vol. 8,*
edited by R. C. Tarazi and J. B. Dunbar.
Raven Press, New York © 1983.

Abnormalities of the Cardiac Sympathetic Nervous System in the Hypertrophied and Failing Heart

James F. Spann

*Section of Cardiology, Department of Medicine, Temple University
Health Sciences Center, Philadelphia, Pennsylvania 19140*

Myocardial stores of norepinephrine (NE) are severely reduced in the hypertrophied heart whether or not congestive failure is present. This reduction was first noted in atrial tissue from patients with congestive heart failure (Fig. 1) (1,2). NE reduction was also found in left ventricular papillary muscles removed from patients at the time of mitral valve replacement for mitral regurgitation with left ventricular failure (2).

There is abundant evidence of such reduction in experimentally induced ventricular hypertrophy in several animal models, with and without congestive heart failure (Fig. 2). In left ventricular hypertrophy and left heart failure produced by constriction of the ascending aorta of the guinea pig (3,4), in right heart failure induced by production of pulmonary stenosis and tricuspid insufficiency in the dog (5), and in right ventricular hypertrophy, with or without heart failure, produced by different degrees of pulmonary arterial constriction in the cat (6), a profound reduction in cardiac norepinephrine concentration and content occurs. Norepinephrine depletion is present in both ventricles, regardless of which ventricle is subjected to the primary hemodynamic burden. The reduced total cardiac content of NE proves that there is a true depletion of catecholamine, rather than dilution of the normal complement of NE by the hypertrophy of the heart.

In one study (7), the time required for depletion of cardiac norepinephrine after imposition of severe ventricular pressure overload was determined in the guinea pig. It was found that average ventricular norepinephrine concentration fell to 22 percent of normal by day 5 after aortic constriction, and remained depressed for the 65-day observation period.

MECHANISMS OF CARDIAC NOREPINEPHRINE DEPLETION

Cardiac sympathetic nerve terminals are complex structures involved in synthesis, uptake, binding, storage, and release of norepinephrine. In ventric-

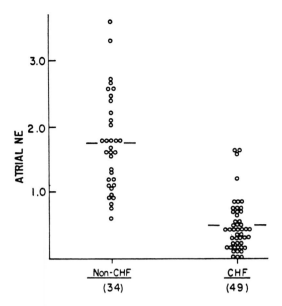

FIG. 1. NE concentrations in biopsy specimens of atrial appendage obtained from 34 patients with no congestive heart failure (Non-CHF) and from 49 patients with congestive heart failure (CHF). (From Chidsey et al., ref. 2, with permission.)

ular hypertrophy and heart failure, at least two defects of the cardiac sympathetic nerves cause NE depletion: A defect in neuronal uptake and binding of NE, and a defect in NE synthesis. In the study by Spann et al. (7), the defect

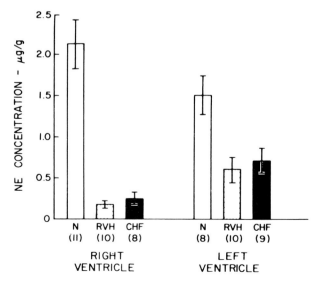

FIG. 2. The average NE concentration of the right and left ventricles of normal cats and cats with right ventricular hypertrophy (RVH) and congestive heart failure (CHF). *Vertical lines with cross bars* = ±1 SEM. Numbers in parentheses: number of animals in each group. (Reprinted from Spann et al., ref. 15, with permission.)

in neuronal uptake and binding was defined by measurement of the NE retained in heart and kidneys, after infusion of non-radioactive L-norepinephrine, in guinea pigs with left ventricular hypertrophy and congestive heart failure compared with NE levels in a control group of normal guinea pigs. In the normal animals, the renal and left and right ventricular concentrations of NE rose to peak values at the completion of the infusion, and the concentrations declined over the ensuing three hours to values that approached the control levels. The increase in ventricular concentrations in the animals with left ventricular hypertrophy and heart failure was minimal, while the renal norepinephrine in this group increased in a manner similar to the normals. When tracer quantities of tritium-labeled DL-norepinephrine were injected into animals with ventricular hypertrophy and failure, a depressed uptake of the tritium-label by the hypertrophied and failing heart was observed. These results were confirmed by Fischer and co-workers (8), who observed a decrease in the uptake of tritiated norepinephrine in the hearts of rats with severe hypertrophy but no congestive heart failure.

To rule out the possibility that the decrease in uptake and binding had been caused by a rapid turnover of infused norepinephrine, the net turnover rate of intraneuronal norepinephrine was investigated by administering a small amount of radioactive norepinephrine to normal guinea pigs and to those with left ventricular hypertrophy and heart failure (7). The turnover rate was determined by monitoring the specific activity in the left ventricles of both groups for 72 hr. In both, the decline of specific activity was complex, and exhibited two exponential components. These findings, similar to the observations of other investigators (9), are compatible with the presence of a multicompartmental distribution of NE. The absolute level of specific activity and the rate of disappearance were essentially identical in both groups, indicating a normal relative turnover rate in the animals with ventricular hypertrophy and failure. Thus, the smaller increment of NE in the heart, following infusion in the animals with hypertrophy and failure, cannot be explained by a more rapid net turnover of NE, but must be interpreted as an abnormality of uptake or binding or both. This defect in uptake or binding is in part responsible for the observed depletion of NE stores in the hypertrophied and failing heart. The presence of a normal net turnover rate in hearts depleted of norepinephrine also indicates that the rate of synthesis in the ventricle must actually be reduced in the group with hypertrophy and heart failure.

A defect in the synthetic pathway for norepinephrine in the failing heart was first reported by Pool and co-workers (10), who demonstrated a severe defect in tyrosine hydroxylase, the rate-limiting enzyme for the synthesis of NE. In the right ventricles of dogs with right ventricular hypertrophy, congestive heart failure, and severe norepinephrine depletion, tyrosine hydroxylase activity was significantly reduced from the normal value of 3.3 ± 0.7 to 0.4 ± 0.1 μmoles/g/hour. Similar reductions in humans have been observed by DiCuatro and co-workers (11) in biopsies of myocardium obtained from patients with hypertrophy and congestive heart failure. DiCuatro et al. also demonstrated a relationship in humans between the extent of cardiac norepinephrine depletion and the extent of reduction of tyrosine hydroxylase activity in the hypertrophied and failing heart. Both NE and tyrosine hydroxylase were more severely reduced in patients with class III and IV heart failure than in patients within class I or II heart failure.

The cardiomyopathic Syrian hamster differs in certain ways from the guinea pig and dog models of hypertrophy and failure, as well as from myocardium obtained from human patients with hypertrophy and failure. This animal shows an increase in the rate constant for cardiac norepinephrine turnover approaching the rate seen with maximum sympathetic stimulation due to immobilization stress (12). Additionally, during heart failure, an increase in the tyrosine hydroxylase activity was noted. The high concentration of dopamine found in the myopathic Syrian hamster implies that, in this animal, the rate-limiting enzyme for NE synthesis in the hypertrophied and failing heart may have been dopamine betahydroxylase (13).

POSSIBLE RELATIONSHIP BETWEEN DEPLETED CARDIAC NOREPINEPHRINE AND DEPRESSED INTRINSIC CONTRACTILE FUNCTION OF THE HYPERTROPHIED AND FAILING HEART

Within a group of pressure-overloaded hypertrophied hearts, there is a pathologic continuum of systolic contractile muscle function that varies from normal in some hearts to depressed in others. The continuum extends from one extreme of normally functioning units of hypertrophied muscle in a pressure-overloaded heart with excessive pump function, across the middle ground of moderately dysfunctioned units of hypertrophied muscle in a pressure-overloaded heart that maintains basic pump function, to the other extreme of severely dysfunctioned units of hypertrophied muscle in a pressure-overloaded heart with poor pump function and congestive failure.

In animal models of experimental pressure-overload, the presence and degree of myocardial contractile dysfunction vary in direct relation to the extent of the overload stress and correlate with the degree of hypertrophy. These relationships can be best demonstrated by subjecting one species of experimental animal to various degrees of overload. Degrees of acute pulmonary artery constriction in the cat have been used in a number of studies in which the right ventricular papillary muscle was isolated and its contractile function analyzed quantitatively. Table 1 provides a summary of the severity of constriction, degree of hypertrophy, and extent of contractile dysfunction in three such studies (14–16). When the pulmonary artery is mildly constricted, hypertrophy is mild and there is no defect of contractile function (14). When the pulmonary artery is moderately constricted, hypertrophy is moderate and there is no heart failure; contractile function is only moderately impaired (15) and may return to normal with time (16). Further, such contractile impairment may be limited to a reduction in isotonic shortening, while isometric tension

TABLE 1. *Relationship of severity and duration of acute pulmonary artery constriction, extent of right ventricular hypertrophy, and degree of right ventricular papillary muscle contractile dysfunction in cat*

Study (ref.)	Degree of PA constriction		CHF	Duration of constriction (weeks)	Extent of hypertrophy: increase RV weight (%)	Contractile function of normal (%)	
	PA band size ID (mm)	Remaining PA lumen (%)				Isotonic velocity	Isometric tension
Pannier (14)	5.0	50	No	4–24	38	100	100
Williams and Potter (16)	4.0	30	No	6	70	74	70
				24	69	100	100
Spann et al. (15)	3.5	20	No	3–12	91	72	85
Spann et al. (15)	2.8	10	Yes	3–13	142	38	38

Abbreviations used: PA, pulmonary artery; CHF, congestive heart failure; ID, internal diameter; RV, right ventricle.

development remains normal (15). When the pulmonary artery is severely constricted, hypertrophy is severe, heart failure occurs, and contractile function is severely impaired as well. The possibility of nonpathophysiologic acute damage imposed by sudden imposition of pressure overload (17) and the return to normal function (16) were demonstrated by Cooper et al. (18), using a chronic progressive pressure-overload model. In this study, kittens were exposed to gradually increasing pressure overload as they grew into an initially nonconstricting band. Right ventricular systolic pressure gradually increased from 25 mm Hg to a stable value of 50 mm Hg at week 16 following placement of the pulmonary artery band. The papillary muscle had reduced contractile function (46 to 72% of normal) at weeks 25 and 60 after the placement of the pulmonary artery band.

The dog is another species of experimental animal in which the ventricle has been subjected to various degrees of pressure overload with various degrees of hypertrophy. In these studies, too, the presence and degree of myocardial contractile dysfunction varied in direct relation to the extent of the overload stress, and they correlate with the degree of hypertrophy. When there is a mild overload, hypertrophy is mild, pump function is increased or normal, and muscle contractile function is normal (6,19,20); when there is more severe overload and more extensive hypertrophy, muscle contractile function is reduced (21).

Similarly, the recent controversy concerning depression of cardiac muscle contractile function of patients with pressure overloaded and hypertrophied hearts appears resolved: Many studies show that contractile function in some patients is normal, in others mildly depressed, and in still others, function is severely depressed. More severe degrees of pressure overload are associated with more severe degrees of ventricular hypertrophy and the presence of muscle dysfunction and congestive heart failure. At least ten recent studies, in which different angiographic and echocardiographic methods of measuring cardiac muscle contractile function have been used, were performed in patients with aortic stenosis or systemic hypertension (11,22–30). Each of these studies used at least two groups of patients with ventricular pressure overload; one group with normal cardiac muscle contractile performance and the other with depressed performance and often heart failure, as well (Fig. 3).

Because cardiac sympathetic nerve activity has positive inotropic effects, it is reasonable to wonder if the depletion of cardiac catecholamines causes the depression of the intrinsic contractile function of the hypertrophied and failing heart. To assess the possibility that the cardiac norepinephrine depletion seen in ventricular hypertrophy and congestive heart failure is also responsible for the intrinsic depression of contractile performance in the failing heart muscle, the contractile state was determined in cardiac muscle removed from experimental animals whose hearts were depleted of NE by a mechanism other than heart failure (4). In 12 cats, cardiac norepinephrine depletion was produced by chronic cardiac denervation, and contractile function of papillary muscles isolated from these hearts was determined. Cardiac norepinephrine concentration in the cardiac-denervated animals was reduced to levels of 0.006 ± 0.003 $\mu g/g$—values even lower than those in the hypertrophy and heart failure groups—but the contractile function of cardiac muscle from the NE-depleted denervated heart was not depressed (Fig. 4). Thus, cardiac norepinephrine stores are not necessary to maintain the basic contractile state of the myocardium, and cardiac norepinephrine depletion that occurs in ventricular hypertrophy and congestive heart failure is not responsible for the intrinsic depression of cardiac contractility in failing heart muscle. These conclusions have been confirmed in a series of experiments in rats (31).

CARDIAC NOREPINEPHRINE DEPLETION AND TRANSMISSION OF CARDIAC SYMPATHETIC NERVE IMPULSES

The possibility that cardiac norepinephrine depletion interferes with the transmission of sympathetic impulses to the failing heart was examined by Covell et al. (32), using dogs with severe cardiac norepinephrine depletion, right ventricular hypertrophy, and right heart failure due to tricuspid insufficiency and pulmonary stenosis. The chronotropic and inotropic responses to graded stimulation of the sympathetic nerves in six dogs with right ventricular hypertrophy and chronic right ventricular failure were compared with the responses of 13 normal animals. In dogs with heart failure, heart rate and right ventricular contractile force response to stimulation of the right cardioaccelerator nerve were sharply reduced. However, myocardium of dogs with heart failure responded normally to the direct effects of exogenously administered NE. These observations demonstrate that the quantity of neurotransmitter released per nerve impulse is dramatically reduced by the cardiac norepinephrine depletion that accompanies experimental ventricular hypertrophy and heart failure.

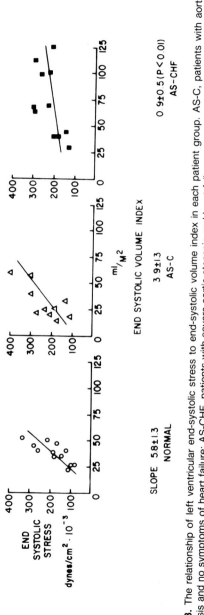

FIG. 3. The relationship of left ventricular end-systolic stress to end-systolic volume index in each patient group. AS-C, patients with aortic stenosis and no symptoms of heart failure; AS-CHF, patients with severe aortic stenosis and heart failure symptoms. The individual points are shown for each patient. *Sloping solid lines* through the points are the linear regressions. The slope of these linear regressions (expressed as ±SE) are shown below each group. P value denotes the significant difference of AS-CHF slope from both AS-C and normal. (Reprinted from Spann et al., ref. 22, with permission.)

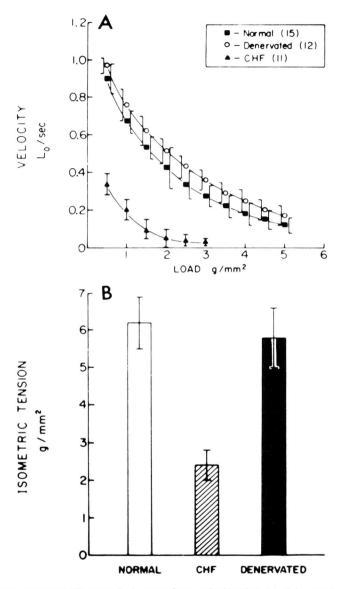

FIG. 4. Ventricular contractile state. **A:** Average force-velocity relation in right ventricular papillary muscles isolated from normal cats (N = 15), from cats with total chronic cardiac denervation (denervated, N = 12), and from cats with congestive heart failure (CHF, N = 11). *Ordinate*: velocity expressed as muscle lengths (L_o)/sec; *abscissa*: total load expressed as g/mm^2; *vertical bars*: ±SEM. **B:** Average maximal active tension, expressed as g/mm, developed at the apex of the length-tension curve in isolated cat right ventricular papillary muscles from same three groups of cats. (From Rutenberg and Spann, ref. 38, with permission.)

Similar results in humans have been reported by Goldstein et al. (23): In 38 patients with heart failure, the reflex chronotropic response to upright tilt and to hypotension induced by nitroglycerin was impaired. Since this abnormality persisted after atropine administration, the sympathetic reflex system of such patients was demonstrably defective.

Thus, sympathetic nervous control of the heart is seriously impaired in the hypertrophied and failing heart, both in experimental animals and in humans (23,32). The heart loses full use of an important mechanism, which, intact, can improve myocardial force development and velocity of contraction, and thus provide compensation for the depression of intrinsic cardiac muscle function.

SUPPORT OF THE HEART AND CIRCULATION BY CIRCULATING NOREPINEPHRINE IN PATIENTS WITH HEART FAILURE

Since a portion of norepinephrine released at the nerve terminals enters the circulating blood, augmented sympathetic activity can be estimated by the extent of increases in arterial plasma norepinephrine concentration that occur with exercise. In normal subjects, moderate muscular exercise causes an elevation of arterial norepinephrine from an average control level of 0.28 μg/L to an exercise level of 0.46 μg/L (30). In patients with congestive heart failure, the resting values of arterial plasma norepinephrine concentration are increased, and moderate exercise elevates the arterial norepinephrine from a control level of 0.36 μg/L to an exercise level of 1.73 μg/L (Fig. 5). Levels in

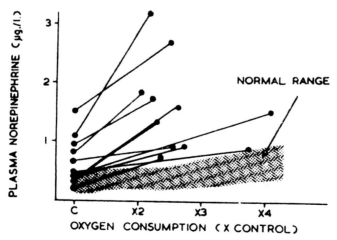

FIG. 5. Changes (from *left circles* to *right circles*) in plasma norepinephrine during exercise in CHF. Oxygen consumption during the exercise period is expressed in multiples of the resting oxygen consumption. C = control or resting values. *Stippled area* = normal range. (Adapted from Braunwald et al., ref. 39, with permission).

patients with heart disease, but without evidence of heart failure, do not differ from normal. These observations of resting plasma norepinephrine concentration elevations in patients with congestive heart failure have recently been confirmed by Thomas and Marks (33). Further, the level of plasma norepinephrine concentration is directly related to the degree of left ventricular dysfunction as indicated by systolic time interval techniques. The excessive augmentation of plasma norepinephrine concentration during exercise in patients with heart failure reflects an increased response of the sympathetic nervous system to exercise. This increased response may have an important supportive effect on hemodynamic function and distribution of blood flow.

The daily urinary excretion of norepinephrine provides an estimate of the total body level of sympathetic activity (2,27). NE excretion averaged 22 μg/day in normal persons and patients with heart disease without congestive failure, but was significantly increased in patients with heart failure (2). Patients with functional class III status (New York Heart Assoc. classification) excreted 46 μg/day, while patients with class IV status excreted 58 μg/day.

Papillary muscles removed from hearts with right ventricular hypertrophy, congestive heart failure, and NE depletion due to pressure overload are supersensitive to the positive inotropic effects of NE (15). Positive chronotropic and inotropic responsiveness of the hypertrophied, failing, and norepinephrine-depleted heart to exogenous norepinephrine was observed in the dog right ventricular model by Covell and co-workers (12). The number of cardiac α_1- and β-adrenoceptors is increased in guinea pigs with ventricular hypertrophy and heart failure due to pressure overload (32).

Because the circulating arterial norepinephrine concentration is increased in heart failure, and because the failing heart muscle is not only responsive to exogenous NE but may even be supersensitive to its positive inotropic and chronotropic effects, the circulating catecholamines play an important role in supporting the contractile function of the failing heart. Agents that block the cardiac β-sympathetic receptor sites may intensify congestive heart failure. Clinical experience with propranolol, a β-adrenergic receptor blocking agent, has shown that in certain patients with advanced cardiac disease, congestive heart failure can appear or increase if propranolol is administered (34).

PREVENTION OF CARDIAC NOREPINEPHRINE DEPLETION IN VENTRICULAR HYPERTROPHY AND FAILURE

Sole and co-workers (12) found that ganglionic blockade of cardiomyopathic Syrian hamsters completely restored the levels of cardiac norepinephrine to control values. They postulate that the ganglionic blockade prevented the progressive increase in cardiac sympathetic tone, which, they believe, was causing a decrease in cardiac norepinephrine. To prove their hypothesis, however, an increased turnover of cardiac norepinephrine is necessary, and such a turnover has been demonstrated only in the cardiomyopathic Syrian hamster and not in other animal models.

When digoxin is administered to cats prior to banding of the pulmonary artery, and continued after the imposition of this pressure overload, the reduced contractile function and reduced myosin adenosine triphosphatase (ATPase) activity usually seen in such hearts does not occur. However, the use of digoxin does not prevent the cardiac catecholamine depletion caused by this pressure-overload lesion (Fig. 6) (35).

REVERSAL OF CARDIAC NOREPINEPHRINE DEPLETION FOLLOWING RELIEF OF CARDIAC HYPERTROPHY AND FAILURE

There has been limited study to determine whether relief of overload on the heart, with resultant relief of hypertrophy and failure, also relieves cardiac norepinephrine depletion. Coulson and co-workers (36) examined the recuperative potential of cat heart subjected to experimental right ventricular pressure overload for a 10- to 14-day period, provoking hypertrophy with and without congestive heart failure. Five groups of cats were studied: a normal control (Normal); a group with a 70% pulmonary artery constriction that produced right ventricular hypertrophy (RVH); a group with an 87% constriction that produced RVH with congestive heart failure (CHF); and two groups that had been similarly subjected to pressure overload but had been allowed a recovery period of 30 days after relief of the pressure overload. Both the 70% RVH and 87% CHF pulmonary constrictions were associated with extensive RVH, depression of myocardial contractile function, and severe reduction of cardiac norepinephrine stores.

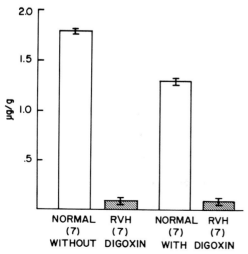

FIG. 6. Right ventricular norepinephrine in four groups of cats: Normal cats that did not receive digoxin; cats that did not receive digoxin before and after being subjected to pulmonary artery banding that caused RVH without failure; normal cats that received digoxin; and cats that received digoxin before and after being subjected to pulmonary artery banding that caused RVH without heart failure. (From Carey et al., ref. 35, with permission.)

In cats in which the RVH had been relieved (Relief-RVH), right ventricular weight and contractile function returned to normal, but the depletion of cardiac catecholamine persisted. Cats with relieved CHF (Relief-CHF) showed persistent depression of contractile function and myocardial norepinephrine depletion, and their right ventricular weight did not return to normal. Cardiac muscle of all pressure-overloaded, nonrelieved hearts (RVH and CHF) showed depressed velocity of shortening and depressed ability to sustain load. Cats with RVH alone regained normal muscle-shortening velocity and load-bearing ability after Relief-RVH, but cardiac muscle from the Relief-CHF group recovered only unloaded shortening velocity, while the ability to sustain load remained depressed. Cardiac catecholamine depletion persisted in both the right and left ventricles of Relief-RVH and Relief-CHF cats. Thus, hypertrophy due to pressure overload in the cat, with or without congestive heart failure, leads to a catecholamine depletion that is not reversed by relief of the overload.

The only other study reported that attempted to determine if there was recuperation of catecholamine deficit in the hypertrophied and failing heart was made by Vogel et al. (37). In two calves with right ventricular hypertrophy and heart failure produced by ligation of one pulmonary artery, while existing at a high altitude, they found that right heart failure and depletion of cardiac catecholamines regressed to normal 30 days after the animals were moved to sea level. It is not known whether cardiac catecholamine depletion returns to normal after relief of overload and heart failure in humans with ventricular hypertrophy and congestive heart failure.

ACKNOWLEDGMENTS

The author wishes to express his appreciation to James A. Weiss, Esq. for editorial assistance and to Maxine Blob for typing the manuscript.

REFERENCES

1. Chidsey, C. A., Braunwald, E., Morrow, A. G., and Mason, D. T. (1963): *New Engl. J. Med.*, 269:653–658.
2. Chidsey, C. A., Braunwald, E., and Morrow, A. G. (1965): *Am. J. Med.*, 39:442–451.
3. Spann, J. F., Chidsey, C. A., and Braunwald, E. (1964): *Science*, 145:1439–1441.
4. Spann, J. F., Jr., Sonnenblick, E. H., Cooper, T., Chidsey, C. A., Willman, V. L., and Braunwald, E. (1966): *Circ. Res.*, 19:317–325.
5. Carabello, A. B., Green, L. H., Grossman, W., Cohn, L. H., Koster, J. K., and Collins, J. Jr. (1980): *Circulation*, 62:42–48.
6. Carabello, B. A., Mee, R., Collins, J. J. Jr., Kloner, R. A., Levin, D., and Grossman, W. (1981): *Am. J. Physiol.*, 240:H80–H86.
7. Spann, J. F., Jr., Chidsey, C. A., Pool, P. E., and Braunwald, E. (1965): *Circ. Res.*, 17:312–320.
8. Fischer, J. E., Horst, W. D., and Kopin, I. J. (1965): *Nature (Lond.)*, 207:951–953.
9. Kopin, I. J., Hertting, G., and Gordon, E. K. (1962): *J. Pharmacol. Exptl. Therap.*, 134:34–40.
10. Pool, P. E., Covell, J. W., Levitt, M., Gibb, J., and Braunwald, E. (1967): *Circ. Res.*, 20:349–353.

11. Dequattro, V., Nagatsu, T., Mendez, A., and Verska, J. (1973): *Cardiovasc. Res.*, 7:344–350.
12. Sole, M. J., Lo, C-M, Laird, C. W., Sonnenblick, E. H., and Wurtman, R. J. (1975): *Circ. Res.*, 37:855–862.
13. Sole, M. J., Kamble, A. B., and Hussain, M. N. (1977): *Circ. Res.*, 41:814–817.
14. Pannier, J. L. (1971): *Arch. Intern. Physiol. Biochim.*, 79:743–752.
15. Spann, J. F., Jr., Buccino, R. A., Sonnenblick, E. H., and Braunwald E. (1967): *Circ. Res.*, 21:341–354.
16. Williams, J. F. Jr., and Potter, R. D. (1974): *J. Clin. Invest.*, 54:1266–1272.
17. Karliner, J. S., Barnes, P., Brown, M., and Dollery, C. (1980): *Euro. J. Pharmacol.* 67:115–118.
18. Cooper, G., IV, Tomanek, R. J., Ehrhardt, J. C., and Marcus, M. L. (1981): *Circ. Res.*, 48:488–497.
19. Sasayama, S., Ross, J., Franklin, D., Bloor, C. M., Bishop, S., and Dilley, R. B. (1975): *Circ. Res.*, 38:172–178.
20. Sasayama, S., Franklin, D., and Ross, J. Jr., (1977): *Am. J. Physiol.*, 232(4):H418–H425.
21. Newman, W. H., and Webb, J. G. (1980): *Am. J. Physiol.*, 238:H134–H143.
22. Spann, J. F., Bove, A. A., Natarajan, G., and Kreulen, T. (1980): *Circulation*, 62:576–582.
23. Huber, D., Grimm, J., Koch, R., and Krayenbuehl, H. P. (1981): *Circulation*, 64:126–134.
24. Chidsey, C. A., Kaiser, G. A., Sonnenblick, E. H., Spann, J. F., and Braunwald, E. (1964): *J. Clin. Invest.*, 43:2386–2393.
25. McDonald, T. C. (1975): *Circulation*, 53:860–864.
26. Levine, H. J., McIntyre, K. M., Lipana, J. C., and Bing, O. H. L. (1970): *Am. J. Med. Sci.*, 259:79–89.
27. Krayenbuehl, H. P., Brunner, H. H., Riedhammer, H. H., Mehmel, H. C., and Senning, A. (1976): *Euro. J. Cardiol.*, 4:123–130.
28. Strauer, B. E. (1978): *Zeit. Kardiol.*, 375–383.
29. Takahashi, M., Sasayama, S., Kawai, C., and Kotoura, H. (1980): *Circulation*, 62:116–126.
30. Karliner, J. S., Williams, D., Corwit, J., Crawford, M. H., and O'Rourke, R. A., (1976): *Br. Heart J.*, 89:1239–1245.
31. Dhalla, N. S., Naidu, J. R., Bhagat, B., and Cristensen, K. (1971): *Cardiovasc. Res.*, 5:376–382.
32. Covell, J. W., Chidsey, C. A., and Braunwald, E. (1966): *Circ. Res.*, 19:51–56.
33. Thomas, J. A., and Marks, B. H. (1978): *Am. J. Cardiol.*, 41:233–243.
34. Stephen, A. (1966): *Am. J. Cardiol.*, 18:463–468.
35. Carey, R. A., Bove, A. A., Coulson, R. L., and Spann, J. F. (1978): *Am. J. Physiol.*, 234(3):H253–H259.
36. Coulson, R. L., Yazdanfar, S., Rubio, E., Bove, A. A., Lemole, G. M., and Spann, J. F. (1977): *Circ. Res.*, 40:41–49.
37. Vogel, J. H. K., Jacobowitz, D., and Chidsey, C. A. (1969): *Circ. Res.*, 24:71–84.
38. Rutenberg, H. L., and Spann, J. F. (1973): *Am. J. Cardiol.*, 32:472–480.
39. Braunwald, E., Ross, J., Jr., and Sonnenblick, E. H. (1976): *Mechanisms of Contraction of Normal and Failing Heart.* Little, Brown, Boston.

Perspectives in Cardiovascular Research, Vol. 8,
edited by R. C. Tarazi and J. B. Dunbar.
Raven Press, New York © 1983.

Myocardial Catecholamines in Hypertensive Ventricular Hypertrophy

Subha Sen and Robert C. Tarazi

Research Division, Cleveland Clinic Foundation, Cleveland, Ohio 44106

The study of cardiac catecholamines has been approached by many investigators with quite different points of view (1). A major effort was aimed at the evaluation of alterations in myocardial catecholamines with the development of cardiac hypertrophy and failure (2–4) and led to better understanding of their role in support of cardiac performance (5). Others investigated cardiac catecholamines as indices of sympathetic activity, to define the role of adrenergic factors in the development of hypertension (6–8). This divergence of interests and aims delayed the awareness of a remarkable contrast between the findings in different types of ventricular hypertrophy (1). Whereas the cardiac hypertrophy of most experimental models (usually banding of the pulmonary artery or aorta) was associated with a reduction, first in myocardial catecholamine concentration and then in myocardial stores, cardiac catecholamines were, by and large, normal in the hypertrophy of the spontaneously hypertensive rat (SHR) (1,6,8).

The documentation of possible differences in cardiac catecholamines in systemic hypertension and other causes of cardiac hypertrophy may have important implications regarding the modulation of myocardial responses, their evolution, and their functional consequences. Unfortunately, the questions cannot be answered by simple comparisons of any two models, one with and the other without hypertension. For one thing, cardiac hypertrophy is not a homogeneous entity; the characteristics of each type vary with the cause of the hypertrophy (9–11). The more appropriate model for arterial hypertension is the hypertrophy consequent to pressure overload, although questions have been recently raised as to whether the cardiac hypertrophy in hypertension is really an exact counterpart of the hypertrophy produced by constriction of the large cardiac vessels (12). Even if these possible differences are minimized, a second difficulty arises from the fact that hypertension itself is not a homogeneous disease, but covers a wide spectrum of entities with different hemodynamic volume and neurohumoral characteristics (13). Although this view is readily accepted in considerations of the pathogenesis of hypertension, it is only recently that it appeared also applicable to its cardiac consequences. This was particularly evident in two aspects: The relation of cardiac hypertrophy to blood pressure levels (14–16) and the variations of myocardial catecholamines in opposite ways in two different models of experimental hypertension.

CARDIAC HYPERTROPHY IN HYPERTENSION

Our studies of hypertensive rats have revealed wide differences among different models in the relationship of blood pressure levels to degree of cardiac hypertrophy (14–16) (Table 1).

Sen et al. (14,15) demonstrated that significant myocardial hypertrophy did occur in the young (three weeks) SHR in the absence of significant hypertension. This lack of correlation between arterial pressure and myocardial mass was confirmed by many other investigators (17–19). Further, the reversal of hypertrophy by antihypertensive therapy in SHR was also shown not to be dependent on blood pressure control alone (14–18).

In marked contrast to these findings was the very close correlation ($r = 0.93$, $p < 0.001$) found between ventricular mass and level of blood pressure in renal hypertensive rats (RHR) (Goldblatt model, two-kidney, one-clipped) both during the development of hypertrophy (15) and with its reversal, either by medical (captopril) or surgical treatment (15,20). More recently, in still another model—this time of acquired and not genetic hypertension [deoxycorticosterone-acetate (DOCA)-salt excession rats]—we found no correlation between ventricular weight and degree of hypertension (21). Thus, ventricular hypertrophy did not follow a simple pattern in its relation to blood pressure levels among various types of genetic and experimental hypertension (22–24). This picture, derived from experimental models, was remarkably similar to the wide diversity of cardiac weight and sizes found among hypertensive patients with apparently similar elevations of blood pressure (25,26).

MYOCARDIAL CATECHOLAMINES IN HYPERTENSIVE CARDIAC HYPERTROPHY

The ventricular hypertrophy consequent upon banding of either the aorta or pulmonary artery seems rather uniform in regard to myocardial catechol-

TABLE 1. *Relation of ventricular weight to blood pressure levels in different models of hypertension*

Group	Ref.	Heart wt/bp (r)
Spontaneous (genetic) hypertension	(14)	0.01
Renovascular hypertension (Goldblatt 2k-1c)[a]	(15)	0.93
DOCA[b]-salt hypertension	(21)	0.02

[a] Two-kidney; one-clipped.
[b] Desoxycorticosterone-acetate.

amines. Fischer (2), Krakoff (27), Spann (28), and their co-workers all reported a reduction in myocardial catecholamines with progressive hypertrophy—even in the absence of decompensation. At first, only the concentration is reduced, while total ventricular stores are normal; eventually, there develops a significant reduction in total myocardial catecholamines in hypertrophied heart (2). In his review of different experimental models, Fanburg (11) concluded that cardiac catecholamines were, as a rule, reduced in experimental myocardial hypertrophy.

In contrast, the picture is quite different in the hypertrophy associated with hypertension. The amount as well as the concentration of cardiac catecholamines varied significantly among three different models of hypertension (Table 2).

In the RHR, findings were essentially similar to those of experimental aortic or pulmonary banding; ventricular catecholamine concentration was reduced ($p < 0.05$) but the total catecholamine content was within normal. In SHR, however, the catecholamine concentration was not significantly different from matched controls, resulting in significantly higher ventricular catecholamine stores.

The DOCA-salt model gave entirely different results from both the SHR and the RHR; it showed a significant reduction in both ventricular concentration and total content of catecholamines. A similar reduction in NE content in the heart of DOCA-salt rats was reported by deChamplain et al. (25). This was related to diminished NE binding in the neural granules and its excessive liberation from the soluble fraction, with enhancement of adrenergic effects of sympathetic stimulation.

MYOCARDIAL CATECHOLAMINES AND REVERSAL OF HYPERTROPHY

The possible influence of myocardial catecholamines on cardiac structural changes can often be studied best during attempts at reversal of cardiac hy-

TABLE 2. *Ventricular norepinephrine (NE) in hypertensive rats*

Group	Ventricular wt (mg)	(mg/g)	Ventricular NE (mg)	(ng/g)
SHR ($N = 30$)	1115	3.45	650	583
	($p < 0.01$)	($p < 0.01$)	($p < 0.01$)	(p:ns)[a]
WKY ($N = 22$)	930	2.6	474	505
RHR ($N = 15$)	1200	3.3	504	420
	($p < 0.01$)	($p < 0.01$)	(p:ns)[a]	($p < 0.05$)
Wistar ($N = 15$)	1000	2.5	540	540
DOCA-salt ($N = 10$)	1220	3.7	322	268
	($p < 0.01$)	($p < 0.001$)	($p < 0.05$)	($p < 0.01$)
Wistar ($N = 10$)	1010	2.8	490	491

[a] ns = not significant.

pertrophy (1). It has been repeatedly shown that the regression of hypertrophy by antihypertensive therapy in SHR did not depend on blood pressure control alone (14,16,18–20,26).

Early studies with three equipotent antihypertensive drugs showed that cardiac weight was reduced only by methyldopa, although hydralazine and minoxidil controlled blood pressure equally if not better (14,26). Three possible factors were postulated as explanations for this divergence in results: (a) alterations in hemodynamic indices other than pressure, (b) variations in catecholamines, and (c) differences in renin response to therapy. None of these factors can be completely discounted at present, although available evidence points to a particularly important role for myocardial catecholamines in the process of reversal of hypertrophy (1,26,30).

The three drugs initially used to control hypertension in SHR could be separated on the basis of their action on both plasma renin activity and adrenergic stimulation (14). The vasodilators (hydralazine and minoxidil) stimulated both, whereas methyldopa reduced them. In an attempt to differentiate between the two neurohumoral influences, we treated the SHR for five weeks, beginning at age three weeks, with a specific angiotensin II (ANG II) antagonist (Sar^1, Ile^8)-ANG II, which led to an increase both in heart weight and blood pressure (31). Therefore, we turned to the normotensive rat (NTR) whose blood pressure was not significantly altered by angiotensin antagonists. Three different angiotensin antagonists were used: (Sar^1, Ile^8)-ANG II, (Sar^1, Ala^8)-ANG II, and (Sar^1, Thr^8)-ANG II (32). The results are summarized in Table 3. Both (Sar^1, Ile^8)-ANG II and (Sar^1, Ala^8)-ANG II resulted in an increase in cardiac mass without a change in blood pressure, whereas the third analog, (Sar^1, Thr^8)-ANG II, altered neither heart weight nor blood pressure.

Of special relevance to this discussion is that, in contrast with the two other analogs, (Sar^1, Thr^8)-ANG II had been shown not to increase adrenal catecholamines (33). Consonant with this, the myocardial catecholamine concentration was increased by (Sar^1, Ile^8)-ANG II but not by (Sar^1, Thr^8)-ANG II injections; further, both the increase in myocardial catecholamines and the increase in ventricular weight produced by the (Sar^1, Ile^8)-ANG II analog could be prevented by bilateral adrenalectomy (32).

TABLE 3. *Chronic administration of ANG II antagonists in NTR*

Treatment (No.)	Absolute ventricular wt (g)	Kidney wt/body wt (mg/g)	bp[a] (mm Hg)
Vehicle (oil) (16)	0.580 ± 0.01	4.20 ± 0.01	125 ± 5
[Sar^1, Ile^8]AII (16)	0.653 ± 0.02[b]	4.16 ± 0.015[c]	127 ± 8[c]
[Sar^1, Ala^8]AII (16)	0.650 ± 0.02[b]	4.00 ± 0.01[c]	127 ± 7[c]
[Sar^1, Thr^8]AII (16)	0.594 ± 0.013[c]	4.10 ± 0.015[c]	120 ± 5[c]

[a] Average of three readings during last week before sacrifice.
[b] p: significance of difference from controls. $p < 0.01$.
[c] p not significant.

These results pointed to the importance of catecholamines in initiating a hypertrophic process with no apparent change in systemic arterial pressure, a concept suggested by Raab (34) and supported by our studies and those of Laks et al. (35). Our results also suggested that catecholamines may play an important role in modulating the cardiac hypertrophy response to blood pressure control. This suggestion was further examined by determining the effects of various antihypertensive drugs on both myocardial catecholamines and ventricular weight and correlating the results with the variations observed in systemic arterial pressure (36).

HYPERTENSIVE DRUG EFFECTS

Experience in SHR

Both methyldopa and hydralazine lowered blood pressure significantly, but ventricular weight was reduced only in rats treated with methyldopa (Fig. 1). Similar results were obtained with other sympatholytics, such as reserpine, whereas minoxidil actually increased ventricular weight despite its excellent control of blood pressure (28). Review of the findings showed that reversal of cardiac hypertrophy was obtained whenever ventricular catecholamines (Vcats) were also reduced; the reversal of hypertrophy had no obvious relationship in these experiments with the degree of blood pressure control (Table 4).

Against this background, the results obtained with propranolol did not seem to fit the expected pattern. Its use alone led to conflicting results—from no significant alteration in ventricular weight (37), to minimal changes (28,29), to prevention of ventricular hypertrophy, at least in young SHR (38). Any effect of propranolol on myocardial catecholamine concentration appeared to have been offset by the uncontrolled hypertension. In order to evaluate the relative role of each factor (pressure load and beta-adrenergic blockade), propranolol was given in varying ratios with hydralazine to SHR. Neither propranolol alone (which reduced myocardial catecholamines but left blood pressure unchanged) nor hydralazine alone (which controlled hypertension but increased myocardial catecholamines) altered ventricular weight significantly (36). Only that ratio of both that reduced blood pressure moderately but also prevented the increase in catecholamines led to significant reversal of cardiac hypertrophy.

These results suggest that at least in SHR myocardial catecholamines play an important role in modulating the cardiac structural responses to variations in blood pressure. A control of both variables was needed in order to reverse ventricular hypertrophy by antihypertensive therapy.

Experience with Renovascular Hypertension

The relationship among heart weight, myocardial catecholamines, and blood pressure appeared quite different in RHR (Goldblatt Hypertension, two-kid-

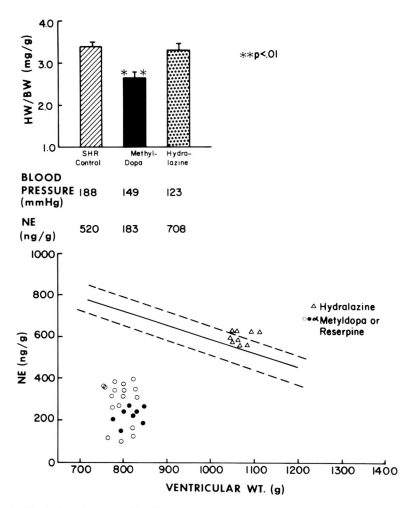

FIG. 1. Effect of treatment on blood pressure, heart weight, and catecholamines in SHR. **Top:** Effect of α-methyldopa and hydralazine on heart weight. **Bottom:** Regression line drawn relating heart weight to myocardial catecholamine concentration; myocardial NE concentration of the treated hearts is plotted against that background. Note: Reversal of hypertrophy was achieved only when NE concentration was reduced (see text for details).

ney, one-clipped). Hypertension was induced in this model by clipping the left renal artery; after four weeks of persistent hypertension, rats were treated by either captopril or left nephrectomy. The results are summarized in Fig. 2. Reversal of hypertrophy occurred whether the myocardial catecholamine concentration was reduced or unaltered. In other studies, Saragoca and Tarazi (20) had also shown, in a similar model, that the reversal of hypertrophy by either surgical or medical treatment was linearly related to the reduction in

TABLE 4. *Effect of antihypertensive therapy on Vcats and cardiac hypertrophy in SHR*

Treatment	bp (mm Hg)	Ventricular wt[a] (mg/g)	Vcats (mg/g)
None	198	3.5	540
Sympatholytics			
α-methyldopa	140[b]	2.8[b]	203[b]
Reserpine	175[b]	3.1[b]	188[b]
Vasodilators			
Hydralazine	120[b]	3.5	718[b]
Minoxidil	118[b]	3.8[b]	—
β-blocker			
Propranolol	118	3.2	451[b]

[a] Ventricular weight calculated relative to body weight (mg/g).
[b] $p < 0.01$ compared to untreated controls.

blood pressure. From this experience, which has been repeatedly confirmed (15,20,39), it seems that in contrast to SHR, the ventricular hypertrophy associated with renovascular hypertension is influenced predominantly by the pressure load. The alterations in myocardial catecholamines in this model are more in line with those observed in banding of the aorta (2).

Experience with Mineralocorticoid Hypertension

The effects of treatment on heart weight, blood pressure, and Vcat concentration in DOCA-hypertensive rats are summarized in Fig. 3. DOCA hypertension was induced by implanting a DOCA pellet (75 mg) in uninephrectomized rats who were also given 1% saline to drink instead of tap water. When hypertension developed after three weeks, rats were treated with the converting enzyme inhibitor, captopril, either alone or in combination with hydrochlorothiazide. Captopril alone failed to reverse hypertrophy or control hypertension. However, the addition of hydrochlorothiazide led to a significant reduction in heart weight as blood pressure fell moderately. In neither case did the myocardial catecholamines change; they were reduced to start with in this model (Table 2) and they remained low irrespective of blood pressure or heart weight variations (Fig. 3).

SUMMARY

The study of myocardial catecholamines revealed a wide spectrum of variations among different types of hypertension. Although ventricular weight was apparently increased equally in renovascular, genetic, and mineralocorticoid hypertension, the concentration of Vcats was slightly reduced in the first, normal in the second, and markedly depressed in the third. The overall picture

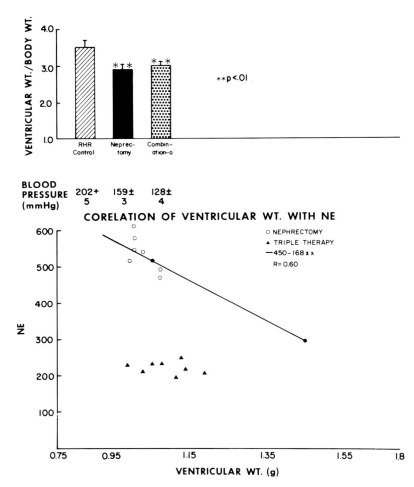

FIG. 2. Effect of treatment on heart weight and catecholamine in RHR. **Top:** Effect of surgical care (nephrectomy) and medical therapy (reserpine, hydralazine, and hydrochlorothiazide) on heart weight. **Bottom:** Regression line drawn from the relationship between heart weight and NE concentration of the heart. *Open circles*, catecholamine concentration in the treated heart; *open triangles*, catecholamine concentration of the heart treated with triple therapy. Reversal was achieved whether NE concentration was lowered or left unchanged.

was, therefore, quite different from the homogenous reduction found by Fischer et al. (2) and Spann et al. (3) in other types of pressure-induced hypertrophy.

In response to therapy, both arterial pressure levels and myocardial catecholamines seemed important in influencing the reversal of hypertrophy in the SHR. In contrast, arterial blood pressure was the dominant factor influencing both the development and reversal of cardiac hypertrophy in the RHR. In the DOCA model, myocardial catecholamines remained low despite blood pressure control and reduction of heart weight.

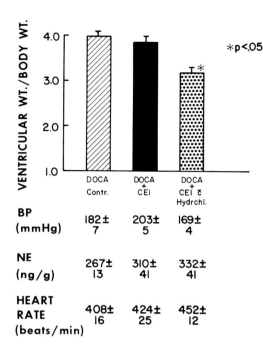

FIG. 3. Effect of treatment on heart weight, blood pressure, and heart rate in DOCA-salt HTR. Converting enzyme inhibition by captopril caused an increase in blood pressure; blood pressure control and reversal of hypertrophy were obtained by combining captopril with a diuretic. This reversal, however, was not associated with any significant change in myocardial catecholamine concentration.

The role of catecholamines in cardiac hypertrophy thus appears more complex than initially thought; more needs to be done in order to unravel the part reflecting the causal disease, the part secondary to the increase in cardiac load, and that part that might play a possible trophic role for the myocardium.

ACKNOWLEDGMENT

This study was supported in part by the National Heart, Lung and Blood Institute (NHLBI-6835).

REFERENCES

1. Tarazi, R. C., and Sen, S. (1979): In: *Catecholamines and the Heart*, edited by K. C. Mezey and A. D. S. Caldwell, pp. 46–57. Academic Press and Royal Society of Medicine, London.
2. Fischer, J. E., Horst, W. D., and Kopin, I. J. (1965): *Nature (Lond.)*, 207:951–953.
3. Spann, J. F., Jr., Chidsey, C. A., Pool, P. E., and Braunwald, E. (1965): *Circ. Res.*, 17:312–317.
4. Pool, P. E., Covell, J. W., Levitt, M., Gibb, J., and Braunwald, E. (1967): *Circ. Res.*, 20:349–353.
5. Braunwald, E., Ross, J., and Sonnenblick, E. H. (1967): In: *Mechanisms of Contraction of the Normal and Failing Heart*, edited by E. Braunwald, pp. 157–163. Little Brown, Boston.
6. Louis, W. J., Krauss, K. R., Kopin, I. H., and Sjoerdsma, A. (1970): *Circ. Res.*, 27:589–594.
7. Yamori, Y. (1972): In: *Spontaneous Hypertension*, edited by K. Okamoto, pp. 59–61. Igaku Shoin, Tokyo.
8. Sjoerdsma, A. (1977): In: *Hypertension*, edited by J. Genest, E. Koiw, and E. Kuchel, pp. 27–30. McGraw-Hill, New York.
9. Skelton, C. L., and Sonnenblick, E. H. (1974): *Circ. Res. (Suppl.)*, II:83–96.

10. Alpert, N. R., Mulieri, L. A., and Litten, R. Z. (1979): *Am. J. Cardiol.*, 44:947–953.
11. Fanburg, B. L. (1970): *N. Engl. J. Med.*, 282:723–732.
12. Tarazi, R. C., and Levy, M. L. (1982): *Hypertension*, 4 (Suppl. II), II-8–II-18.
13. Dustan, H. P., Tarazi, R. C., and Bravo, E. L. (1972): *Am. J. Med.*, 52:610–613.
14. Sen, S., Tarazi, R. C., Khairallah, P. A., and Bumpus, F. M. (1974): *Circ. Res.*, 35:775–781.
15. Sen, S., Tarazi, R. C., and Bumpus, F. M. (1981): *Am. J. Physiol.*, 240:H408–H412.
16. Sen, S., Tarazi, R. C., and Bumpus, F. M. (1976): *Cardiovasc. Res.*, 10:254–261.
17. Cutilleta, A. F., Erinoff, L., and Heller, A. (1977): *Circ. Res.*, 40:428–436.
18. Tomanek, R. J., Davis, J. W., and Anderson, S. C. (1979): *Cardiovasc. Res.*, 13:173–182.
19. Yamori, Y., Morichuzo, M., and Nishio, T. (1979): *Am. J. Cardiol.*, 44:964–969.
20. Saragoca, M. A., and Tarazi, R. C. (1981): *Hypertension*, 3 (Suppl. II), II-171–II-176.
21. Sen, S., and Tarazi, R. C. Submitted for publication.
22. Ehrstrom, M. (1948): *Acta Med. Scand.*, 103:86–93.
23. Grant, R. P. (1953): *Am. Heart. J.*, 46:154–158.
24. Tarazi, R. C., Ferrario, C. M., and Dustan, H. P. (1977): In: *Hypertension Physiopathology and Treatment*, edited by J. Genest, E. Koiw, and O. Kuchel, pp. 738–754. McGraw-Hill, New York.
25. deChamplain, J., Krakoff, L., and Axelrod, J. (1969): *Circ. Res.*, 24:75–92.
26. Sen, S., Tarazi, R. C., and Bumpus, F. M. (1977): *Cardiovasc. Res.*, 11:427–433.
27. Krakoff, L. R., deChamplain, J., and Axelrod, J. (1967): *Circ. Res.*, 21:583–591.
28. Spann, J. F. Jr. (1971): In: *Cardiac Hypertrophy*, edited by N. R. Alpert, pp. 465–481. Academic Press, New York.
29. Pfeffer, J., Pfeffer, M., Fletcher, P., and Braunwald, E. (1980): *Am. J. Cardiol. (Abstract)*, 45:490.
30. Tarazi, R. C., and Sen, S. (1981): In: *The Heart in Hypertension*, edited by B. E. Strauer, pp. 75–87. Springer-Verlag, Berlin.
31. Sen, S., Tarazi, R. C., and Bumpus, F. M. (1975): *Circulation (Abstract)*, 51:98.
32. Sen, S., Tarazi, R. C., and Bumpus, F. M. (1979): *Clin. Sci.*, 56:439–444.
33. Peach, M. J., and Ackerly, J. A. (1976): In: *The Symposium on Pharmacology of Angiotensin, Fed. Proc.*, 35:2502–2512.
34. Raab, W. (1953): *Hormonal and Neurogenic Disorders.* Williams and Wilkins, Baltimore.
35. Laks, M. M., Morady, F., and Swan, H. J. C. (1973): *Chest*, 64:75–78.
36. Sen, S., and Tarazi, R. C. (1983): *Am. J. Physiol.*, 244:H97–H101.
37. Pfeffer, M. A., Pfeffer, J. M., Weiss, A. K., and Frohlich, E. D. (1977): *Am. J. Physiol.*, 232:H639–H644.
38. Weiss, L. (1978): *Cardiovascular Res.*, 12:635–638.
39. Wicker, P., Tarazi, R. C., and El-Khair, M. (1981): *Clin. Res. (Abstract)*, 29:250A.

*Perspectives in Cardiovascular
Research, Vol. 8,*
edited by R. C. Tarazi and J. B. Dunbar.
Raven Press, New York © 1983.

Adaptation of Arterial Vasculature to Increased Pressure and Factors Modifying the Response

Rosemary D. Bevan

*Department of Pharmacology, School of Medicine, Center for Health Sciences,
University of California at Los Angeles, Los Angeles, California 90024*

A progressive increase in peripheral vascular resistance is associated with the development and maintenance of hypertension, and is of primary importance in the sustained elevation of arterial pressure. This increase in resistance involves both structural and functional changes in the vasculature, the nature and relative importance of which seem to vary with the etiology, duration, and height of the pressure elevation. In essential or primary hypertension, found in the majority of human subjects with elevated pressure, derangements in both heart and resistance vessels are early manifestations and have been detected in children and young people (40). A detailed analysis of alterations in blood vessels in human hypertension is not available, although many morphologic studies indicate similar structural features in human disease and animal experimental models. There is, at the moment, no reason to question that our understanding of how blood vessels function and how they are altered in disease, derived from animal studies, is not relevant to the human condition.

Hypertension may be induced in animals by perturbation in many different systems involved in blood pressure regulation. A broad classification of those factors affecting the vasculature that may be of etiological significance include circulating blood volume, neurogenic influences, and circulating substances causing constriction of vascular smooth muscle. Although each of these are associated with their own characteristic changes in the structure and function of the circulation, which may in part be due to the age of onset and the rate of rise and absolute height of the blood pressure elevation, there are certain characteristic changes common to all. Additional problems of animal models, however, are (a) that functional changes are observed that may or may not be relevant to the hypertensive process, and (b) that differences among species may exist. Although alterations in both veins and arteries have been described in hypertension, analytical studies have been focused mainly on the latter. Arteries that can be viewed by the naked eye become thicker, stiffer, and more tortuous. Although the entire arterial tree contributes to the total peripheral resistance, the smallest arteries and arterioles, particularly those with one to three or four vascular smooth muscle (VSM) layers are thought to be the major contributors. Recently developed technology has made it possible to begin to study directly sequential changes in resistance vessels. Previous studies on the conduit arteries have furnished important information concerning the pathophysiology of hypertension, and this has served to direct the thrust of research and the approach to be adopted in the study of resistance vessels. However, there are important differences that caution a simple extrapolation from large to small vessels.

Almost all arteries and muscular veins are innervated by the sympathetic nervous system, which is the main neurogenic regulator of vascular tone (4). Nerve stimulation elicits, in comparison to the large arteries, a proportionately larger response with a lower threshold and steeper frequency–response curve in the small arteries. These small vessels show increased spontaneous rhythmic activity and/or possibly maintained tone, the basis of which is not understood. Myogenic spread of activation is probably greater in smaller arterioles and is possibly due to an increase in gap junctions between muscle cells. There are increased numbers of myoendothelial junctions. It is very possible that there are different types of mature VSM cells. Changes in shape of the smooth muscle (SM) and endothelial cells in the wall become more important in influencing resistance to flow when lumen diameter is small and intravascular pressure is low. There are regional differences not only in the structure of vessels in the microcirculation (2,60), but also in functional characteristics including response to neurohumoral substances such as catecholamines, angiotensin, and certain types and number of receptors and dilator mechanisms. The terminal arterioles are particularly influenced by the metabolism of the organ they supply.

There is little evidence at present for a primary change in vascular smooth muscle alone, which is responsible for pressure elevation—although membrane abnormalities in a number of mesenchymal derived tissues have been detected in the prehypertensive phase of genetic forms of hypertension, both human and animal (25,26,52). The response of the vascular wall is thought to be adaptive, but this question is by no means closed.

This chapter is concerned only with adaptive changes and some of the factors influencing them. Many papers could be cited in support, but this is not an extensive review and only a few will be mentioned to illustrate points, particularly precise morphometric or analytical studies which have focused on important observations of earlier investigators. Adaptive changes to intraluminal pressure elevation may be classified as alterations in wall thickness and length, lumen diameter, and physical and functional properties. Changes in VSM cells occupy the central role in this process because of their contractile and synthetic properties, which include the formation of collagen, elastin, and glycosaminoglycans. However, all three layers of the vascular wall, the endothelium, the media containing vascular smooth muscle, and the adventitia consisting of fibroblasts, nerve terminals, collagen, and elastin, are altered in hypertension.

ADAPTIVE VASCULAR CHANGES

Changes in Wall Thickness and Length

It is generally recognized that arterial wall mass is greater in vessels exposed to increased wall stress. In a study of hypertension induced two weeks previously by partial abdominal aortic constriction (PAAC) distal to the celiac artery, the wall thickness of the basilar artery of the rabbit was shown to correlate positively with mean arterial pressure (3b). In this study, the conduit arteries also increased in length (3a). The latter feature could contribute to both increased wall mass and resistance in smaller vessels. Such changes are difficult to identify and quantitate in the microcirculation, due to the variability of branching patterns and wall dimensions. All cells in the arterial wall contribute to the increased mass (11,36,56), but the VSM cells are predominant. The latter show hypertrophy (36,49) and hyperplasia (19,5,21,45) when exposed to a sustained increase in pressure. When the same vascular bed is compared in the same species but in different models of hypertension, e.g., SHR and 1-kidney 1-clip, the pressure distribution differs also, and this should be reflected in the site of adaptive changes. Studies of the microcirculation indicate this. Collagen, elastin, and glycosaminoglycans accumulate and, in some forms of hypertension, an increase in water content occurs, although its precise distribution has not been defined (61). Detailed analyses have been made of structural changes in conduit vessels, but there are no comparable studies on resistance vessels. It is not yet possible to differentiate distinctive sequences of events in the vasculature during the time course of development and maintenance of hypertension in the various animal models because studies, particularly of the microcirculation, are incomplete. Of all the animal models, the spontaneously hypertensive rat (SHR) has been the most extensively studied, as it is thought to most closely resemble human essential hypertension.

The ultrastructural features of hypertrophied VSM cells in the early phases of hypertension include increased nuclear size (36) and, in the SHR aorta, increased nuclear deoxyribonucleic acid (DNA) content associated with polyploidy (51). The enlarged cytoplasmic volume contains increased numbers of rough endoplasmic reticulum, mitochondria, Golgi apparatus, and myofilaments (36,49). An analysis of actin, myosin, and intermediate filament content and ratios has not been made in arteries. The augmented synthetic activity in VSM is expressed in increased uptake of amino acid precursors of structural proteins (7,49). An expansion in volume of the extracellular compartments containing other major structural components of the arterial wall, the connective tissue proteins, progresses with the duration of hypertension. Changes have been analyzed and quantitated in the media of conduit, but not resistance, vessels. The structural framework and relative composition of the media in normal vessels differs markedly in different parts of the vasculature and is probably dependent on hemodynamic factors and age. Absolute amounts of elastin, collagen, and glycosaminoglycans are usually considered to be increased in chronic hypertension in both large and small arteries compared with controls of similar age, sex, and weight. Elastic laminae are thickened in the aorta, a typical response of these SM cells to an increase in pressure even in normal growth (38). In the smaller arteries and arterioles, reduplications of the internal elastic lamina occur frequently. By quantitative analysis, collagen has been found to be increased in the aorta (62) and small arteries (58). Some investigators, however, have detected a decrease in collagen content of hypertensive conduit vessels despite increased stiffness and change in physical properties (18,26). The bases for these differences may be times of sampling, models of hypertension, or analytical methods. Whether or not the type of collagen formed differs in hypertension or the process of cross-linking is enhanced is not known. The mechanisms for gene selection of collagen are easily influenced by environmental factors in tissue culture, although this has not been demonstrated with VSM cells. The effect of increased scleroprotein content in the adventitial layer of the artery wall on vascular properties of functional significance has not been defined.

Changes in Lumen Diameter

Examination of the morphologic changes in resistance vessels has demonstrated a reduction in lumen diameter in association with increased wall thickness, even in the absence of a new subendothelial layer, which denotes damage to the vessel wall. In-depth studies of resistance vessels by *in vivo* and *in vitro* approaches are predominately of the SHR in 2 regional beds: muscular and mesenteric. Investigators are agreed that a structural difference exists in the microcirculation of the SHR compared to the Wistar-Kyoto rat (WKY), but are not in agreement on the sites and causes of the major increase in resistance, or whether or not the capillary pressures are normal. An early structural phenomenon, observed at 4 to 6 weeks of age in the SHR in comparison to WKY, is a reduction in lumen size of small mesenteric resistance vessels of 150 μM (43b) and 100 to 20 μM (34) and 50 to 5 μM muscular arterioles (64), although systemic pressure is significantly higher. Zweifach et al. (64) observed that all arteriolar vessels showed some increased resistance, the greatest increases occurring in the smallest arterioles of less than 30 μM. By 12 weeks of age, changes were more pronounced, and the greatest resistance was in vessels up to 40 μM. The cause of the resistance increase in the microcirculation during the early evolution of hypertension in the SHR is speculative. However, at 12 weeks of age, when SHR blood pressure elevation is almost completed, luminal dilation of the small arteriolar vessels has been seen, compared to WKY (31,33,64), but these contain a higher pressure in the SHR. However, in a larger sized artery in the mesentery, 150 μM internal diameter, Mulvany et al. (43b) still found reduced lumen diameter at 12 weeks of age measured *in vitro* at a comparable pressure to WKY and in addition an increase in wall thickness. This is in agreement with the morphometric studies of Limas and co-workers (39) in the SHR renal vascular bed, which indicated progressive reduction of lumen diameter in arterioles 30 to 100 μM in diameter associated with progressive increases in wall thickness with age—detectable from approximately 10 weeks of age, when systemic pressure was markedly elevated in comparison to the WKY. This is illustrated in Fig. 1. Similar changes in vessels of this size include those from the mesenteric (34), coronary (48), and cerebral vessels (30). By contrast, conduit vessels tend to dilate with sustained hypertension (11,36).

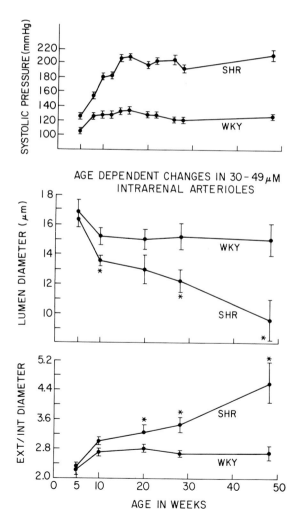

FIG. 1. Age-dependent changes in the lumen diameter and the ratio of external diameter to lumen diameter of intrarenal arterial vessels 30 to 49 μM (range of external diameter) of SHR and WKY rats. The course of mean systolic blood pressure of SHR's and WKY rat is shown. Mean $\pm$ SE, N = 10 to 20; $p < 0.05$ to 0.01, as determined by Student's t-test. (From ref. 39, with permission.)

Reduced Numbers of Arterioles

A number of investigators consider that a reduced number of terminal and precapillary arterioles partially accounts for the elevated pressure in the SHR (13,31,33). A genetic form of hypertension developing during the rapid growth phase of an animal may not be typical of all forms of the disease. Preliminary evidence for this comes from *in vivo* studies of the microcirculation in muscles of a volume-dependent model of hypertension, the 1-kidney Goldblatt rat in which the pressure distribution differs and specific arteriolar lumen diameters are reduced (43b,54). Increased wall/lumen ratios tend to restrict blood flow even at full relaxation, and any vasoconstrictor stimulus would be more effective in increasing resistance. Thus, both phenomena would tend towards the same end result. Structural adaptation can occur rapidly in arteries, and has been shown to parallel the rise in pressure in the rabbit with partial aortic constriction (5,11). These changes affect the arterial wall in the region of the carotid and aortic baroreceptors, and would be expected to blunt homeostatic reflex vascular control.

Changes in Physical Properties of Arteries

Arteries in hypertension are characteristically stiffer, i.e., exhibit decreased compliance when fully relaxed. Figure 2 is essentially a passive stress–strain curve of an elastic and muscular artery in the SHR and WKY at 20 weeks of age, illustrating that the hypertensive arteries are stiffer, the elastic artery more so than the muscular. It is usually thought that the scleroproteins, elastin and

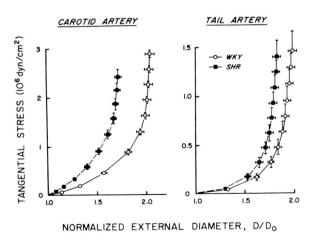

FIG. 2. Summary of passive tangential stress-normalized external diameter curves for arteries from the two animal groups, SHR and WKY. Diameter was normalized by dividing by the value of the passive external diameter at zero mm Hg (D_0). (Adapted from ref. 18, by permission from the American Heart Association.)

collagen, are responsible for the passive properties of the artery wall based on the study of a normal vessel by Roach and Burton (55). This point needs to be reevaluated to determine whether altered VSM cells in hypertension can also contribute to the passive stiffness.

Changes in Functional Properties

The increased muscle mass in arteries in hypertension has functional importance. Reactivity or contractility—the capacity of the vessel wall to develop force, its response to a vasoconstrictor agent—is elevated in hypertension. Increased contractility in large and small muscular arteries has been shown to be directly related to increased muscle mass (3a,18,44), but in contrast, decreased contractility has been observed in some conduit vessels (29,58). Based on studies of human and animal models, Folkow and co-workers (23) have emphasized the importance of the increased wall/lumen ratio of resistance vessels coupled with decreased relaxed diameter in the maintenance of elevated blood pressure and increased reactivity.

In the ear artery of the PAAC rabbit, the wall thickness increased in proportion to pressure rise, and there was a positive association between wall thickness and response to adrenergic nerve stimulation. The implication is that there may be associated changes in neuronal function and that the artery *in vivo* would constrict more in response to nerve activation (3b).

Many functional abnormalities of VSM and its sympathetic innervation have been described in experimental hypertension. They differ with the animal model, and conflicting opinions exist. It is not yet clear how the alterations in vascular smooth muscle activation mechanisms are related to the hypertension, if they precede or are secondary to the increased wall stress. Such changes are discussed in some detail in the literature (6,14). Briefly, they include an increased sensitivity to vasoactive agents, which varies with the type of hypertension, changes in membrane permeability so that the active and/or passive transport of ions is altered, change in electrolyte composition of cells, abnormal calcium handling and impaired relaxation.

Since the reports published (see refs. above), further evidence has accrued in support of changes in membrane permeability to cations in circulating red and white cells, VSM, and adipocytes in hypertension. Although the changes described are in different mechanisms, they all involve a defective handling of Na^+ that may potentially lead to its accumulation in the cell, with resulting heightened reactivity. It is not clear if there is any relationship or common feature between the different membrane mechanisms implicated. No direct studies of VSM in humans are available.

Briefly, the changes in membrane handling of monovalent cations in hypertension recently described are as follows.

There is an inherited abnormal erythrocyte Na-K cotransport system which may be a characteristic of essential hypertension (26). A similar defect has been found in the SHR (52). The mechanism of Na–K cotransport involves associated movements of solute and water and may influence regulation of cell volume. This transport may be affected by membrane potential.

Changes have been noted in cellular handling of Na as reflected by an increase in a specific $Na^+(Li_i^+\text{-}Na_o^+)$ countertransport system in erythrocytes of hypertensive patients (16) and also in a $K_i^+\text{-}Na_o^+$ countertransport system.

The activity and regulation of Na–K adenosine triphosphatase (ATPase), the enzyme responsible for the active transport of Na and K across the cell membrane, is an active area of investigation at present. Based on the earlier work of Dahl and Haddy and Overbeck (28), it has been postulated that the rise in blood pressure in essential hypertension may be partly due to an increase in a circulating ouabain-like substance that inhibits the Na–K pump and promotes excretion of sodium in the kidney. However, by its action on sympathetic nerve terminals and the VSM, it is responsible for an increase in vascular tone. The pump is electrogenic and therefore a regulator of VSM membrane potential.

In a small group of hypertensive patients the active transport of Na in white and red blood cells was found by Poston et al. (53) to be impaired by a circulating factor in the serum of these patients. There is supporting evidence from a number of investigative groups for an increased concentration of a Na-K-ATPase inhibitor in the plasma of patients with essential hypertension.

In the rat, in experimental hypertension associated with reduced renal capacity, increased salt sensitivity or low renin hypertension, a circulating factor with a ouabain-like suppression of the vascular Na-K pump has been described by Haddy et al. (28). However, in the SHR, the smooth muscle membrane is more "leaky" to ions and the activity of the Na-K pump is increased (24,35). It is postulated that Na^+ plays a central role in the pathogenesis of hypertension, but the exact mechanism of this action is not clear.

SOME FACTORS INFLUENCING THE NATURE AND SIZE OF THE VASCULAR CHANGES IN HYPERTENSION

Time Course and Height of Arterial Pressure Rise

A survey of various experimental models indicates that there is an acute phase of arterial pressure rise followed by a subsequent plateau phase at a sustained elevated level. The acute phase may be measured in hours; for example, when angiotensin-induced, or after lesions of the nucleus tractus solitarii; or in days to weeks, as in aortic constriction, desoxycorticosterone acid (DOCA) salt, and renal insufficiency forms; or in months, as in the case of the SHR. When the increase in pressure outstrips the ability of the vessels to adapt, there results degrees of damage commensurate with the rapidity of elevation and the height of sustained arterial pressure. There may be a critical level of pressure above which the endothelium is unable to function adequately. The endothelial cells in vessels exposed to an acute increased wall stress have an increased number of pinocytic vesicles, probably denoting enhanced permeability (46,62); an enhanced rate of turnover of endothelial cells occurs as well (56). These two factors may be related to the appearance of a subintimal pathological accumulation of cells and scleroprotein, reducing the lumen diameter and contributing to wall rigidity. The common pattern of injury includes VSM cell necrosis, plasmatic vasculosis, and fibrin deposition, with an ensuing inflammatory response resulting in perivascular and subendothelial fibrosis, VSM proliferation and hyalinization. A comparison of pathological changes in the vasculature in angiotensin-induced hypertension and the SHR illustrates this point. The pathological changes occurring in the heart and coronary arteries of the former associated with rapid elevation of systolic and diastolic pressures to high levels are described by Engler et al. (20) and Bhan and co-workers (12). In the SHR with a relatively slow elevation in pressure occurring during the growth phase, pathological changes in arteries are not detected until relatively high sustained levels are reached, and then they only progress slowly.

Duration of Pressure Elevation

There is evidence that the time course and duration of the various changes in the vasculature during the course of development and the subsequent maintenance of hypertension differ (8,63). This is illustrated in Fig. 3, derived from a study of the PAAC rabbit. Following the aortic constriction, arterial pressure in proximal arteries rises acutely and reaches a plateau. During the acute phase, complex structural and functional changes occur in the VSM and its sympathetic innervation, probably representing a cellular response to the increased intramural pressure (3). The arterial wall enters a new equilibrium phase after the arterial pressure reaches the plateau. Some of the changes disappear and are therefore transient, but the increase in arterial wall mass contributed by muscle and extracellular constituents persists, resulting in increased contractility and stiffness of the wall. During the ensuing months of sustained hypertension, the arterial wall is not entirely static. In addition to aging phenomena, there is further evidence of structural adaptation. The time course of these changes and their importance differs in arteries from different vascular beds. For instance, in the PAAC rabbit the wall thickness and lumen diameter of the muscular basilar artery changes during the phases depicted in Fig. 3. In the acute phase, wall thickness increased, correlating with the arterial pressure, but lumen diameter did not change. By 8 months, internal diameter was increased after complete relaxation, correlating with the pressure. Wall thickness was unrelated to hypertension at this time. This indicates that some adaptive changes may take a long time, and reflects a remodeling of the vascular wall.

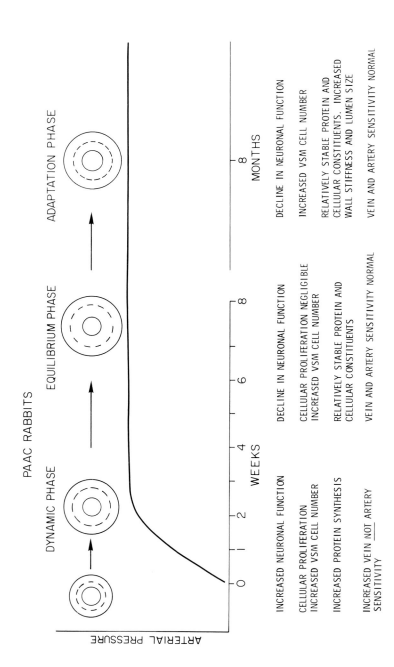

FIG. 3. Diagrammatic representation of three phases discernable from studies of the changes in some structural and functional parameters of VSM cells in selected conduit arteries and large veins in response to elevation in arterial pressure in PAAC rabbits, 2 weeks, and 2 and 8 months following the constriction. For further details see text.

Age of Onset of Hypertension

Some of the changes in the vasculature of the SHR, with its genetic basis for elevated pressure, are structurally and functionally unique. It is not yet clear whether some of these are due to the elevation of pressure at an early age, which continues to rise during the growth phase of the animal. There are no detailed comparable studies of induced hypertension at an early age. Knowledge of the development, maturation, and interrelationship of systems involved in blood pressure control is incomplete; little is known about the development of the microcirculation and factors that influence it. It seems that the structural development of the microcirculation in the SHR is different from its control, the WKY.

During the dynamic phase of growth, conduit arteries increase in length, wall thickness, and internal diameter, implying continuous structural remodeling. VSM cells increase in size and number, the microfilament content of cells increases, while rough endoplasmic reticulum content declines (17). Growing tissues have a higher metabolic rate than mature ones. Elastin and collagen synthesis and degradation rates decline with increasing age (37,47). Cellular aging shifts collagen synthesis to a more stable form, so that cross-linking increases. During growth, the vasculature becomes innervated by the sympathetic nervous system (15), the neuroeffector system matures, and sympathetic fibers acquire the ability to conduct high frequency impulses (57). The developing vasculature might be expected to be more susceptible to modification by environmental factors including trophic substances, humoral status, and sympathetic nerve traffic, and possibly is more easily adaptable to elevated pressure, providing it is not excessive.

Sympathetic Innervation

Although reducing the level of sympathetic control is important in the treatment of hypertension in man, and prevents or modifies development of experimental hypertension depending on the model, any specific effects on the hypertensive vascular wall are difficult to distinguish from those due to reduction of arterial pressure itself. VSM cells deprived of sympathetic innervation develop nonspecific supersensitivity to agonists (22) and reduction in resting membrane potential associated with reduced activity of the Na-K pump (1).

In the rabbit, the effect of chronic loss of sympathetic innervation has been examined in one central ear artery and compared with the normal contralateral vessel (9). Arteries were studied *in vitro* 8 weeks after denervation of 3 age groups: growing (4 weeks), young adult (10 weeks), and adult (more than 16 weeks). As can be seen in Fig. 4, an age-related complex effect on structure and reactivity were found. Significant reductions in tissue weight, force of maximum contraction, and sensitivity to norepinephrine occurred in all

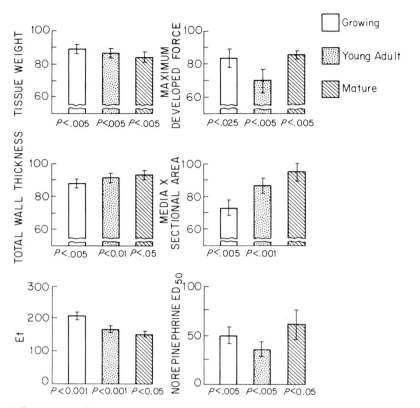

FIG. 4. Parameters of isolated denervated ring segments of ear arteries from rabbits of three age groups are expressed as a percentage of their innervated controls. A unilateral superior cervical ganglionectomy was performed 8 weeks prior to testing. Et: tangential modulus of elasticity at internal circumference equivalent to 80 mm Hg. P: comparisons between denervated and innervated vessels using paired *t*-test. *Brackets* = SEM (N = 8–14). For further details, see text. (Data from ref. 9, with permission.)

groups. Age-related differences were found, however, in the cross-sectional area of the media and the passive mechanical properties of the wall. There was less muscle, and the wall was stiffer, possibly indicating a change in the collagen content, in vessels denervated during the growth phase. Similar results were obtained following preganglionic denervation when the nerves remain *in situ* but are nonfunctional (10).

It would appear that the sympathetic innervation, besides regulating vascular tone, can have a complex "trophic" effect on VSM metabolism, which depends on the passage of nerve impulses. This may be the neurotransmitter itself or another unidentified trophic substance released by nerve activity. Trophic substances are known to affect cell size also, but that was not examined in this experiment. Alternatively, the activity level of the VSM, which can be influenced by tension on the vessel wall, circulating factors, e.g., angiotensin II, catecholamines, as well as the sympathetic nervous system, may be the important modulator of cell metabolism. The precise effect of a sustained increase in sympathetic activity on the vascular wall has not yet been documented.

Angiotensin

Angiotensin II can affect the vasculature by a direct vasoconstrictor action on the VSM in the vessel wall or by increasing the level or efficacy of sympathetic nerve activity. It is difficult to distinguish the effects of such actions on the vasculature from those secondary to an acute elevation of pressure due to vasoconstriction or from an increased permeability associated with its administration. If its effect on VSM, which ranges from "trophic" to "injurious," is concentration-dependent, it should be demonstrated that any prescribed action is specific and not a common property of other substances. Angiotensin infusions have been shown to cause increased protein and DNA synthesis in cells of the vascular wall and heart (20).

The preceding findings are selective. Many other factors undoubtedly modify the response to increased tension on the arterial wall. Sex hormones are important, but comparatively little is known concerning their mode of action.

WHAT IS THE STIMULUS TO ADAPTIVE CHANGE?

In the PAAC rabbit, hypertension, which is probably volume-dependent, develops only proximal to the constriction. Arterial pressure is normal distally. Only arteries exposed to the increased wall stress develop the characteristics of hypertensive vessels. In Fig. 5, the time course of the percentage of VSM cells synthesizing DNA (the labeling index) seen in transverse sections of the arteries 2 hr after a single pulse of ^{3}H-thymidine is shown for both an elastic and muscular artery exposed to the increased wall tension. The mitotic index was also increased, indicating that the cells are proliferating. There is a close similarity to the time course of this change and arterial pressure rise. This also applied to other parameters of change (some of which are detailed in Fig. 3). Distal arteries did not differ from controls.

The most likely stimulus to adaptation in this experimental model was an increase in wall tension, as the response was seen in arteries with no evidence of injury as viewed by the light microscope. The uptake of radioactively-labeled thymidine and proline, precursors of cell division and protein synthesis, respectively, has been found to be tension-dependent in an *in vitro* culture system of the rabbit ear artery (32). A circulating factor would have affected proximal and distal arteries equally, unless it was only operative in conjunction with the sustained increase in wall tension. However, there is the possibility that "growth factors," such as platelet-derived growth factor and somatomedins, are present in the plasma; they, in association with increased tension or increased wall permeability described in the acute phase of hypertension (46,62),

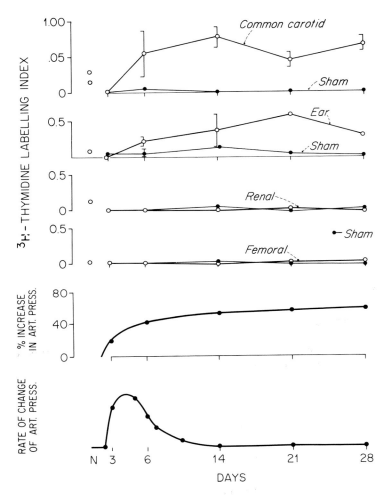

FIG. 5. Time course of ³H-thymidine labelling indices of VSM cells in the media of an elastic (common carotid) and muscular (ear) artery proximal to the constriction in the PAAC rabbit and arteries distal (renal and femoral) to the constriction and sham-operated controls. The time course of the mean arterial pressure and the rate of change of arterial pressure are also shown. *Brackets:* mean ± SE, *N* = 3–4 for hypertensive rabbits at each time period; shams are the mean of two observations.

may initiate the complex events leading to cell hypertrophy and proliferation. Polypeptide growth factors are known to stimulate an increase in cell size and/ or number. Cells usually require prolonged exposure to trophic factors for them to be effective. It would seem feasible that prolonged elevation of vasoconstrictor substances, such as catecholamines and angiotensin in insufficient concentration to cause cell damage, might have a trophic effect on VSM cells.

Another important factor responsible for proliferation of components of the artery wall is injury, in relation to hypertension, probably due to excessive distension or vasoconstriction. This initiates an inflammatory response and proliferation of cells of the wall with subsequent increase of scleroprotein.

Additional factors undoubtedly influence the adaptive changes of the vasculature. Certainly many different factors are known to influence VSM cell proliferation.

REVERSIBILITY OF ADAPTIVE CHANGES

Reduction of chronically elevated pressure can, in some cases, occur rapidly after removal of the cause. This must imply a rapidly reversible functional or structural alteration in VSM. Structural alterations that could reverse rapidly are elevated water content or proteins with a rapid turnover rate that would probably be produced by hypertrophied cells adapting to the increased pressure load.

In the rat 2-kidney 1-clip Goldblatt hypertension, removal of the clip after 3 to 4 weeks reduced arterial pressure to normal and reversed structural change (41), but complete reversal did not occur in either parameter after the blood pressure had been elevated for 4 months (42). This indicated that some new factor was in operation affecting the function of the VSM or that irreversible structural changes had occurred. Reversibility of hypertrophic muscle readily occurs in the absence of the stimulus in heart and skeletal muscle but has not been adequately studied in blood vessels. Although it is known that in the normal adult VSM cells there exists a relatively stable population in conduit arteries, there is no information on the turnover rate in hypertension. The rapidity of reversal of hyperplasia is not known.

In hypertension, elastin, collagen, and cell debris accumulate in the arterial wall. Elastin and collagen have slow turnover rates decreasing further with age; with increasing age, there is a shift in the production of labile polymers to stable polymers of collagen. A distinction must be made between the reversibility of elevated pressure and the reversibility of the adaptive changes in the arterial wall. It is unlikely that the arterial wall structure will return to normal once the scleroprotein content has increased unless the metabolism of these compounds can be altered. Collagen metabolism in blood vessels in hypertension is an important area to study.

REFERENCES

1. Abel, P. W., Urquilla, P. R., Goto, K., Westfall, D. P., Robinson, R. L., and Fleming, W. W. (1981): *J. Pharmacol. Exp. Ther.*, 217:430–439.
2. Anderson, B. G., and Anderson, W. D. (1981): *Biomed Res. (Suppl.)*, 2:209–217.
3a. Bevan, J. A., Bevan, R. D., Chang, P. C., Pegram, B. L., Purdy, R. E., and Su, C. (1975): *Circ. Res.*, 37:183–190.
3b. Bevan, R. D., Purdy, R. E., Su, C., and Bevan, J. A. (1975): *Circ. Res.*, 37:503–508.

4. Bevan, J. A., Bevan, R. D., and Duckles, S. P. (1980): In: *Vascular Smooth Muscle, Handbook of Physiology, Vol. II*, edited by D. F. Bohr, A. P. Somlyo, and H. V. Sparks, pp. 515–566. American Physiology Society, Baltimore.
5. Bevan, R. D. (1976): *Blood Vessels*, 13:100–128.
6. Bevan, R. D. (1980): In: *Report of the Hypertension Task Force*, Vol. 4, DWEW publication No. (NIH)79-1627.
7. Bevan, R. D., Eggena, P., Hume, W. R., Lais, L. T., Van Marthens, E., and Bevan, J. A. (1979): *Clin. Sci. (Suppl.)*, 57:7s–9s.
8. Bevan, R. D., Eggena, P., Wyatt, R., Hume, W. R., and Van Marthens, E. (1980): *Hypertension*, 2:63–72.
9. Bevan, R. D., and Tsuru, H. (1981): *Circ. Res.*, 49:478–485.
10. Bevan, R. D., and Tsuru, H. (1981): In: *Disturbance in Neurogenic Control of the Circulation*, edited by F. M. Aboud, H. A. Fozzard, J. P. Gilmore, and A. J. Reis, pp. 153–160. American Physiological Society, Baltimore.
11. Bevan, R. D., Van Marthens, E., and Bevan, J. (1976): *Circ. Res. (Suppl.)*, 38:58–62.
12. Bhan, R. D., Giacomelli, F., and Wiener, J. (1978): *Exp. Mol. Pathol.*, 29:66–81.
13. Bohlen, H. G., Gore, R. W., and Hutchins, P. M. (1971): *Microvasc. Res.*, 13:125–130.
14. Bohr, D. F. (1979): In: *Report of the Hypertension Task Force*, Vol. 5, DWEW publication No. (NIH)79-1627, Bethesda, Maryland.
15. Burnstock, G., and Costá, M. (1975): *Adrenergic Neurons*. Wiley, New York.
16. Canessa, M., Adragna, N., Solomon, H. S., Connolly, T. M., and Tosteson, D. C. (1980): *N. Engl. J. Med.*, 302:772–776.
17. Cliff, W. J. (1976): *Blood Vessels*. Cambridge University Press, London.
18. Cox, R. H. (1981): *Hypertension*, 3:485–495.
19. Crane, W. A. J., and Dutta, L. P. (1963): *J. Path. Bact.*, 86:83–97.
20. Engler, E., Matthias, D., and Becker, C. H. (1980): *Exp. Pathol.*, 18:37–51.
21. Fernandez, D., and Crane, W. A. J. (1970): *J. Pathol.*, 100:307–316.
22. Fleming, W. W. (1968): *J. Pharmacol. Exp. Ther.*, 162:277–285.
23. Folkow, B. (1978): *Clin. Sci. Mol. Med.*, 55:3s–22s.
24. Friedman, S. M., and Friedman, C. L. (1976): *Circ. Res.*, 39:433–441.
25. Friedman, S. M., Nakashima, M., McIndoe, R. A., and Friedman, C. L. (1976): *Experientia*, 32:476–478.
26. Garay, R. P., Elghozi, J-L., Dagher, G., and Meyer, P. (1980): *N. Engl. J. Med.*, 302:769–771.
27. Greenwald, S. E., and Berry, C. L. (1978): *Cardiovasc. Res.*, 12:364–372.
28. Haddy, F. J., Pamnani, M. B., and Clough, D. L. (1980): *Cardiovascular Review & Reports*, 1:376–385.
29. Hansen, T. R., Abrams, G. D., and Bohr, D. F. (1974): *Circ. Res. (Suppl.)*, 34–35:I101–I107.
30. Hart, M. D., Heistad, D. D., and Brody, M. J. (1980): *Hypertension*, 2:419–423.
31. Henrich, H., Hertel, R., and Assmann, R. (1978): *Pflügers Arch.*, 375:153–159.
32. Hume, W. R. (1980): *Hypertension*, 2:738–743.
33. Hutchins, P. M., and Darnell, A. E. (1974): *Circ. Res. (Suppl.)*, 34:I–161.
34. Ichijima, K. (1969) *Japan. Circ. J.*, 33:785–810.
35. Jones, A. W. (1973): *Circ. Res.*, 33:563–772.
36. Jurukova, Z., Hadjisky, P., Renais, J., and Scebat, L. (1976): *Path. Europ.*, 11:105–115.
37. Kao, K. T., Hilker, M., and McGovack, T. H. (1961): *Proc. Soc. Exp. Biol. Med.*, 106:335–341.
38. Leung, D. Y. M., Glagov, S., and Mathews, M. B. (1977): *Circ. Res.*, 41:316–323.
39. Limas, C., Westrum, B., and Limas, C. (1980): *Am. J. Pathol.*, 98:357–384.
40. Lund-Johansen, P. (1980): *Clin. Sci.*, 59:343s–354s.
41. Lundgren, Y. (1974): *Acta Physiol. Scand.*, 91:275–285.
42. Lundgren, Y., and Weiss, L. (1979): *Clin. Sci. (Suppl.)*, 57:19s–21s.
43a. Meininger, G. A., Harris, P. D., Joshua, I. G., Miller, F. N., and Wiegman, D. L. (1981): *Microcirc.*, 1:237–254.
43b. Mulvany, M. J., Aalkjaer, C., and Christensen, J. (1980): *Hypertension*, 2:664–671.
44. Mulvany, M. J., and Halpern, W. (1977): *Circ. Res.*, 41:19–26.
45. Mulvany, M. J., Hansen, P. K., and Aalkjaer, C. (1978): *Circ. Res.*, 43:854–864.
46. Nag, S., Robertson, D. M., and Dinsdale, H. B. (1980): *Acta Neuropathol. (Berl.)*, 52:27–34.

47. Newman, R. A., and Langner, R. O. (1975): *Conn. Tis. Tes.*, 3:231–236.
48. Ohtaka, M. (1980): *Japan. Circ. J.*, 44:283–293.
49. Olivetti, G., Anversa, P., Melissari, M., and Loud, A. V. (1980): *Lab. Invest.*, 42:559–565.
50. Ooshima, A., Fuller, G. C., Cardinale, G., Spector, S., and Udenfriend, S. (1975): *Proc. Natl. Acad. Sci. USA*, 71:3019–3023.
51. Owens, G. K., Cornhill, J. F., and Schwartz, S. M. (1981): *Fed. Proc.*, 40:614.
52. Postnov, Y. V., Orlov, S. N., Shevchenko, A., and Adler, A. M. (1977): *Pflügers Arch.*, 371:263–269.
53. Poston, L., Sewell, R. B., Wilkinson, S. P., Richardson, P. J., Williams, R., Clarkson, E. M., MacGregor, G. A., and De Wardener, H. E. (1981): *Br. Med. J.*, 282:847–849.
54. Prewitt, R. L., Chen, I. I. H., and Dowell, R. (1982): *Am. J. Physiol.*, 243:H243–H251.
55. Roach, M. R., and Burton, A. C. (1957): *Can. J. Biochem. Physiol.*, 35:681–690.
56. Schwartz, S. M., and Benditt, E. P. (1977): *Circ. Res.*, 41:248–255.
57. Schwieler, G. H., Douglas, J. S., and Bouhuys, A. (1970): *Am. J. Physiol.*, 219:391–397.
58. Shibata, S., Kurahashi, K., and Kuchii, M. (1973): *J. Pharmacol. Exp. Ther.*, 185:406–417.
59. Spector, S., Ooshima, A., Iwatsuki, K., Fuller, G., Cardinale, G., and Udenfriend, S. (1978): *Blood Vessels*, 15:176–182.
60. Suwa, N., and Takahashi, T. (1971): *Morphological and Morphometrical Analysis of Circulation in Hypertension and Ischemic Kidney*. Urban & Schwarzenberg, Berlin.
61. Tobian, L., and Redleaf P. D. (1958): *Am. J. Physiol.*, 192:325–330.
62. Wiener, J., Lattes, R. G., Meltzer, B. G., and Spiro, D. (1969): *Am. J. Pathol.*, 54:187–207.
63. Wolinsky, H. (1972): *Circ. Res.*, 30:301–309.
64. Zweifach, B. W., Kovalcheck, S., De Lano, F., and Chen, P. (1981): *Hypertension*, 3:601–614.

Perspectives in Cardiovascular
Research, Vol. 8,
edited by R. C. Tarazi and J. B. Dunbar.
Raven Press, New York © 1983.

Angiotensin and Myocardial Protein Synthesis

Philip A. Khairallah and Jan Kanabus

*Department of Cardiovascular Research, Division of Research,
Cleveland Clinic Foundation, Cleveland, Ohio 44106*

Twenty-five years after the octapeptide angiotensin II was made available synthetically (1,2), it has been shown to have multiple biological actions, many of which have a rapid onset and short duration after a single administration of the peptide (3,4). This has been attributed to angiotensin interacting with specific angiotensin receptor sites, leading to diverse physiological manifestations, in many instances involving calcium ions (3,4). There are, however, some actions of angiotensin that have much slower onset and more prolonged action. The action that has been studied most is the stimulation of the biosynthesis of aldosterone, in particular the first step, the conversion of cholesterol to pregnenolone. It has been shown that aldosterone biosynthesis induced by angiotensin II (5,6), PGA_1 (7,8), and adrenocorticotropin hormone (ACTH) (6) is blocked by inhibitors of messenger ribonucleic acid (mRNA) translation, namely cycloheximide and puromycin, but not by actinomysin D, an inhibitor of transcription of deoxyribonucleic acid (DNA) (8,9). These drug effects have been interpreted as indications that angiotensin stimulation leads to a protein synthetic step required for the conversion of cholesterol to pregnenolone. The mechanism of action, however, is not clear-cut since the maximum effects of angiotensin on adrenal protein synthesis require 30 to 90 min, while steroidogenesis occurs within 3 to 5 min. Thus, the likelihood is that both the protein synthetic step and the aldosterone biosynthesis occur simultaneously, but may not be causally linked. On the other hand, the chronic effects of the renin–angiotensin system and aldosterone biosynthesis may involve an increased synthesis of an enzyme protein (5).

Munday and co-workers (10,11), studying angiotensin stimulated fluid and sodium transport by the rat jejunum, demonstrated that these effects can be inhibited by cyclophosphamide, an inhibitor of mRNA translation, but not by actinomysin D, again implicating protein synthesis (12).

There are some other effects of angiotensin II that cannot easily be explained. In 1971, we demonstrated that 5 to 10 ng of either tritiated angiotensin or ^{14}C-labeled angiotensin rapidly injected into the left ventricle of adult rats led to a preferential localization of radioactivity in the nuclear zone of vascular and cardiac muscle cells (13). This localization of radioactivity could be prevented by prior administration of a 1,000-fold excess of nonlabeled angiotensin. At the time, it was proposed that, in addition to its effects on cell mitosis, one of the indirect effects of the peptide might be a stimulation of mRNA and protein synthesis. Ganten (14) demonstrated that angiotensin II caused proliferative changes in cultured fibroblasts in arterial smooth muscle cells, and Simonian and Gill (15) demonstrated similar effects in bovine adrenal cortical cells in culture as well as an increased DNA synthesis.

Because of these findings, an attempt was made to see whether angiotensin would also stimulate protein synthesis in the rat heart (16). We incubated isolated rat atria with tritiated uridine or thymidine or with ^{14}C-isoleucine for 2 hr at 37°C, the atria were then homogenized in ice cold perchloric acid, and the DNA, RNA and protein separated and counted. Angiotensin I or angiotensin II were added to the incubation medium at concentrations of 1 to 62.5 ng/ml. In another series of experiments, bilaterally adrenalectomized female rats were anesthetized with urethane and tritiated uridine, and thymidine and ^{14}C-isoleucine were administered intravenously together with peptides. Organs were removed at the end of 2 hr, RNA, DNA, and protein isolated, and radioactivity measured. Organs studied included uterus, spleen, brain, liver, kidney, and both atria and ventricles. In the isolated rat atria, angiotensin II increased the turnover of thymidine, but did not change total DNA content, while in the *in vivo* experiments, where angiotensin was infused at 45 ng/kg/min for 30 min followed by saline infusion for 90 min, turnover of DNA was increased in the atria and ventricles as well as in the renal medulla and renal cortex. There was also a total DNA increase in the atria, renal medulla, and renal cortex. Other tissues showed no changes. Studies on RNA showed that specific activity and, therefore, turnover of RNA was increased with 10 ng/ml angiotensin in the isolated atria; in addition, total RNA content was increased by 10, 25, and 62.5 ng with angiotensin II. The decapeptide had approximately 20 to 25% activity of the octapeptide. When angiotensin was given intravenously, there was significant increase in the incorporation of uridine into RNA in spleen, atrium, ventricles, renal cortex, brain, and liver. There was also a significant increase in total RNA content in all the organs measured except the uterus. Actinomysin D, at a concentration of 1 µg/ml, completely inhibited the effect of 10 ng/ml angiotensin II, both on the incorporation and net RNA content of isolated atria, as well as in the *in vivo* studies following angiotensin infusion. Thus, there were some indications that angiotensin could stimulate certain steps leading to protein biosynthesis in myocardial cells. Similar results were reported by Roth and Hughes (17), using guinea pig atria, but could not be confirmed by Hill et al. (18), using atria from male rats instead of female rats that were used in our early work.

The question as to whether or not angiotensin and certain angiotensin analogs stimulate protein synthesis leading to cardiac hypertrophy was recently posed again. Sen et al. (19) reported that when male rats (Kyoto Wistar strain) were administered angiotensin antagonists (Sar[1], Ile[8])AII and (Sar[1], Ala[8])AII subcutaneously (s.c.) at a dose of 100 μg every 8 hr for 4 weeks, they developed significant increase in heart weight. On the other hand, (Sar^1, Thr^8)AII, another angiotensin II antagonist, did not produce cardiac hypertrophy. Another difference between the two angiotensin antagonists was that (Sar^1, Ile^8)AII and (Sar^1, Ala^8)AII caused a significant increase in catecholamine concentration in the myocardium, while (Sar^1, Thr^8)AII did not. Finally, they demonstrated that cardiac hypertrophy by (Sar^1, Ile^8)AII was prevented by bilateral adrenalectomy, thus suggesting an important role for catecholamines in mediating the peptide stimulus to cardiac hypertrophy.

Due to these previous findings, we decided to reinvestigate the mechanisms by which angiotensin and its analogs stimulate cardiac hypertrophy. We assumed that indications of stimulation of protein biosynthesis over a short period of time is one of the early signs of development of cardiac hypertrophy, recognizing that measurement of biosynthesis alone may not give a full explanation, since turnover of myocardial proteins must also play an important role. Experiments were designed to focus on the initial steps leading to protein biosynthesis in cardiac hypertrophy and thus were planned for 2 and 6 days only. For purposes of comparison, norepinephrine (NE) and epinephrine were administered to detect the involvement of the catecholamines and possible interaction of catecholamines and angiotensin.

METHODS

Male Sprague-Dawley rats weighing 200 to 250 g were given standard laboratory chow and water *ad libitum*. Drugs were administered s.c. by osmotic minipumps (model 2001, Alza Corp.), and the dosage was calculated assuming an infusion rate of 0.9 μl/hr, as estimated by the pump manufacturer, based on an estimated subcutaneous temperature of 33 to 34°C at the site of the minipump. The drugs administered and the dosages were as follows: epinephrine 3 to 100 nmol/hr; NE 40 to 150 nmol/hr; angiotensin 20.9 to 5.0 nmol/hr; (Sar^1, Ile^8)AII 0.9 to 1.5 nmol/hr; and (Sar^1, Thr^8)AII 0.9 to 15.0 nmol/hr. Since animals gained weight constantly, the exact dosages were calculated based on the body weight at the time of decapitation. Blood pressure was measured by the tail-cuff method of Friedman and Freed (20), starting 1 to 2 weeks before beginning the infusions. Blood pressure measurements were done twice a week and then once just prior to sacrifice in the 2-day infusion experiments, and once on day 3 and then just prior to sacrifice in the 6-day experiments. Control animals received minipumps filled with sterile distilled water. To study mechanisms by which catecholamines and the angiotensin peptides initiated cardiac hypertrophy, phenoxybenzamine, an α-adrenergic blocking agent, was given s.c. at 1.25 mg/animal/day on days -1, 0, 2, 4, and 6, with the last dose given 4 to 6 hr before sacrifice. Saline injections were used as placebo controls. *d,l*-propranolol was given in the drinking water at a concentration of 750 mg/l. Animals were allowed to drink *ad libitum*, which usually averaged 35 ml/day, equivalent to a daily dose of propranolol of between 85 and 130 mg/kg depending upon the body weight of the animal. Propranolol administration was started 2 days before implantation of the minipump, and β-adrenergic blockade was confirmed by a significant decrease in heart rate within 24 hr and a significant decrease in plasma renin activity from 15 ng angiotensin II per ml/hr to 4 ng/ml/hr. Also at the time of sacrifice, plasma propranolol levels were measured by the spectrofluorometric method of Vasiliades et al. (20a).

At the end of the experiments, rats were weighed, decapitated, and trunk blood collected in a heparanized beaker on ice for subsequent determinations of plasma renin activity and propranolol levels. The chest was opened, hearts rapidly removed, and rinsed with ice-cold saline to eliminate as much blood as possible. Large vessels and atria were carefully removed and discarded, the left ventricle opened, and the whole heart blotted dry and weighed. The right ventricle was then separated from the left ventricle with the intraventricular septum kept part of the left ventricle. Pieces of the right and left ventricle, including intraventricular septum, were removed, weighed again, and placed in 4 ml ice-cold ethanol. These samples were used for chemical analysis, while the remainder of the two ventricles were dried at 120°C to constant weight. The pre-weighed samples of the ventricles were left in ice-cold ethanol for 16 hr and then homogenized in an all-glass homogenizer. The suspension was transferred to centrifuge tubes, the homogenizer washed with 2 ml ethanol and 2 ml water, and the solutions were combined. Ethanol-insoluble material was collected by centrifugation and the pellet was extracted sequentially with 3 ml each of 0.2 N perchloric acid at 4°C, 1 N perchloric acid at 80°C for 30 min, and then 0.1 N sodium hydroxide (NaOH). After each extraction, the samples were centrifuged and reextracted once. The extract with 0.2 N perchloric acid was discarded. The extract with 1 N perchloric acid at 80°C was used for nucleotide determination, and the extract with NaOH was used for protein determination. Nucleotide determinations were carried out according to the methods of Schneider (21), using orcinol to detect ribose and diphenylamine to detect deoxyribose. Protein determination was according to Lowry et al. (22), using purified serum albumin as a standard.

RESULTS

Both epinephrine and NE significantly increased ventricular weight, both in the 2-day ($p = 0.0001$) and the 6-day ($p = 0.0001$) experiments, while angiotensin significantly increased ventricular weight only in the 6-day experiments ($p = 0.0001$) (Fig. 1). In all instances, ventricular weight increased at doses of agonists that also increased blood pressure. At subpressor dosages of epinephrine, NE, or angiotensin, no change in heart weight occurred by 6 days of infusion. An analysis of the regression line of ventricular weight and dose of agonist administered indicated that angiotensin was approximately 25 times

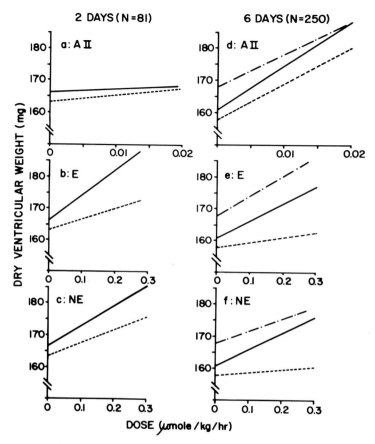

FIG. 1. Linear regression analysis of changes in dry ventricular weights as a function of the dose of agonists infused for 2 or 6 days. *Solid lines*, agonist dose; *dashed lines*, agonist plus propranolol; *dashed and dotted lines*, agonist plus phenoxybenzamine.

more potent than epinephrine or NE on a molar basis ($p = 0.0001$). Since percent dry weight in all hearts, whether treated or untreated, did not change, this increase in heart size was measurable either as total heart weight or as dry ventricular weight (Fig. 1). When phenoxybenzamine was administered to these rats there was no effect on cardiomegaly following epinephrine, NE, or angiotensin. However, phenoxybenzamine in itself increased heart weight in control animals approximately 30 mg (7 mg dry weight) ($p = 0.001$). Thus, at all levels of catecholamine or peptide administration in the phenoxybenzamine treated animals, heart weight was higher than in nonphenoxybenzamine animals, yet the increment per dose of agonist remained the same. This picture was very different following administration of propranolol. This β-adrenergic antagonist abolished any increase in heart weight following administration of epinephrine or NE, but it had no effect on the increase in heart weight following administration of angiotensin or the angiotensin analog (Sar[1], Ile[8])AII. At the dose of propranolol used, there was a significant decrease in heart rate but no change in blood pressure. With phenoxybenzamine, there was essentially no change in heart rate; blood pressure was reduced, but not to normal, following catecholamine infusions, with no change in blood pressure following angiotensin infusions. Administration of (Sar[1], Ile[8])AII increased blood pressure minimally (approximately 6 mm), but not significantly. There were no changes in heart rate.

(Sar[1], Ile[8])AII at 13.0 nmol/hr produced a significant increase in heart weight (Fig. 2), while (Sar[1], Thr[8])AII at 13 nmol/hr caused a slight but barely significant increase ($p = 0.1$). In an attempt to see whether or not responses to angiotensin were mediated by angiotensin receptors, angiotensin II at 4.33 nmol/hr was infused together with (Sar[1], Ile[8])AII at 13 nmol/hr or (Sar[1], Thr[8])AII at 13 nmol/hr. Both of these peptides significantly reduced the pressor responses to AII. As can be seen in Fig. 2, (Sar[1], Thr[8])AII had no effect at all on the heart weight responses to angiotensin, while (Sar[1], Ile[8])AII slightly de-

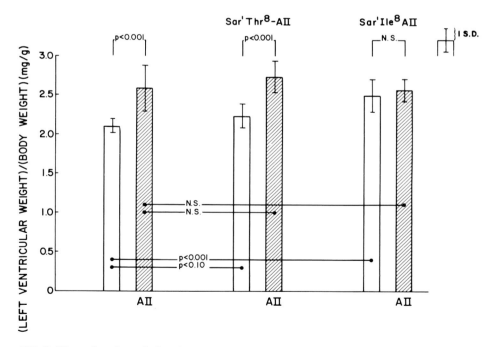

FIG. 2. Effect of angiotensin II and its analogs on left ventricular weight/body weight ratio. **First column:** saline control; **second column:** angiotensin II, 4.33 nmol/hr; **third column:** (Sar[1], Thr[8])AII, 13 nmol/hr; **fourth column:** (Sar[1], Thr[8])AII, 13 nmol/hr, and AII, 4.33 nmol/hr; **fifth column:** (Sar[1], Ile[8])AII, 13 nmol/hr; **sixth column:** (Sar[1], Ile[8])AII, 13 nmol/hr, and AII, 4.33 nmol/hr.

creased the degree of hypertrophy, but this was not significantly different from AII alone.

Total NaOH extractable proteins tended to decrease slightly in both the 2- and 6-day experiments when expressed as protein concentration/mg ventricular weight, but when expressed as total ventricular protein per heart, the increase was similar to that of dry ventricular weight (Fig. 1). Total protein content also mimicked dry ventricular weight in those rats treated with phenoxybenzamine or with propranolol. RNA concentration was significantly increased in the ventricles with both epinephrine and NE in the 2-day experiments, while in the 6-day experiments RNA concentration was only slightly increased following epinephrine and showed a slight decrease following NE. On the other hand, angiotensin II administration had no effect on RNA concentration in the 2-day experiments, although in the 6-day experiments a small but significant increase was observed. Total ventricular RNA followed similar patterns; propranolol and phenoxybenzamine had no consistent effect on these responses. With both catecholamines there was a greater increase in the 2-day experiments than in the 6-day experiments, while with angiotensin II there was only an increase in the 6-day experiments with essentially no change in the 2-day experiments.

Concentrations of DNA decreased significantly in both ventricles following the administration of epinephrine (Fig. 3). Total tissue DNA was similar to control values: Although tissue concentration decreased, heart weight increased. With NE, there was a slight decrease in DNA concentration in the left ventricle and no change in the right ventricle. However, total tissue DNA was significantly increased both at day 2 ($p = 0.0004$) and at day 6 ($p = 0.0001$). With the administration of angiotensin II, there was an increased DNA concentration ($p = 0.03$) in the 2-day experiments with no change in total tissue DNA in the 6-day experiments. Responses to adrenergic blocking agents on total DNA were small and insignificant.

DISCUSSION

Cardiac hypertrophy has been recognized for some time to be a non-homogenous entity. It can develop from many causes, and different forms of cardiac hypertrophy manifest themselves by different biochemical, functional, and anatomical characteristics (23). The striking findings in our experiments are the rapidity of the development of hypertrophy and the fact that increased heart weight following the administration of catecholamines is blocked by propranolol, but hypertrophy following administration of angiotensin is not blocked.

The rapid onset of hypertrophy was manifest in our experiments, since after 2 days of both epinephrine or NE administration heart weight increased as did the concentration of RNA. With angiotensin, however, there were no changes in the 2-day experiments, but both heart weight and RNA concentration in-

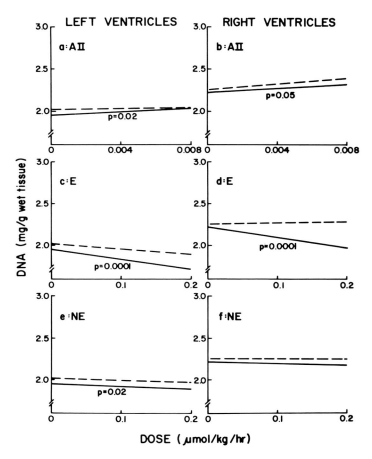

FIG. 3. Linear regression analysis of changes in DNA concentration as a function of doses of agonists infused for 2 days. *Solid line*, agonist alone; *dashed line*, agonist plus proopranolol.

creases occurred in the 6-day experiments. This rapid onset following cate-cholamine administration was first reported by Stanton et al. (24), who showed that significant cardiomegaly occurred in rats receiving isoproterenol after 48 hr (5 mg/kg s.c. twice a day). Other investigators, however, could produce cardiac hypertrophy following low doses of isoproterenol (0.08 to 1.25 mg/kg) (25), and these changes occurred within 12 hr or less. They also demonstrated that the increase in cardiac weight is due to increased protein synthesis and not water accumulation, that it is associated with increased cardiac DNA and RNA, and that these changes could be prevented by β-adrenergic block-ade (26–27).

Our results are very similar in many respects. Following administration of epinephrine, there was increased protein content within 2 days, indicated by an increased dry ventricular weight. There was no change in water content of the ventricles. Also, within 2 days there was an increased concentration of RNA with a markedly increased total RNA content. However, by 6 days, both the RNA concentration and content, although still increased, were less than the 2-day response; DNA content of the heart did not change. These findings can be explained by epinephrine, acting through β-adrenergic receptors, initiating protein biosynthesis by stimulating RNA formation. By 6 days, the stimulus to RNA formation, although still present, showed a somewhat lesser response. DNA concentration decreased and total ventricular DNA remained the same, indicating that the heart underwent pure hypertrophy, each cell becoming larger with no increase in the number of cells. Responses to NE, on the other hand, were somewhat different. Within 2 days, there was an increased heart weight, increased total ventricular protein content, and an increased RNA concentration and total content. By 6 days, however, RNA concentration decreased somewhat, so that total RNA content was only marginally increased. On the other hand, DNA concentration did not change, so that total DNA content increased. These findings can best be explained by NE interacting with β-adrenergic receptors, since its response can be blocked by propranolol, stimulating protein synthesis rapidly within 2 days, but at the same time stimulating DNA formation consistent with production of new cells, possibly connective tissue. Other factors could be an increase in the frequency of polyploidy, an infiltration of inflammatory cells, or finally, an increase in mitochondrial DNA. None of these possibilities can be ruled out at present.

Responses to angiotensin are somewhat different. First of all, the time course seems to be much slower than response to the catecholamines, since essentially no changes were observed in the 2-day experiments; but within 6 days, there was an increased protein content, increased heart weight, and increased RNA concentration and content. These effects of angiotensin and some of the angiotensin analogs were not mediated by β-adrenergic receptors, possibly indicating no interaction between angiotensin and myocardial catecholamines, at least in the short-term initiation experiments. Responses to angiotensin, however, also did not seem to involve angiotensin receptors, since angiotensin antagonists that block the pressor responses to the infused peptide did not block the hypertrophic responses. One possible explanation is that the peptide angiotensin is internalized and rapidly localized on nuclei (13), which also could explain why DNA content increased in the 2-day experiments but was back to normal in the 6-day experiments. At these doses of angiotensin there was no evidence of infiltration of inflammatory cells (*preliminary observations*).

In our experiments, cardiac hypertrophy could not be produced with subpressor doses of angiotensin II, epinephrine, or NE within the 6 days of the experimental period. Other investigators, however, were able to produce left ventricular hypertrophy in dogs receiving continuous infusions of small subpressor doses of norepinephrine for periods of 6 to 63 weeks (28). Phenoxybenzamine, which diminished the pressor responses to epinephrine and NE, although not abolishing them totally, had no effect on the degree of cardiac hypertrophy, while propranolol, which had no effect at all on blood pressure, abolished the hypertrophic responses to epinephrine and NE. Finally, (Sar^1, Ile^8)AII, one of the angiotensin antagonists that produced cardiac hypertrophy, did so with a minimal, nonsignificant elevation of blood pressure. Thus, one has to conclude that there is no direct relationship between the degree of cardiac hypertrophy and the degree of elevation of blood pressure, leading to a strengthening of the hypothesis that the catecholamines and angiotensin might be "myocardial hypertrophy hormones," the messenger linking the stimulus of physical stress on the heart to the metabolic hypertrophic responses of the myocardium (29). Raab (30) argued 28 years ago that cardiac hypertrophy was not a mechanical response to cardiac load but the result of complex hormonal and adrenergic factors, and our results fully support this conclusion.

ACKNOWLEDGMENTS

This research was supported in part by NIH grant 6835. Data were partially analyzed using the PROPHET computer system supported in part by the Biotechnology Resources Program, Division of Research Resources, National Institutes of Health.

REFERENCES

 1. Bumpus, F. M., Schwarz, H., and Page, I. H. (1975): *Science*, 125:3253–3255.
 2. Rittel, W., Iselin, B., Kappeler, H., Riniker, B., and Schwyzer, R. (1974): *Helv. Chim. Acta*, 40:614–624.
 3. Regoli, D., Park, W. K., and Rioux, F. (1974): *Pharmacol. Rev.*, 26:69–124.
 4. Peach, M. J. (1977): *Physiol. Rev.*, 57:313–370.
 5. Aguilera, G., and Marusic, E. T. (1971): *Endocrinol.* 89:1524–1529.
 6. Kaplan, N. M., and Bartter, F. C. (1962): *J. Clin. Invest.* 41:715–724.
 7. Fishman, M. P., Littenberg, G. D., Brooker, G. (1972): *Circ. Res. (Suppl.)*, 31:II19–II35.
 8. Saruta, T., and Kaplan, N. M. (1972): *J. Clin. Invest.*, 51:2246–2251.
 9. Saruta, T., Cook, R., and Kaplan, N. M. (1972): *J. Clin. Invest.*, 51:2239–2245.
10. Munday, K. A., Parsons, B. J., and Poat, J. A. (1972): *J. Physiol.*, 224:195–206.
11. Bolton, J. E., Munday, K. A., Parsons, B. J., and York, B. G. (1975): *J. Physiol.*, 253:411–428.
12. Bolton, J. E., Munday, K. A., and Parsons, B. J. (1977): *J. Endocr.*, 74:213–221.
13. Robertson, A. L., and Khairallah, P. A. (1971): *Science*, 172:1138–1139.
14. Ganten, D., Schelling, P., and Flugel, R. M. (1975): *Intern. Res. Comm. Med. Sci.*, 3:327.
15. Simonian, M. H., and Gill, G. (1979): *Endocrinol.*, 104:588–595.
16. Khairallah, P. A., Robertson, A. C., and Davilla, D. (1972): In: *Hypertension '72*, edited by J. Genest and E. Koiw, pp. 212–220. Springer-Verlag, New York.
17. Roth, R. H., and Hughes, J. (1972): *Biochem. Pharmacol.*, 21:3182–3186.
18. Hill, R. N., Severs, W. B., and Liu, P. K. (1975): *Proc. Soc. Exp. Biol. Med.*, 148:418–419.
19. Sen, S., Tarazi, R. C., and Bumpus, F. M. (1979): *Clin. Sci.*, 56:439–443.
20. Friedman, M., and Freed, S. (1949): *Proc. Soc. Exp. Biol. Med.*, 70:670–672.
20a. Vasiliades, J., Turner, T., and Owens, C. (1978): *Am. J. Clin. Pathol.*, 70:793–799.
21. Schneider, W. C. (1957): In: *Methods of Enzymology* edited by S. P. Colowick and N. O. Kaplan, pp. 680–684. Academic Press, New York.

22. Lowry, C. M., Rosebrough, N. J., Farr, A. L., and Randall, R. J. (1951): *J. Biol. Chem.*, 193:265–275.
23. Skelton, C. L., and Sonnenblick, E. M. (1974): *Suppl., Circ. Res.* 35:83–96.
24. Stanton, H. C., Brenner, G., and Mayfield, E. R. (1969): *Amer. Heart J.*, 77:72–80.
25. Szabo, J., Csaky, L., and Szegi, J. (1975): *Acta Physiol. Acad. Sci. Hungary*, 46:281–285.
26. Szabo, J., Nosztray, K., Csaky, L., and Szegi, J. (1976): *Acta Physiol. Acad. Sci. Hungary*, 48:79–80.
27. Pagano, V. T., and Inchiosa, M. A. (1977): *Life Sciences*, 21:619–624.
28. Laks, M. M., Morady, F., and Swan, H. J. C. (1973): *Chest*, 64:75–78.
29. Tarazi, R. C., and Sen, S. (1979): In: *The Royal Society of Medicine International Congress and Symposium, Series No. 8*, edited by K. C. Mezey and A. D. S. Caldwell, pp. 47–57. Academic Press, London.
30. Raab, W. (1953): *Hormonal and Neurogenic Cardiovascular Disorders.* Williams & Wilkins, Baltimore.

*Perspectives in Cardiovascular
Research, Vol. 8,*
edited by R. C. Tarazi and J. B. Dunbar.
Raven Press, New York © 1983.

Conclusion and Future Directions

Robert C. Tarazi and *John B. Dunbar

*Research Division, Cleveland Clinic Foundation, Cleveland, Ohio 44106;
*Hypertension and Kidney Diseases Branch, Division of Heart and
Vascular Diseases, National Heart, Lung, and Blood Institute,
National Institutes of Health, Bethesda, Maryland 20205*

Hypertension is the most common antecedent of left ventricular hypertrophy and congestive heart failure, at least in the United States and Westernized countries. It is surprising, therefore, that cardiac studies in hypertension have lagged behind studies of myocardial hypertrophy in other diseases. In part, this is because hypertension research has been principally concerned with control of the peripheral vessels, since increased systemic resistance is the hemodynamic hallmark of the disease. Little attention has been given to the heart because it appeared to play a minor role in hypertension development (only recently have these views been somewhat altered). There were, in addition, ethical and practical difficulties in using the available invasive methods in what was essentially an asymptomatic disorder. Therefore, most of our knowledge concerning the heart in hypertension had to be derived from studies of other types of diseases.

Translation from one field to another, however, has been proven unacceptable because of the heterogeneity of cardiac hypertrophy, which is now widely documented. Even within a specific type of hypertrophy, e.g., pressure overload, significant differences in effect on hypertrophy and function can be found between systemic hypertension and other conditions such as valvular stenosis and coarctation of the aorta. These differences can be ascribed to a variety of factors, such as duration of the pressure load, natural history of the disease, influence of the arterial system and reflected waves on aortic impedance, and magnitude of the driving head of coronary perfusion. The study of left ventricular hypertrophy in hypertension is particularly important because the full spectrum of the cardiac (as opposed to hemodynamic) effects of therapy have yet to be determined. Further, it has recently been found that left ventricular hypertrophy is not a late development of advanced disease but, rather, a common occurrence early in the evolution of hypertension, presenting in adolescents with borderline blood pressure elevations.

There are other factors that attest to the importance of studies of left ventricular failure in hypertension. Among them are the methodological advances achieved in the past few years allowing accurate quantification of left ventricular hypertrophy by noninvasive means; the result has been a marked expansion of the concept of hypertrophy in hypertension (e.g., not all patients have developed the expected left ventricular concentric hypertrophy). Another factor indicating the need for further studies is that various types of cardiac alterations have been documented—such as asymmetric septal thickening, eccentric hypertrophy, and alterations in ventricular compliance—even in the absence of definite evidence of increase in ventricular mass. Further, it has been documented both in man and experimental animals that the reversal of hypertrophy is not a simple consequence of the lowering of blood pressure. From studies undertaken at many centers, evidence has accumulated that drugs that are equipotent in lowering blood pressure have differential effects on the structure of the cardiovascular system.

The question of whether or not hypertrophy benefits the patient has acquired a wider and more practical—even urgent—dimension. The demonstration that hypertrophy can be reversed if the proper drugs are used, together with the finding that hypertrophy can occur in early hypertension, present new questions. Should antihypertensive therapy be dictated only by blood pressure levels, or should it make one of its aims the reversal of cardiovascular structural changes? Should no attempt be made to reverse the hypertrophy if it is "adequate or appropriate" to the load? (Adequate hypertrophy is the type that leaves cardiac performance unchanged or even improved, possibly because of parallel changes in left ventricular wall thickness and cavity diameter.) An important need in that regard is to determine if alterations in cardiac mass are associated with similar changes in the structure of arteries—both the large arteries and resistance vessels. Hypertension is a systemic disease, and its evolution will depend as much on its cardiac aspects as on the structural alterations it induces in peripheral vessels. Some studies have suggested that cardiac and vascular hypertrophy develop in parallel with evolution of the disease and will respond in parallel to antihypertensive measures. Others suggest that the hyperplasia that characterizes vascular responses to increased load is a different mechanism from the hypertrophy occurring in myocardial cells, and it is not certain that the reversal of cardiac hypertrophy will be associated with the same changes in resistance vessels.

Many studies, therefore, are needed in the field of hypertensive hypertrophy, both in experimental and clinical situations. The steering committee responsible for arranging the symposium from which this book originated felt the following lines of investigation would prove productive. The Committee wished to acknowledge that these are personal recommendations and points of view that reflect their interests, preferences, and biases. The list is in no particular order, and the suggestions by no means exhaust the many opportunities for productive research. Finally, the listing does not necessarily reflect the interests of the National Heart, Lung, and Blood Institute.

1. Studies of cardiac hypertrophy in models of hypertension of long duration are of great interest; a combination of etiologies, such as hypertension plus coronary artery disease or diabetes, would be especially important for study.

2. Better definition of methods for diagnosis and quantitation of left ventricular mass and function is needed for use in man. This is important because the reported prevalence of asymmetric hypertrophy in the United States differs markedly from that in Europe. The exact prevalence of eccentric hypertrophy in hypertension is not known. The role of socioeconomic factors in furthering marked hypertrophy or leading to the more deleterious combination of dilation and hypertrophy also needs definition. The availability of noninvasive methods to quantitate left ventricular mass and calculate the ratio of the wall thickness to cavity diameter should allow the development of the data needed for future investigation.

3. Studies of catecholamine turnover in the myocardium are important because of the reported differences between hypertensive and nonhypertensive hypertrophy, and because present knowledge deals only with myocardial catecholamine concentrations. A highly suggestive body of evidence has been developed recently to the effect that adrenergic influences play a role in modulating structural responses of the heart and resistance vessels to hypertension. The evidence, however, is still circumstantial, and more definitive studies are desirable.

4. Coronary blood flow disturbances appear to be basically different in different types of hypertrophy, depending on the magnitude of the driving head of pressure in the coronary bed; studies of the effects of blood pressure control on coronary flow are needed.

5. The study of myocardial metabolism has been undertaken mostly in nonhypertensive conditions. It is important to ascertain whether substrates and types of proteins (both contractile and noncontractile) are different between genetic and nongenetic forms of hypertension. Evidence has been developed that protease activities are greatly increased in the myocardium during the development of hypertensive hypertrophy. The systems responsible for the increased activity and their involvement in controlling the rate of proteolysis need to be further defined, since an imbalance in them can account for changes in cardiac muscle size and protein composition, and result in changes in contractile activity and metabolic function.

6. Recent studies of myosin isoenzymes have been productive in revealing the ways in which the heart adapts to various loads, with slower isoenzymes developing under conditions of pressure overload. This new field of investigation may permit more direct study of cardiac hypertrophy as an adaptive response, with the possible evolution of the hypertrophy towards a favorable or unfavorable performance. It also becomes important to determine the extent of dynamic changes in these enzymes, if the cause of the hypertrophy is controlled or eradicated. At a more fundamental level, the mechanisms regulating myocardial calcium kinetics need to be determined because of the recent emphasis on the use of calcium entry blockers in everyday therapy for hypertension, coronary artery disease and, possibly, hypertrophic cardiomyopathy.

7. The fibrous skeleton of the heart, as regards typing and morphology of collagen, its influences on the diastolic and systolic functions of the heart, and

the role of collagen in the evolution of hypertensive hypertrophy and genesis of heart failure, requires examination. This field is of particular importance because the complex network of collagen bundles in the heart, which interconnects the myocytes and capillaries and orders the myocytes into groups, is altered in disease states. There is as yet no organized body of information to relate abnormalities of the connective tissue to altered ventricular function in cardiac hypertrophy. Closely linked to the study of the connective tissue is the evaluation of the "nonmuscle space" in the heart, particularly in regard to the organization of the microvascular bed, the lymphatics, and connective tissue matrix. The relationship of capillary surface area/unit tissue should be determined because diffusion distances appear to be unimportant in the production of progressive myocardial cell loss.

8. Reversal of hypertrophy remains the common goal of all these studies, all of which have to be performed during the development, but also after the reversal, of hypertrophy. Biochemical studies have suggested that collagen concentration might be selectively increased following reversal of most, but not all, hypertrophy. The effects of reversal on cardiac performance have yet to be defined. The available studies are few in number, and it has been reported that the intact heart *in situ* becomes more sensitive to acute pressure changes after reversal of hypertrophy than either the normal or hypertrophic heart, in contrast to the return to normal of myocardial mechanics (in papillary muscle studies). Data are just beginning to emerge regarding reversible versus irreversible wall alterations in hypertrophy and further work is required to determine the reasons for the irreversible state.

9. The transition from compensated hypertrophy to heart failure still remains largely a mystery. Even though epidemiologic studies show hypertension to be the most frequent concomitant of heart failure, clinicians find many patients to be asymptomatic—even after many years of hypertension and hypertrophy. Also, the rapid transition in spontaneously hypertensive rats, from a condition of almost normal cardiac performance to markedly diminished performance after the age of eighteen to twenty-four months, still has not been adequately explained. A plea is made for further studies defining this all important event in the evolution of cardiac diseases.

Subject Index

Actin
  myosin interactions, thyrotoxicity,
    75–77
  polymorphic characteristics, 10
Actinomyosin D, angiotensin inhibition,
  338
Action potentials, renal hypertension,
  220–224
Active muscle properties
  hypertension and hypertension
    reversal, 183, 185–187
  isolated cardiac muscle, 168–169
  pressure overload, 169–177
Actomyosin, heat production,
  isomyosins, 163–165
Actomyosin ATPase
  hypertension and hypertension
    reversal, 186–190
  stress effects, 15, 17–18
Acute reversible pressure overload
  as hypertrophy model, 129–134,
    138–142
  methods, 124, 126–127
Adenosine, vasodilation, 267–270
Adenosine diphosphate
  creatine kinase system, 146–148
  growing hearts, DNA, 8
Adenosine triphosphate, see ATP
Adventitial surface, arteries,
  hypertension, 60–61
Afferent sympathetic fibers, 235–245
Afterload increments
  aortic bands versus SHR, 171–172,
    175
  pressure overload model, 141
Afterpotentials, renal hypertension,
  230–232
Age effects
  cardiac hypertrophy, 6–7
  hypertension onset, 329
  myocyte size estimates,
    cardiomegaly, 46–48
  spontaneous hypertensive rats, 176
  sympathetic innervation, 329–330
  thyroid hormone hypertrophy, 77–79
    isomyosin profile, 87–88

Aging, thyroid hormone effects, 77–79
Aldosterone synthesis, angiotensin, 337
Alpha receptors
  cardiac reflexes, 235–236
  heart failure, norepinephrine, 304
Angiotensin
  hypertension damage mediation,
    69–71
    vasculature, 331–332
  hypertrophy stimulus, 22–23
  myocardial protein synthesis,
    337–346
  vascular pathology, 327
  ventricular weight, 340–345
Angiotensin antagonists
  cardiac hypertrophy, 338–339
  heart weight, 342–343, 346
  hypertension, 312–313
Angiotension analogs, 312–313,
    338–339, 342–343
Anoxia, arteriole lesions, 69–70
Anterior ventricular wall, 264–265
Antihypertensives
  and blood pressure, catecholamines,
    310, 313–317
  indications for use, 350
  mechanism of action, catecholamines,
    312
  ventricular weight, SHR, 199
Aortic banding
  catecholamine levels, 310–311, 315
  mechanics effect, versus SHR,
    169–177
  myocardial blood flow, 262, 263–270
  myocardial growth, 7
Aortic stenosis
  collagen network, 53
  and coronary circulation, 279–282
  myocardial blood flow, 262–263
  myocardial contraction, 299–301
  ventricular hypertrophy,
    morphometry, 28–33
Aorto-caval fistula, cardiomegaly, 46
Arrhythmia, afterpotentials, 231–232
Arterial contraction, hypertension, 325
Arterial pressure

Arterial pressure *(contd.)*
  aortic stenosis effect, 281
  baroreceptors, 238, 242–244
  and catecholamines, hypertrophy,
    313–317
  hypertension adaptation, 326–327
  reversibility, 333
  time course, 326–328
  and ventricular dysfunction, SHR,
    197–198
  and ventricular weight, 198–199
Arteries
  hypertension adaptation, 319–333
  wall thickness, 321–322, 326–328
    sympathic innervation, 325
Arterioles
  adaptive changes, 319–333
  morphology, 65–69, 322–323
  peripheral resistance, 319–320
Asymmetric hypertrophy, 211, 351
Atherosclerosis, collagen, 54, 56
ATP
  activity in hypertrophy, 22–23
  creatine phosphate balance, 145–154
    nuclear magnetic resonance,
      151–154
ATP regenerating systems, 120
ATPase, sarcoplasmic reticulum
    111–112
Atrium
  angiotensin effect, proteins, 338
  cardiac reflexes, receptors, 237,
    243–244
  isomyosins, 9
  myosin characteristics, 75, 83
Autonomic factors, *see* Sympathetic
    nerves
Autopsy studies, ischemia, 287–288

BAPN (Betaminoprorionitrile), 168
Baroreceptors, cardiac function,
    238–244
Basal laminae, hypertension, 64–66
BB-creatine kinase, 146, 149
Beta-adrenoreceptors
  cardiac reflex role, 235–236
  heart failure, norepinephrine, 304
  hypertrophy stimulus, 22–23
  ventricular weight role, 313
    angiotensin interactions, 341–346
Betaminoprorionitrile, 168

Biochemical analysis, myocytes, 41–42,
    45–48
Blood flow
  cardiac development, 5
  hypertrophy stimulus, 24
  left ventricular hypertrophy, 261–271
Blood flow velocity, 280–281
Blood pressure, catecholamines; *see*
    Hypertension
Body weight
  hypertension and hypertension
    reversal, 181–183
  renal hypertension, 220
    versus aortic banding, 170, 176

Ca^{2+}
  action potential effect, hypertension,
    222, 231
  hypertrophied myocytes, 35
  relaxation impairment mechanism,
    212
  sarcoplasmic reticulum activity,
    111–115
    hemodynamic overload, 133
    hypertrophy, 115–121
    transport, 113–114
Ca^{2+}-ATPase
  sarcoplasmic reticulum, 111–121
  v_1 myosin, thyrotoxicity, 75–77
Capillaries
  collagen connections, 50–51, 53
  hypertension effect, ventricles,
    62–63, 70
  hypertrophy adaptations,
    morphometry, 29–32, 36
Capillary density
  hypertrophy adaptation,
    morphometry, 29–30
  and oxygen transport, 249–259
  pressure load, 274
Capillary growth factor, 259
Capillary lumen, 61–63
Capillary luminal surface density,
    29–30
Capillary luminal volume density,
    29–30
Capillary:myocyte ratio, 32
Capillary reserve, 249–259
Captopril, 315
Cardiac development
  cell differentiation, 2–3

embryogenesis, 2–5
neonates, 5–8
Cardiac hypertrophy; *see also*
  Myocardial hypertrophy
  adaptation versus myopathy, SHR,
    193–199
  angiotensin effects, 339–346
  capillary reserve, 249–259
  catecholamine levels, 310–311
  cell size, methods, 41–48
  in chronic ischemia, 287–293
    pathophysiology, 291
  collagen alterations, 49–56
  coronary circulation abnormalities,
    273–283
  creatine kinase system, 145–154
  future research directions, 349–352
  growth characteristics, 1–10
  myocardial compliance, 211–216
  myosin isoenzymes, review, 73–80
  myosin isoenzymes, thermodynamics,
    157–165
  oxygen transport, 249–259
  sarcoplasmic reticulum, 111–121
Cardiac mass; *see also* Mass-to-volume
    ratio
  and blood pressure, hypertension, 310
  coronary vascular growth, 274–275
  ischemia effect, 288–289
Cardiac motion, microcirculation, 251
Cardiac output, SHR, 195–199
Cardiac pacing
  coronary circulation, 276
  myocardial blood flow, 266–270
Cardiac performance, SHR, 194–199
Cardiac reflexes, 235–245
Cardiac volume, 206–208; *see also*
  Volume overload
Cardiomegaly, experimental, 41–48
Cardiomyopathic hamster, 117
Cardiomyopathy
  collagen alterations, 56
  diastole impairment, 212–213
  human heart effect, 206–207
  spontaneous hypertensive rat,
    193–199
Cat, right ventricular hypertrophy, 124
Cathecholamines
  versus angiotensin, ventricular weight,
    340–346
  future research directions, 351
  heart failure and hypertrophy,
    295–306

hypertensive ventricular hypertrophy,
    309–317
  reversal, 311–313
  vasculature adaptation, 332
C_{eff} (effective membrane capacity), 228,
    232
Cell death, myocardial embryogenesis,
    5
Cellular hyperplasia
  experimental cardiomegaly, 48
  morphometry, 32–35
Cellular hypertrophy
  model dependence, 127–130, 136
    pressure overload, 130, 136
    volume overload, 127
  morphometry, 32–35, 41–48
Chalones, hypertrophy stimulus, 24
Chromatin
  high mobility group proteins, 105–
    106
  RNA regulation, 99–101, 103–106
  structure, 102–103, 105
Chronic progressive pressure overload
  as hypertrophy model, 134–142
  methods, 125–127
Collagen
  aorta constriction versus SHR model,
    216
  cardiac hypertrophy, alterations, 49–
    56
  future research directions, 351–352
  hypertension effect, humans, 208–
    209
  myocardial mechanics, 167–168
  vascular smooth muscle cells, 322
    age factors, 329
    reversibility, 333
Compliance; *see also* Ventricular com-
    pliance
  hypertensive rat arteries, 324–325
  myocardial hypertrophy, 211–216
Congestive heart failure
  neural reflexes, 243–244
  norepinephrine levels, 296–306
Connective tissue
  aorta-constriction versus SHR model,
    216
  collagen alterations, 49–56
  hypertension effect, humans, 208–
    209
  hypertrophy adaptation, morphometry
    32–33
  myocardial mechanics role, 167–168

Contraction, *see* Myocardial contraction
Contraction duration, 183–184, 190
Coronary artery disease
  heart weight, autopsy, 288
  hypertrophy effect, 59–71, 287–306
Coronary artery stenosis
  cardiac mass correlation, 288–289
  chamber weight, hypoxia, 292
Coronary circulation
  future research directions, 351
  hypertrophy abnormalities, 273–283
    humans, 281
  structural alterations, 273–274
Coronary occlusion
  hyperemic response, humans 280
  and hypertrophy, death incidence,
    276–278
  sympathetic nerve activity, 241
Coronary reserve capacity
  neonates, right ventricle, 279
  pressure overload, humans, 279–283
  volume induced hypertrophy, 270,
    275–278
Coronary vascular resistance
  cardiac mass effect, 274–275
  left ventricular hypertrophy, 267
Coronary velocity, occlusion, 280–281
Creatine isozymes, 145–154
Creatine kinase system, 145–154
  basic characteristics, 145–147
  hypertrophy stimulus, 23
  in spontaneously hypertensive rat,
    145–154
    nuclear magnetic resonance,
      151–154
Creatine phosphate, 146–154
Cross-bridge cycling, 163–164
Cross-sections, myocytes, 42–43, 45–
  48
Cyclic AMP
  calcium transport, sarcoplasmic
    reticulum, 114
  hypertrophy mechanism, 22–23
Cyclophosphamide, 337
Cytodifferentiation, cardiac develop-
  ment, 2–3
Cytoplasmic RNA polymerase, 95–96

DEAE-Sephadex columns, RNA,
  96–97

Deoxycorticosterone-acetate, 310–311,
  315–317
Developed tension, 183–187; *see also*
  Tension
Developmental effects, *see* Age effects
DFMO (α-Difluoromethylornithine),
  103
Diabetes
  isomyosin changes, thyroid, 78–79
  myocardial changes, hypertrophy,
    17–18
Diastole
  collagen struts, 51–52, 55
  and compliance, 211–216
  coronary disease effect, 289
  exercise effects, 264
  heart rate, 266, 270
  after polarizations, hypertension, 232
  receptor effects, LV, 237–238
  sarcoplasmic reticulum, overload,
    116, 119–120
α-Difluoromethylornithine, 103
Digoxin, catecholamine levels, 305
DNA
  angiotensin effect, 338, 343–346
  catecholamine effect, 343–345
  developing myocytes, 4, 8
  myocyte size estimation, 41–42
  RNA synthesis regulation, 93–94,
    104
    nonhistone proteins, 100–101
    structure, 102–103
  smooth muscle hypertrophy, 32
  time course, 331–332
DNA polymerase-α, neonates, 8
DNase, 103–105
DOCA (Deoxycorticosterone-acetate),
  310–311, 315–317
Dog
  capillary reserve, 252–255
  sarcoplasmic reticulum, hyper-
    thyroidism, 118
"Down" regulation, isomyosin, 79
Duration of contraction, 183–184, 190

Eccentric hypertrophy, 211, 351
EDTA activity, isomyosins, 75, 77
Effective membrane capacity, 228, 232
Ejection fraction
  coronary artery disease, 289
  heart failure, receptors, 243

left ventricle, 194–199
Elastic lamella, 62–65, 322
"Electrical diastole", 230
Electrical properties, ventricle, 219–232
Electrocardiographic measurements, 228–230
Embolism, sympathetic nerves, 241
Embryogenesis, cardiac development, 2–5
Endocardial region
  action potentials, LV, 225–228
  blood flow, 265–270
  electrocardiography, 229
  hypertrophy adaptation, 27–31
morphometry, hypertension, 60–62, 70
Endoplasmic reticulum, myocytes, 35, 38
Endothelium
  arterial pressure, 327
  cellular morphometry, 32–33, 38
  hypertension effects, morphometry, 61, 63–67, 69–70
Energetics, hypertrophy
  creatine kinase system, 145–154
    nuclear magnetic resonance, 151–154
  model dependence, 123–142
  stimulus characteristics, 22–23
  transport system, diagram, 147
Engaged RNA polymerase, 98
Epicardium
  action potentials, LV, 225–228
  blood flow, LV, 265–270
  electrocardiography, 229
  hypertension effects, morphometry, 60–62, 64, 68
  hypertrophy adaptations, 27–28
Epinephrine
  DNA regulation, growing hearts, 8
  ventricular weight, 340–346
Erythrocytes, capillary density measurement, 249–250
Exercise
  coronary circulation, 276
  myocardial blood flow, 263–265
  myocardial changes, hypertrophy, 17–18
  norepinephrine levels, heart failure, 303–304
  sarcoplasmic reticulum effects, 118–119
Experimental cardiomegaly, 41–48; *see*

also Cardiac hypertrophy

Feedback, cardiac reflexes, 236–237, 239, 243–244
Fibroblasts, hypertrophy adaptation, 38
Fibrosis, 216
Filling rate, ventricle, 213–214
Force development
  stress effects, 14–15
  thyroxine and pressure hypertrophy, 162
    isomyosin, thermomechanics, 162–165
Force-shortening relationships, models, 128–132, 136–137
Force-velocity relationships
  aortic bands versus SHR, 171–172, 175–176
  denervation effect, 302
  hypertension and hypertension reversal, 183, 185–190
  model dependence, overload, 128–132, 136–137
"Free" RNA polymerase, 98

Ganglionic blockade, catecholamines, 304–305
Gene expression
  heart growth regulation, 8–10
  isomyosins, 91
  protein synthesis, hypertrophy, 93–94
Genetic hypertension, *see* Spontaneous hypertensive rats
Genetic program, myocyte proliferation, 7–8
Goldblatt rat, 324, 333
Golden hamsters, *see* Hamsters
Gradual pressure overloading
  contractile performance, 189
  renal hypertension, electrophysiology, 220
  spontaneous hypertensive rats, 197–198
  ventricular mass, 141
Growth factors, 331–333; *see also* Protein factors

Hamsters
  collagen network, 52
  norepinephrine levels, 298, 304
  sarcoplasmic reticulum, cardio-myopathy, 117

Heart failure
　neural reflexes, 243–244
　sympathetic nerves, 295–306
Heart rate
　myocardial blood flow effect,
　　266–270
　norepinephrine depletion, 300
　sympathetic nerves, 236–240
Heart weight
　angiotensin and catecholamines, 340–
　　346
　aortic bands versus hypertensive rats,
　　170, 176
　chronic ischemia, 287–288, 290
　DOCA-hypertension reversal, 315
　hypertension and hypertension
　　reversal, 181–183
　renal hypertension, 60, 220
Heat production, hypertrophy models,
　162
Heavy chains, myosin, *see* Myosin
　heavy chains
Heavy Meromyosin (HMM), 76–77
Hemodynamic overload
　isomyosins, thyroid hormone, 78–79
　model dependence, 123–142
　right ventricular hypertrophy,
　　123–138
Hemodynamics
　cardiac development, 5–6
　normotensive versus SHR, 196
　right ventricle, hypertrophy models,
　　123–142
High mobility group proteins, 105–106
Histometric methods, myocytes, 42–48
Histone proteins
　DNA relationship, 102–103
　RNA regulation, chromatin, 99–106
Humans
　coronary circulation, 279–283
　hypertrophy mechanics and structure,
　　201–209
　isomyosin up-regulation potential, 79
　sarcoplasmic reticulum, 116–117
　thyroid hormone effect, isomyosin, 74
Hydralazine, 199, 312–316
Hydrochlorothiazide, 315–316
Hydrostatic pressure, mRNA synthesis,
　22
Hydroxyproline, pressure overload, 136
Hyperemia, *see* Reactive hyperemia
Hyperoxemia, recruitment, 254

Hyperplastic lesions, epicardial arteries,
　64–69
Hypertension; *see also* Hypertensive
　hypertrophy
　arterial vasculature adaptation,
　　319–333
　cardiac receptor reflexes, 244
Hypertensive hypertrophy; *see also*
　Renal hypertension hypertrophy
　age factors, 329
　arterial vasculature adaptation,
　　319–333
　cardiac receptor reflexes, 244
　catecholamines, 309–317
　collagen alterations, 53–54, 329
　contractile alterations, 179–191
　　model advantages, 189
　　reversal effects, 179–191
　coronary circuit adaptation, 59–71
　electrophysiology, 219–232
　human heart, mechanics and
　　structure, 205–208
　research directions, 350–352
　ventricular effects, morphometry, 27–
　　28
Hyperthyroidism; *see also* Thyroid
　hormone
　myocardial changes, 17–18
　nonhistone protein chromatin, 102
　RNA polymerase, 96–98
　sarcoplasmic reticulum function,
　　117–119
　onset factors, 119
Hypertrophic cardiomyopathy,
　212–214; *see also* Cardiomyopathy
Hypertrophy, *see specific types*
Hypoxemia
　coronary disease hypertrophy
　　mechanism, 292–293
　recruitment, 254

Infarction, cardiac reflexes, 240–243
Intercapillary distance, 252–259, 293
Interstitium
　hypertension effect, volume, 61–63,
　　70
　ventricular hypertrophy effects,
　　27–28, 32
Intimal thickening, arteries, 64–66, 69
Intramural arteries, hypertension,
　68–70

Intramyocardial arteries, 60–61, 63–66, 68–69
Intrarenal arterioles, 323
Ion transport
  creatine kinase, 146–147
  smooth muscle cells, hypertension, 325–326
Ionic strengths
  action potentials, 222
Heavy Meromyosin, thyrotoxicity, 77
Ischemia
  arteriole lesions, hypertension, 69–70
  and cardiac hypertrophy, 287–293
  cardiac reflexes, 240–243
  and cardiomyopathy, 287
  left ventricular hypertrophy, 261–271
  relaxation impairment, 212
Isolated muscle mechanics
  active properties, 168–169
    model comparison, 169–177
  method evaluation, 174–175
  normotensive versus SHR, 194–196
  passive properties, 167–168
Isolation technique, myocytes, 42, 45–48
Isometric contraction
  aortic bands versus hypertensive rats, 170–171
  denervation, 302
  hypertension and hypertension reversal, 183–185
  model dependence, overload, 128–142
  pulmonary artery banding, 298–299
  thyroxine and pressure hypertrophy, heat, 161–165
Isomyosins, *see* Myosin isoenzymes
Isoproteins, heart growth, genes, 9
Isoproterenol
  cardiac hypertrophy inducement, 344
  nucleoprotein phosphorylation, 102–103
Isotonic contractions
  aortic bands versus SHR, 171–172, 175–176
  hypertension and hypertension reversal, 183, 185–190
  model dependence, overload, 127–142
  pulmonary artery banding, 298–299

K$^+$, *see* Potassium

Kidney weight, 181–183
Kyoto Wistar rats
  high mobility protein, 105–106
  myocardial chromatin, hypertrophy, 104–105

Lamella, arteries, hypertension, 62–65, 322
LaPlace equation, 13–14
Left ventricle, *see* Ventricle, left
Length-tension relationship, 183, 185
Longitudinal sections, myocytes, 44–48
Looping, cardiac embryogenesis, 3–4
Lumen
  endothelial blebs, 67
  resistance vessels, diameter, 322–323, 327–328

Magnesium, sarcoplasmic reticulum, 111–113
Man, *see* Humans
Mannitol, thermomechanics, calcium, 160
Mass-to-volume ratio
  coronary artery disease effect, 289, 292
  human heart disease, 206–207
Maximum velocity of shortening, *see* Velocity of shortening
MB creatine kinase, 146, 149, 151
Mechanics, *see* Myocardial mechanics
Membrane potentials
  renal hypertension, 219–232
  smooth muscle cells, hypertension, 325–326
Mesenteric resistance vessels, 322–323
Methoxamine, stroke volume, 195–198
Methyldopa, 312–314
Mg^{2+}, sarcoplasmic reticulum, 111–113
Mg-ATPase activity, 75–76
Midwall region, myoctyes, 46–48
Mineralocorticoid hypertension, 315–317
Minimal coronary resistance
  heart rate, 267
  pressure overload hypertrophy, 276
Minoxidil, 312–313
Mitochondria
  creatine kinase isozyme, 146–149,151
  hypertension effects, myocardium, 67–68
  hypertrophied myocytes, 35–38

Mitochondria *(contd.)*
oxygen, 30–31
hypertrophied smooth muscle cells,
321
oxygen consumption, model
dependence, 129, 133, 135
hypertensive rats versus aortic bands,
171, 173, 176
myofibrillar ratio, 176
MM-creatine kinase, 146, 149, 151
Models
hypertrophied myocardium,
evaluation, 123–142
ventricular hypertrophy,
methodology, 13–19
Modulus of elasticity, *see* Stress-strain
relationship
Monoclonal antibodies, myosin heavy
chains, 85–86, 90
Morphometric studies, 27–38
Muscle length, 183–184
Muscle weight, 183–184
MVO_2, *see* Oxygen consumption
Myelinated fibers, cardiac reflexes,
235–245
Myocardial compliance, 211–216; *see
also* Compliance
Myocardial contraction
hypertension and hypertension
reversal, 179–191
hypertrophy effects, 14–18
duration of contraction, 183–184,
190
model dependence, 123–142
norepinephrine depletion, 298–306
oxygen gradients, 258
receptor effects, feedback, 239
Myocardial development, 3–5
Myocardial hypertrophy; *see also*
Ventricle, left, hypertrophy
mechanics and structure, humans,
201–209
model dependence, function,
123–142
models and methods, 13–19, 41–48
mechanics, 167–177
physiological stimulus, 21–25
pressure overload models, 167–177
RNA synthesis control, 93–106
Myocardial infarction
coronary occlusion and hypertrophy,
276–278

hypertrophied myocardium effect,
292–293
Myocardial mechanics
basic concepts, 13–15, 167–169,
201–204
human hypertrophied myocardium,
201–209
hypertension and hypertension
reversal, 179–191
isomyosin effects, 157–165
pressure overload, two models,
167–177
Myocardial oxygen consumption, *see*
Oxygen consumption
Myocardial perfusion, 261–172,
275–276
Myocardial stress, 13–14, 21–25; *see
also* Stress-strain relationship
Myocardial wall thickness, 14–15; *see
also* Ventricular wall thickness
Myocyte nuclear profiles, 44–45
Myocytes; *see also* Cellular
hypertrophy
collagen connections, hypertrophy,
50–56
embryogenesis, 2–5
in experimental cardiomegaly, size,
41–48
hypertrophy adapation, morphometry,
27–33, 41–48
surface to volume ratio, 33–34
model dependence, hypertrophy, 136
postnatal development, 5–8
DNA polymerase-α, 8
volume composition, hypertension,
61–62
Myofibrils
aortic bands versus SHR, 171,
173–174, 176
mitochondria ratio, 176
creatine kinase, 146–147
embryogenesis, 2–4
hypertrophied myocytes, 34–35,
37–38
Myofilaments
hypertension effects, arterioles, 67
hypertrophied myocytes, 37
smooth muscle cells, 321
Myoglobin, oxygen transport, 257–258
Myopathy, *see* Cardiomyopathy
Myosin; *see also* Myosin isoenzymes
cross-bridge cycling, heat,

isomyosins, 163–164
enzymatic properties, thyrotoxicity, 75
in hypertrophy, review, 73–80
structural polymorphism, 9–10
thyroid hormone effects, neonates,
83–91
Myosin ATPase, thyroid hormone
effect, 73–75, 78
Myosin heavy chains
molecular changes, thyroid, neonates,
83–91
monoclonal antibody separation,
85–86
peptide maps, 87
synthesis rates, thyroid hypertrophy,
88
Myosin isoenzymes, 73–80
enzymatic properties, 75–77
future research directions, 351
hypertrophy effect, 15
brief review, 73–80
structural polymorphism, 9–10
thermomechanical economy,
157–165
thyroid hormone effects, 73–77,
83–91
neonates, 83–91
synthesis rate, 88–89

Na$^+$
action potentials, hypertension, 222
smooth muscle cells, hypertension,
325–326
Na$^+$-K$^+$ pump
repolarization time course, 224, 227
smooth muscle cells, hypertension,
326
Necrosis
hypertension effect, 64–68, 70
hypertrophy stimulus, 24–25
Neonates
heart, 5–8
myocyte size, cardiomegaly, 47
pressure-overload, circulation,
278–279
Nephrectomy, hypertension
normalization, 179–191
"Nicking", DNase, 105
"No-reflow" phenomenon, 69
Nonhistone proteins, 99–106
animal models, 101–106
RNA regulation, chromatin, 99–101

Norepinephrine
versus angiotension, ventricular
weight, 340–346
antihypertensive effects, 313–317
hypertensive rats, 311
in hypertrophy and heart failure, 295–
306
depressed contraction, 298–302
hypertrophy stimulus, 22–23
vascular wall, hypertension, 329–331
Normotensive rats
angiotensin II antagonists, 312
cardiac receptor reflexes, 244
creatine kinase activity, 150–151
pressure overload, two models,
169–175
Nuclear magnetic resonance, 148–154
Nuclear profiles, myocytes, 44–45
Nucleases, myocardial chromatin, 105
Nucleolar RNA polymerase, properties,
95–96
Nucleoplasmic RNA polymerase,
properties, 95–96
Nucleosome
characterization, 102
RNA synthesis relationship, 103

"**Off**" actomyosin state, 163–164
Oligomycin, mitochrondrial respiration,
133, 135
"On" force producing state, 163–164
Ouabain, Na-K pump, 326
Oxygen consumption
and blood flow, 262–263
in heart failure, norepinephrine, 303–
304
microcirculation, 249–259
mitochondria usage, hypertrophy, 36
papillary muscles, model dependence,
126–138
pressure overload, 129–131,
133–134, 136–138
volume overload, 126–127
Oxygen transport
capillary density, 253
normal and hypertrophied hearts,
249–259

P-31 NMR spectroscopy, 153–154
Papillary muscle
action potentials, hypertension,
220–232

Papillary muscle *(contd.)*
   contraction defects, norepinephrine,
      298–302
   hypertension and hypertension
      reversal, 183–190
   hypertrophy effects, model
      dependence, 127, 130
      pressure overload, 130, 133,
        136–137
      volume overload, 127
   normotensive versus SHR,
      mechanics, 194–196
   sarcoplasmic reticulum kinetics, 117
   thyroxine and pressure hypertrophy,
      161
   ventricular hypertrophy,
      morphometry, 27–37
Partial abdominal aortic constriction,
   321, 325–333
Partial pressure of oxygen
   capillary density determinant, 253
   hypertrophy, myoglobin, 257–258
Passive muscle properties
   hypertension and hypertension
      reversal, 183, 185
   hypertensive rat arteries, 324–325
   isolated cardiac muscle, 167–168
Passive electrical properties, 227–228
Peak velocity, coronary occlusion, 280–
   281
Peptide maps, myosin heavy chains, 87,
   89
Perimysium, heart, 51–52
Phenoxybenzamine, 341–343
Phosphoenolpyruvate, 120
Phospholambam, 114
Phosphorylation
   creatine kinase system, 147–148, 154
   myocyte nuclei, DNase digestion,
      103–104
   nonhistone proteins, RNA synthesis,
      101
   sarcoplasmic reticulum function,
      113–114
   thyrotoxicosis, myosin, 75
Physical training, 118–119; *see also*
   Exercise
Physiologic hypertrophy, 117; *see also*
   Hyperthyroidism
Pinocytotic vesicles
   cellular hypertrophy, 38
   hypertension, 327

Polarographic myography, 126
Polymerases, *see* RNA polymerase
Posterior ventricular wall, 264–265
Potassium
   action potential duration, 227
   smooth muscle cells, 326
Pressure overload hypertrophy
   versus beta-adrenergic blockade, 313
   chronic renal hypertension model,
      189
   contraction defects, norepinephrine,
      298–302, 305–306
   coronary circulation effect, 275–277
      humans, 279–283
   human heart, 205–208
   ventricular hypertrophy, 13–18
      morphometry, 32, 35–36
   ventricular relaxation, 213
      stiffness, 215–216
Proline uptake, hypertension, 331–332
Propranolol
   angiotensin interaction, 341–346
   catecholamine actions, 313
Prostaglandin synthesis, 22–24
Protein factors
   arterial adaptation, hypertension,
      331–333
   RNA polymerase stimulation, 99
Protein kinase
   calcium transport, 114, 118
   nonhistone protein phosphorylation,
      101–102
Protein synthesis
   angiotensin, 337–346
   future research directions, 351
Pulmonary artery banding
   catecholamine levels, 310–311
   contraction defects, norepinephrine,
      298–302
      hypertrophy reversal, 305–306
   hemodynamic overload, 124–142
   ventricular stiffness, 215–216
Pyknosis, smooth muscle cells, 67

QRS properties, 228–230
Quick release technique, 175

Rabbit
   arterial adaptations, hypertension,
      PAAC, 321, 325–333
   isomyosin up-regulation, 79

sarcoplasmic reticulum, 115–116, 118
thyroid hormone effect, isomyosin, 74
Rat
  capillary reserve, 252–259
  collagen network, 52
  sarcoplasmic reticulum, 115–116, 118
  thyroid hormone effect, isomyosin, 74, 79
Reactive hyperemia
  blood flow increase, 263
  occlusion effect, 279–281
  right ventricular hypertrophy, 282
Receptors, cardiac reflexes, 235–245
Recruitment
  hyperemia, capillary bed, 259
  hypoxemia and hyperoxemia, 252, 254
Reflexes, cardiac, 235–245
Relaxation, left ventricle, 212–213
Renal arterioles, 323
Renal hypertension hypertrophy
  arterial and myocardial effect, 60–71
  blood presure-ventricular mass correlation, 310
  cardiac receptor reflexes, 244
  catecholamine levels, 311, 313–315
  contractile alterations, and reversal, 179–191
    model advantages, 189
  and coronary occlusion, death, 276–278
  electrical effects, ventricles, 219–232
  ischemia interactions, 293
  myocardial blood flow, 262
  ventricular effects, morphometry, 27–28
Repolarization, action potentials, 220–232
Reserpine, 313–314
Reset mechanisms, heart failure, 243–244
Resting oxygen consumption, 259
Resting tension, 183–187
Right ventricle, *see* Ventricle, right
  angiotensin, 337–338, 343–346
  catecholamines, 343–344
  hypertrophied myocardium, 93–106
  pressure effects, myocardium, 22
RNA polymerase
  nucleosome regulation, 103

RNA synthesis, hypertrophy, 95–99
  T_3 effects, engaged-to-free ratio, 98
Running-induced hypertrophy, 118–119
Ruthenium red, 133, 135

Salt hypertension
  catecholamine levels, 311
  ventricular weight correlation, 310
Sar[1], Ile[8], *see* Angiotensin antagonists
Sarcolemma, myocyte hypertrophy, 34–35, 37
Sarcomeres
  hypertension effect, subendocardium, 67–68
  stress effect, 17
Sarcoplasmic reticulum
  cardiac hypertrophy effect, 111–121
  characterization, 111–112
  hemodynamic overload, 133
  myocyte hypertrophy adaptation, 35
Saturation transfer NMR, 153–154
Scleroproteins, *see* Collagen
Shortening, 127–132, 136–137; *see also* Velocity of shortening
Sigma factor, 99
Smooth muscle cells, *see* Vascular smooth muscle cells
Sodium, *see* Na
Species effects, *see specific species*
Spontaneous hypertensive rats
  active and passive stiffness, 168
  versus aorta constriction, collagen, 216
  arterial compliance, 324–325
  arterial vasculature adaptation, 321–333
  cardiac receptor reflexes, 244
  catecholamine levels, 311–312
    antihypertensives, 313
  creatine kinase system, 145–154
  hypertrophy, adaptation or myopathy, 193–199
  and hypertrophy, hypertension absence, 310
  lumen diameter, 322–323
  mechanics effect, versus aortic banding, 169–177
  microcirculation, wall thickness, 321–322
  myocardial chromatin, 104–106
  pressure overload model appropriateness, 142

Spontaneous hypertensive rats *(contd.)*
  sarcoplasmic reticulum, 116
  transcribing RNA polymerases,
    97–98
  vascular pathology, 327
ST wave, renal hypertension, 228–229
Stiffness
  hypertensive arteries, 230, 324–325
    time course, 328
  hypertrophy model effect, 167–168
  pulmonary artery banding, 215–216
Strain, myocardial, 204–205
Stress-strain relationship
  human myocardium, 201–209
  hypertensive rat arteries, 324–325
  pulmonary artery banding, 215–216
Strobed light, microcirculation, 251
Stroke volume, 194–199
Subendocardial region
  collagen increase, 54–55
  myocardial blood flow, 262–270
  myocyte size estimation, 46–48
  renal hypertension effect, 60, 68, 70
Subendothelial space, arteries, 64–66
Sudden cardiac death, 276–277
Supravalvular aortic stenosis, 262–270
Supravalvular pulmonary obstruction,
  278
Sympathetic nerves
  cardiac reflexes, 235–245
  hypertensive vascular wall, 329–331
  hypertrophy and heart failure,
    295–306
Systole
  cardiac damage, hypertension, 70–71
  collagen struts, 51–52
  diastole relation, hypertrophy,
    211–214
  heart rate effect, 266
  hypertension and hypertension
    reversal, 181–183
  myocardial blood flow changes, 262–
    264, 266
    exercise, 264
  thyroxine and pressure hypertrophy,
    161
  wall stress and strain, 204–205
    diseased human heart, 205–208
Systolic overload, 115–116, 119

T-system
  electrical properties, 232

myocyte hypertrophy adaptation,
  34–35
T wave, renal hypertension, 228–230
T_3, *see* Triiodothyronine-induced
  hypertrophy
T_4, *see* Thyroxine-induced hypertrophy
Tachycardia, coronary circulation, 276
TEA (Tetraethylammonium), 222, 231
Tension
  aortic bands versus SHR, 170–177
  arterial adaptation stimulus, 331
  electrical aspects, hypertension, 231–
    232
  hypertension and hypertension
    reversal, 183–190
  isomyosin effects, thermomechanics,
    159
  model dependence, hypertrophy,
    128–134, 136
Tension-dependent heat
  actomyosin, 163–164
  measurement, 159–160
Tetraethylammonium, 222, 231
Thymidine
  angiotensin, 338
  in hypertension, uptake, 331–332
Thyroid hormone; *see also*
    Hyperthyroidism
  heart effects, 77–79
  isomyosin, 73–79
  myosin heavy chain molecules, 83–91
  sarcoplasmic reticulum function, 118
Thyrotoxic myosin, 75–77, 86
Thyroxine-induced hypertrophy
  developmental changes, 88
  isomyosin effects, 78, 90
    thermomechanicals, 157–165
  nonhistone protein chromatin activity,
    102
  sarcoplasmic reticulum function, 118
Time course
  angiotensin and catecholamine
    effects, 345
  arterial pressure, hypertension,
    326–328
Time to peak shortening, 183, 185, 187
Time to peak tension
  aortic bands versus SHR, 170–171,
    175
  hypertension and hypertension
    reversal, 183–185
Tissue adaptations, ventricles, 27–28

Tissue hormone, hypertrophy stimulus, 24
Transcapillary oxygen, 258–259
Transcription, genes
histone and nonhistone proteins, 99–100, 104
hypertrophy, 94–97
Transmembrane action potentials, 220–224
"Trap-door" mechanism, 70
Triiodothyronine-induced hypertrophy
developmental changes, 88, 91
nucleoprotein phosphorylation, 102–103
RNA polymerase activity, 96–97
Troponin, 10
Tyrosine hydroxylase, 297–298

Unilateral nephrectomy, 179–191
"Up" regulation, isomyosin, 79
Uridine, angiotensin effect, 338
Uridine ratios, RNA polymerase, 96

V_1 and V_3 isomyosins; *see also* Myosin heavy chains
age effects, 77–78, 88
enzymatic properties, thyrotoxicity, 75–77
monoclonal antibody separation, 85–86
myosin heavy chain relationship, 85–91
structure, 74
thermomechanical economy effect, 157–165
thyroid hormone effect, 74–80
neonates, 83–91
synthesis, 88, 90
V_2 isomyosin
monoclonal antibody separation, 85–86
myosin heavy chain relationship, 85–91
structure, 74
thyroid hormone effect, 74
Vagal nerve, cardiac reflexes, 235–245
Vascular resistance, 319–320
Vascular smooth muscle cells
hypertension adaptation, 319–333
reversibility, 333
stimulus, 331–333
time course, 323–333

membrane permeability, 325
morphology, coronary arteries, 62–69
wall thickness ultrastructure, 321–322
Vascular wall, 319–333
Vasodilation, 263, 267–270
Velocity of shortening
aortic bands versus SHR, 171–172, 175–176
denervation effect, 302
hypertension and hypertension reversal, 183, 185
model dependence, 127–132, 136–137
stress effects, 14–15, 17–18
Ventricle, left
capillary reserve components, 252–253, 255
coronary disease effects, function, 288–290
neonatal development, 6
receptor activity, 237–245
Ventricle, left, hypertrophy
aortic banded versus hypertensive rats, 170–171, 173
cardiomyopathy, SHR, 193–199
catecholamines, 309–312
coronary circulation interactions, 275–280
directions for research, 349–352
electrical properties, renal hypertension, 219–232
Ventricle, left, hypertrophy
ischemia effect, 288–293
mitochondrial creatine kinase system, 151
morphometric studies, 27–38
myocardial blood flow, 261–271
pressure overload models, 141–142
receptors, cardiac reflexes, 237–245
relaxation impairment, 212–213
renal hypertension effect, 60
sarcoplasmic reticulum kinetics, 117
subendocardial necrosis cause, 70
volume composition, 60–62
wall force and stress, 201–208
Ventricle, right
capillary reserve components, 252–253
contractile and energetic function, 123–142
coronary circulation, 278–279

Ventricle, right *(contd.)*
  humans, 282–283
  electrophysiology, model weaknesses, 219
  hemodynamic hypertrophy, 123–142
  neonatal development, 6
  norepinephrine levels, 296–300, 305–306
  thyroxine and pressure hypertrophy, 161
Ventricular compliance
  cardiac hypertrophy, 214–216
  coronary artery disease, 289
Ventricular fibrillation, 276–277
Ventricular hypertrophy; *see also* Ventricle, left, hypertrophy
  collagen network, 49–56
  models and methods, 13–19
  morphometric studies, 27–38, 41–48
  myocardial blood flow, 261–271
  pressure overload models, 141–142
  right ventricle, *see* Ventricle, right
  sarcoplasmic reticulum kinetics, 117
Ventricular performance, 194–199
Ventricular volume, *see* Volume overload
Ventricular wall
  blood flow abnormalities, 264–270
  coronary artery disease effect, 288–291
  hypertrophy stimulus, tension, 21

  myocyte-collagen connections, 51–52
  stress and strain, 201–208
Ventricular wall thickness
  coronary artery disease, 290–291
  diseased human heart, 206
  physiologic stimulus, 25
  renal hypertension effect, 60
Ventricular weight
  angiotensin and catecholamines, 340–346
  antihypertensives, 313–314, 316
  and arterial pressure, SHR, 198–199
Volume overload
  coronary circulation, 277–280
    humans, 282
  diastolic abnormalities, 215
  as model, evaluation, 127–129, 138–142
    method, 124, 126–127
  models and methods, 13–15, 17

Wall force, 201–203; *see also* Ventricular wall
Wall/lumen ratio, 273, 324–325
Wall stress; *see also* Ventricular wall
  myocardium, 203–204
  thickness adaptation, 321–322
Wall tension, *see* Tension

Z-lines, myocytes, 67–68